RESPONDING
TO CAIRO

RESPONDING TO CAIRO

Case studies of changing practice in reproductive health and family planning

Nicole Haberland
Diana Measham

Editors

POPULATION COUNCIL NEW YORK

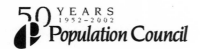

The Population Council is an international, nonprofit, nongovernmental organization that seeks to improve the well-being and reproductive health of current and future generations around the world and to help achieve a humane, equitable, and sustainable balance between people and resources. The Council conducts biomedical, social science, and public health research and helps build research capacities in developing countries. Established in 1952, the Council is governed by an international board of trustees. Its New York headquarters supports a global network of regional and country offices.

Population Council
One Dag Hammarskjold Plaza
New York, New York 10017 USA
telephone: 212-339-0500
fax: 212-755-6052
e-mail: pubinfo@popcouncil.org
http://www.popcouncil.org

Library of Congress Cataloging-in-Publication Data

Responding to Cairo : case studies of changing practice in reproductive health and family planning / editors, Nicole Haberland, Diana Measham.
      p. cm.
   Includes bibliographical references.
   ISBN 0-87834-106-4
      1. Birth control—Case studies. 2. Reproductive health—Case studies. I. Haberland, Nicole. II. Measham, Diana M.

   HQ766 .R4485 2002
   363.9′6—dc21   2002016967

To Lila, Max, Michaela, and Sam

Contents

Foreword   xi
George F. Brown

Acknowledgments   xv

1   Introduction   1
         Nicole Haberland and Diana Measham

Part I   Moving National Health and Family Planning
**   Systems Toward a Client Center**
2   Dismantling India's Contraceptive Target System:
         An Overview and Three Case Studies   25
         Nirmala Murthy, Lakshmi Ramachandar, Pertti Pelto,
         and Akhila Vasan
3   Offering a Choice of Contraceptive Methods in
         Deqing County, China: Changing Practice in the
         Family Planning Program Since 1995   58
         Baochang Gu, Ruth Simmons, and Diana Szatkowski
4   Transforming Reproductive Health Services in South Africa:
         Women's Health Advocates and Government in Partnership   74
         Sharon Fonn and Khin San Tint

Part II   Reorienting Programs to Meet the Needs of
**   Clients and Health Workers**
5   Learning About Clients' Needs: Family Planning
         Field Workers in the Philippines   99
         Anrudh Jain, Saumya RamaRao, Marilou Costello,
         Marlina Lacuesta, and Napoleon Amoyen
6   Empowering Frontline Staff to Improve the Quality of
         Family Planning Services: A Case Study in Tanzania   114
         Maj-Britt Dohlie, Erin Mielke, Grace Wambwa,
         and Anatole Rukonge

Part III   Addressing Sexuality, Gender, and Partners in Services

7   "When I Talk About Sexuality, I Use Myself
        as an Example": Sexuality Counseling and
        Family Planning in Colombia   133
        Bonnie Shepard

8   Coming to Terms with Politics and Gender:
        The Evolution of an Adolescent Reproductive
        Health Program in Nigeria   149
        Adenike O. Esiet and Corinne Whitaker

9   Talking About Sex in a Conservative Setting:
        An Experiment in Egypt   168
        Nahla Abdel-Tawab, Laila Nawar, Hala Youssef,
        and Dale Huntington

10   Recovery from Abortion and Miscarriage in Egypt:
        Does Counseling Husbands Help?   186
        Nahla Abdel-Tawab, Dale Huntington,
        Ezzeldin Osman, Hala Youssef, and Laila Nawar

11   Promoting Postpartum Health in Turkey:
        The Role of the Father   205
        Janet Molzan Turan, Hacer Nalbant, Ayşen Bulut,
        W. Henry Mosley, and Gülbin Gökçay

Part IV   Addressing Neglected Reproductive Health Concerns

12   A Hospital in Nigeria Reinvents Its
        Reproductive Health Care System   223
        Oladapo Shittu, Dennis I. Ifenne, and Charlotte Hord

13   Improving Postabortion Care in a
        Public Hospital in Mexico   236
        Ana Langer, Angela Heimburger, Cecilia García-Barrios,
        and Beverly Winikoff

14   Addressing Gender Violence in a Reproductive
        and Sexual Health Program in Venezuela   257
        Alessandra C. Guedes, Lynne Stevens, Judith F. Helzner,
        and Susana Medina

15   Sexual Risk, Sexually Transmitted Infections, and
        Contraceptive Options: Empowering Women in
        Mexico with Information and Choice   274
        Christiana Coggins and Angela Heimburger

16   Pitfalls and Possibilities: Managing RTIs in Family
        Planning and General Reproductive Health Services   292
        Nicole Haberland, B. Ndugga Maggwa,
        Christopher Elias, and Diana Measham

Part V **Working with Communities and Women to**
        Improve Reproductive Health and Rights

17   How a Family Planning Association Turned
        Its Approach to Sexual Health on Its Head:
        Collaborating with Communities in Belize   321
        Lucella Campbell and Mervin Lambey

18   "Let's Be Citizens, Not Patients!":
        Women's Groups in Peru Assert Their Right
        to High-Quality Reproductive Health Care   339
        Bonnie Shepard

19   Action Research to Enhance Reproductive
        Choice in a Brazilian Municipality:
        The Santa Barbara Project   355
        Margarita Díaz, Ruth Simmons, Juan Díaz,
        Francisco Cabral, Debora Bossemeyer,
        Maria Yolanda Makuch, and Laura Ghiron

20   ReproSalud: Feminism Meets USAID in Peru   376
        Debbie Rogow and Susan Wood

21   "If Many Push Together, It Can Be Done":
        Reproductive Health and Women's Savings
        and Credit in Nepal   395
        Tom Arens, Denise Caudill, Saraswati Gautam,
        Nicole Haberland, and Gopal Nakarmi

22   Mobilizing Communities to End Violence
        Against Women in Tanzania   415
        Lori S. Michau, Dipak Naker, and Zahara Swalehe

23   Protecting and Empowering Girls: Confronting the
        Roots of Female Genital Cutting in Kenya   434
        Asha Mohamud, Samson Radeny, Nancy Yinger,
        Zipporah Kittony, and Karin Ringheim

Contributors   459

Foreword

The extraordinary recommendations of the International Conference on Population and Development, held in Cairo in September 1994, represent a sea change in the way population and reproductive health problems are conceptualized. A wide range of national population policy pronouncements, organizational changes, and program interventions in many countries have been guided by these recommendations in the ensuing years. The Programme of Action, signed by 179 governments, remains a landmark document. It provides a broad framework for a new approach to delivering reproductive health services in a comprehensive, user-friendly fashion, with respect for reproductive rights, and rejects the demographically driven, top-down approach that has been the hallmark of many family planning programs for the past four decades.

Since 1994 a major challenge has been to translate the Programme of Action into effective reproductive health services that satisfy the needs of women and men. This has often required removing demographic targets, overturning traditional patterns of family planning service provision, and introducing entirely new and comprehensive services to address many reproductive health concerns, such as sexually transmitted infections, violence against women, maternal mortality and morbidity, and abortion. It has been clear from the beginning that there is no simple road map, no single approach. Experimentation is essential, coupled with careful evaluation and monitoring.

These changes are not easily made. Governments must engage in sometimes-difficult debates to formulate and approve new policies. Decades of top-down, autocratic service systems cannot be changed overnight. Providers with deep-seated attitudes and behaviors regarding their clients need to be retrained and better supervised, and new categories of community health care providers must be created. Communities themselves need to be mobilized to become active participants in meeting their own reproductive health needs. Health officials must develop novel ways of evaluating the performance of workers who, in many cases, are no longer assessed according to the number of clients accepting contraceptives.

The case studies in this book represent the most comprehensive effort since the Cairo conference to examine in detail many of the most promising practical efforts to translate the Programme of Action into reproductive health programs and services that respond directly to the needs of women in the developing world. Their geographic and programmatic range is remarkable: from national policy and program changes in China and India to community-based projects in Peru; from shifts in national policy to grassroots projects on neglected issues such as postabortion care and involving men as partners; and from innovations in service delivery to efforts to challenge gender power norms in the community.

The case studies highlight the varied programmatic innovations that have been initiated throughout the developing world. Many demonstrate success in empowering women and communities to seek and obtain comprehensive reproductive health services. Major shifts in national policies have been encouraging. Yet the difficulties that remain in changing hierarchical and demographically driven policies and programs are enormous. The challenge to authority and tradition posed by women's empowerment remains at the heart of this resistance to change. The hopes and promises of the Programme of Action are gradually being realized, but no one should have illusions that all of its goals are in sight. These case studies offer hope, fresh ideas, and sobering insights into the challenges that lie ahead. They provide rich, practical information on both successes and failures.

Although each of the projects surveyed has been evaluated to some degree, evaluation in general remains a critical challenge. No longer can the traditional measures of contraceptive prevalence or fertility reduction adequately encompass the goals of the Cairo recommendations. Although work is proceeding on developing new indicators for assessing progress toward reproductive health goals, comprehensive evaluation methods remain elusive.

Another fundamental concern is that most reproductive health interventions are carried out on a small scale and are infrequently replicated or scaled up to the national level. Years of work lie ahead in advocating national policy changes, rethinking programmatic strategies, and implementing effective programs at the community level. Far more resources are needed, from both national and international sources. It will be an enormous challenge to maintain the commitment and dedication to the common goals of the Cairo conference throughout the world.

Yet, much has been accomplished, and it is evident that the broad concept of a client-oriented approach to reproductive health is increasingly accepted as the norm. As I look back over the four decades of my own work in this field, the change is truly remarkable. Beginning in Tunisia in 1964, I was engaged in helping establish national family planning programs. In the 1960s many countries were beginning to focus on rapid population growth and the need to lower birth rates and were paying only lip service to women's health needs. Men, for the most part, were ignored. The immediate measures of success were acceptance of family planning services and contraceptive prevalence. It was inevitable that this top-down demographic approach brought little or no community involvement and no attention to maternal mortality, reproductive tract infections, and many other health problems. Women's empowerment was virtually an unknown concept, or was considered irrelevant.

Tunisia was an interesting exception. After independence in 1956, President Bourguiba initiated far-ranging social policy changes to improve the status of women by educating girls; liberalizing marriage, divorce, and inheritance laws; improving women's health services; and initiating family planning services that included access to abortion and sterilization, both unique in the Arab world at that time. The results were impressive, with increased age at marriage, higher levels of education for girls, and increased contraceptive prevalence.

I was lucky to start my reproductive health career in such an enlightened setting, although I confess that my own viewpoint, and that of my employer, the Population Council, were sharply focused on contraceptive acceptance and the introduction of the "hot" contraceptive of the day, the Lippes Loop IUD. We were less enlightened than Tunisia!

Curiously, Tunisia's example was not emulated in other countries. A single-minded focus on fertility reduction through increased contraceptive prevalence was almost universally the norm from the 1960s to the mid-1990s. Looking back, there is no doubt in my mind that, had the Tunisian model been applied more widely, the world would have achieved far more in improving the lives of women and men, and there would still have been a significant change in fertility behavior.

During the past four decades, policies and programs have gradually undergone a shift toward greater sensitivity to women's needs, improved quality of care, and the incorporation of a user perspective in family planning programs. I was fortunate to work closely with many colleagues at the Population Council and in sister institutions who initiated many of these changes. But the changes were slow and were sometimes reversed, and the underlying demographic paradigm remained. Improving quality of care was "too expensive," counseling and informed consent "too difficult," and attention to broader reproductive health needs "not feasible." Reproductive rights could not be addressed. Educating girls and improving the status of women were outside the purview of the family planning establishment.

The Cairo conference and the tireless efforts of women's health advocates leading up to it resulted in a profound and essential breakthrough. Reproductive health

and rights and improving the status of women became centerpieces of the new paradigm. It seems that a great hurdle has been overcome, and that there will be no turning back. And yet challenges remain. Efforts by conservative governments and groups
to revise and even overturn elements of the Cairo agenda have been made repeatedly.
Vigilance and persistence are critical in ensuring that the new paradigm will become a
practical reality.

   This book demonstrates how the international efforts initiated in the 1960s
have been transformed in the new millennium. It provides a key benchmark in the
long passage toward the achievement of a humane, client-oriented approach to reproductive health and rights, sexuality, and women's empowerment.

GEORGE F. BROWN
The Rockefeller Foundation

Acknowledgments

This book is the realization of the extraordinary vision of Judith Bruce, director of the Population Council's Gender, Family, and Development Program. We thank her for serving as our inspiration and our compass, and for her steadfast support and friendship.

Transforming Judith's idea into a 23-chapter volume leaves us indebted to many, many people in almost 20 countries. First and foremost, we thank the policymakers, program managers, women's health activists, service providers, and women and men who conceived of and carried out these efforts to realize the goals outlined in 1994 in Cairo. We applaud their vision and tenacity in working to overcome the many remaining obstacles to change. We thank the passionate and patient authors of each chapter, who worked tirelessly to document their own efforts and those of their colleagues so that others may learn from their successes and their mistakes. We aimed to transcend the typical project reporting style commonly used in this field to bring readers a narrative tale, told from a range of perspectives and with a clear sense of what came before and what came after. We also wanted to convey a clear sense of what worked and what did not. Staying true to these goals required an extraordinary level of editorial collaboration, drafting, and redrafting—and in some cases original research. We are extremely grateful to all the authors for embarking on this journey with us and seeing it through to its conclusion.

We owe enormous thanks to Debbie Rogow for her creative vision and unwavering collegiality—her storytelling magic touched most of these chapters. Elizabeth McGrory and Judith Anderson Outlaw also played key roles in shaping several of the chapters. We are very grateful for their insight, good humor, and unsurpassed editorial skill.

We thank our core review team—Adrienne Germain, Barbara Ibrahim, Purnima Mane, and Kirsten Moore—who took a great deal of time to share their expertise on the content of specific chapters and ask us tough but essential questions. Similarly, we thank Ayo Ajayi, Maria de Bruyn, Deborah Burgess, Mary Catlin, Charlotte Hord, Anrudh Jain, Joan Kaufman, Saroj Pachauri, Elizabeth Shrader, Janneke van de Wijgert, and Beverly Winikoff for sharing their substantial technical expertise. Carmen Barroso and Ruth Dixon-Mueller also deserve many thanks for their thorough review of the manuscript and their extremely helpful comments, queries, and suggestions on individual chapters and on the book overall.

We thank Robert Heidel, Jared Stamm, and Christina Tse in the Population Council's Publications Office for their painstaking copyediting and creative graphics work, and for their patience, commitment, and flexibility during the final months of production.

We thank Rachel Goldberg, Carey Meyers, Diane Rubino, and Anna Stumpf, who played critical research, editorial assistance, and preproduction roles. Special thanks to Erica Chong, whose organizational skill, editorial assistance, and calm during the final stages of this project have been invaluable.

We are very grateful to the Pew Charitable Trusts for allowing us to reprogram other grant funding in order to launch this project. We also thank the Ford Foundation for its generous and flexible financial support throughout, and the Population Council for filling in the gaps.

Finally, we thank our families. Our final review of the final chapter of this book was undertaken while Nicole nursed week-old Michaela and Diana allowed 18-month-old Lila to scribble on her pants with a pen. This moment crystallized for us the challenge of working motherhood, which began for us with the launch of this project. We gave birth to three beautiful children while conceptualizing and editing this book—Lila, Max, and Michaela—and five-year-old Sam was only a few months old when Judith first floated the idea. We thank them all—and our ever-patient and supportive husbands, Andrew and Ben—for bringing us so much joy and helping us keep things in perspective. Our parents—Peter and Anke, Tony and Carol—have also helped us navigate both our careers and our family life and have always been there to step in when the two collide. For this, and their unwavering support and guidance, we thank them.

February 2002

NICOLE HABERLAND
DIANA MEASHAM

1

Introduction

Nicole Haberland and Diana Measham

The 1994 International Conference on Population and Development (ICPD) in Cairo codified views long advocated by women's health activists the world over. Their humanistic and feminist goals became cornerstones of Cairo's landmark accord, which recognized the rights of all people to reproductive health, called for special attention to women's empowerment and clients' needs, and repudiated reliance on contraceptive services as the tool for achieving demographic targets (United Nations 1995). The ratification of the ICPD Programme of Action marked a turning point in the history of the population field—one that brought reproductive health and women's rights to the forefront of the international population agenda.

Five years after the ICPD, reproductive health and population professionals reconvened at a follow-up conference, ICPD+5, to assess their progress toward implementing the ICPD agenda and lessons learned regarding how best to do so. While the ICPD drew attention to the limitations of service-delivery systems and outlined next steps in general terms, directions for implementation were vague. Given this fact and the many policy, funding, and programmatic measures that needed to be set in place to effect the changes called for in Cairo, few measurable improvements could be reported at ICPD+5. At both the ICPD and ICPD+5, calls were issued for the development of case material—concrete documentation of changes in the field.

This volume adds this new dimension of analysis to the body of material documenting efforts to realize the ICPD agenda. The case studies in this book examine past and present practice in a variety of settings, highlighting changes, however incremental they may be. Drawn from 22 projects in 18 developing countries, they present the stories of policymakers, program managers, health workers, health advocates, and clients. The case studies comprise a set of illustrative examples. Our belief is that by looking at noteworthy projects in depth, we can provide guidance to others grappling with how best to implement the ICPD agenda in specific settings. Have we made progress in implementing this agenda? The case studies profiled here indicate a qualified "yes." Many challenges remain; at the same time, some seminal changes in policy and practice have taken place, notably the following:

- The two largest countries in the world, India and China, have abolished or modified population policies that were hostile to individuals'—especially women's—rights and freedom of choice. Nonetheless, strong pressures to achieve demographic goals by promoting contraceptive use persist in some settings.

- Decisionmakers in some settings have increased their willingness to regard sexuality as a legitimate part of reproductive health care and to incorporate attention to it into programs. However, mechanisms to address underlying issues of gender and power in the context of reproductive health care remain elusive, largely because attitudes, norms, and behaviors in this area are deeply entrenched. Concerted, long-term efforts are required to eliminate these ingrained obstacles to change.

- There is now widespread acceptance of the benefits of integrating and expanding services to meet a wider range of reproductive health needs. Efforts to broaden the content of services have met with considerable success, often at low or no additional cost. Progress in this area has been enhanced by some technological innovations (e.g., the development and distribution of manual vacuum aspiration) and has been hindered by some technological gaps (e.g., the lack of simple, low-cost diagnostic tools for most RTIs and of female-controlled microbicides for prevention of HIV and other STIs). Efforts to develop and improve reproductive health technologies must be accorded much higher priority and investment.

- The social and economic antecedents of women's reproductive health problems can be successfully addressed and overcome. Efforts to empower women as health care consumers, equal partners in sexual relationships, and important members of their families and communities are feasible and desired. To be effective, such efforts require working closely with women themselves and stepping outside clinic walls. Failure to address the socioeconomic underpinnings of reproductive health problems can prevent service-delivery interventions from fully achieving their goals.

Other themes and lessons learned post-ICPD abound. Many are detailed in this volume. Together, the case studies represent a rich and growing body of experience that can help to provide direction, fresh ideas, and cautions as we move forward.

OVERVIEW

The Cairo accord called for profound changes at multiple levels of systems, as well as in communities. Accordingly, this book is structured around five main themes. We begin in Part I with government systems in which both subtle and overt changes in population and health policy have taken place. Chapters in this section address the field-level effects of national policy change in three countries that are important in terms of their size, history, and the scope of their reproductive health problems: India, China, and South Africa.

The chapters in Parts II–IV of this book focus on innovations in service delivery—the level at which most policy changes ultimately affect clients. These innovations encompass three critical areas: reorienting health workers to provide more client-centered services; expanding providers' capacity to deal with underlying issues of sexuality, gender, and partner relations; and broadening the constellation of services to include neglected reproductive health concerns.

In Part V we turn to the community level, where the objective is particularly daunting: changing the gender norms and power relations that lie at the root of many reproductive health problems. Despite the challenges, notable efforts have been made to empower women, to involve community members in designing and improving reproductive health services, and to combat violence against women and girls.

The remainder of this Introduction provides an overview of the book rather than a comprehensive summary of its chapters. We invite the reader to delve further into the richness of the case studies themselves.

Part I: Moving National Health and Family Planning Systems Toward a Client Center

Violations of women's reproductive rights have occurred throughout the world, but some of the most widely condemned took place in India under its contraceptive target system, in China under its birth planning program, and in South Africa under apartheid. Following the Cairo conference, policies that permitted abuse in these settings were abandoned or modified. In 1996 India abolished its contraceptive target system. In 1995 China initiated an experiment to improve quality of care, including the expansion of contraceptive choice. And in 1994 South Africa ended apartheid and in the ensuing years began restructuring its health care system to overcome decades of racism and neglect of primary care, including reproductive health care.

In each setting, change in national-level policy was necessary before meaningful change could occur in service-delivery systems. While national policy change sets the stage, responsibility for the details of implementation typically falls to officials at the state, province, county, and district levels. What techniques have been used to implement national policy changes? What has happened locally since these historic changes were initiated?

In Chapter 2 Murthy and colleagues examine the measures that were developed to replace the contraceptive target system in India. Under that system, each state was directed to recruit a certain number of "contraceptive acceptors" per year. Health workers were assigned specific recruitment targets for contraceptive acceptors, primarily for sterilization. Pressure to meet sterilization targets was particularly high. Health and other government workers were offered incentives to recruit sterilization candidates, and women received incentives to undergo the procedure. Contraceptive targets led to a range of well-documented abuses, including denial of informed consent and involuntary sterilization.

When India's contraceptive target system was officially abolished, a huge bureaucratic apparatus geared toward achieving specific targets had to be radically reoriented. State-level officials were left to determine how to carry out the central government's proposed new approach, which called for community needs assessments and attention to a broader range of reproductive health concerns. Implementation of this policy change has, therefore, been strikingly variable.[1] Murthy and colleagues documented this variation through intensive fieldwork in three districts of two states, Karnataka and Tamil Nadu. The authors report that since centrally set contraceptive targets were removed, health workers have begun assessing community needs and developing their own targets for the provision of contraceptives and a range of previously neglected reproductive health services.

One unanticipated consequence of the changes documented in this chapter is a considerable increase in the workloads of female health workers as they seek to attend to more clients and address a wider array of reproductive health concerns. In some instances, workers have taken on this new workload eagerly because they had a role in determining it. These workers have become known as advocates for broader community needs rather than promoters of sterilization.

In districts where providers report the most success in the transition from the target system, supervisors generally support the changes and treat workers with respect. In other districts, workers' own performance goals are summarily supplanted by the targets of mid-level supervisors who continue to be concerned about what they perceive to be enduring high-level demands for "demographic achievements."

Chapter 3 documents a quality-of-care experiment in Deqing County, China. In this case study, Gu and colleagues describe a nominally less radical policy shift than in India, but one that may presage more dramatic change ahead. China's one-child policy, enacted in 1979, remains in force; however, public dissatisfaction with the policy is building, and inroads are being made by way of changes at the service-delivery level. In its strictest form, the one-child policy is generally accompanied by severe limitations on contraceptive choice. After their first birth, women are expected to have an intrauterine device (IUD) inserted; after a second birth—permitted if the couple's first child is female, for example—women are supposed to be sterilized. The experiment documented by Gu and colleagues does not address the broader one-child policy; rather, it introduces more contraceptive choice within the context of that policy. In Deqing County women are allowed to choose from among five contraceptive methods; they are no longer required to accept the IUD or sterilization based on parity; and method switching is allowed. The experiment also offers somewhat more client-centered follow-up care, and seeks to improve the relationship between workers and clients.

Various systems were restructured as part of the Deqing County experiment, and some of these changes had more tangible effects than others. For example, the "childbirth permit" that couples previously had been expected to obtain was changed to a "childbearing service certificate." This certificate is now delivered to the couple by the village family planning worker, and it includes a checklist of reproductive health services to which the couple are entitled. While the document's name change reflects new, client-centered aims, it still serves to "manage" births by documenting, tracking, and limiting the number of children couples have.

Continuing limits on the overall number of births, and corresponding rewards for achieving demographic goals, made mid-level officials in Deqing wary of the new focus on informed choice. Special care was taken to assuage these fears by undertaking small-scale trials before the experiment was scaled up. These trials demonstrated that most women continued to choose sterilization or the IUD, even when given other contraceptive options. This suggests that women may not have exercised their option to adopt user-controlled methods in the face of stiff penalties for unauthorized pregnancies.

In Chapter 4 Fonn and Tint describe a remarkable partnership between the South African government and a women's health organization. The Transformation of Reproductive Health Services Project aimed to improve the government's largely dysfunctional health system by making existing services more client-centered, and to set the stage for expanded reproductive health services. The project was conducted in three provinces. The underlying principle was that discrete reproductive health services could not be layered onto the public health system until the latter had undergone significant reform.

The health system inherited by the post-apartheid government was fragmented, focused on tertiary care, and gave priority to providing health care to whites. Waiting times were long, supplies inadequate, provider–client interactions deficient, and providers poorly supervised. Despite these deficits, both the newly independent government and nongovernmental organizations (NGOs) shared an optimistic outlook that contributed to an unusually collaborative approach.

Project staff recognized the importance of engaging staff and officials at all levels of the health care system. These parties were included in diagnostic research to pinpoint problems in the country's splintered health care infrastructure. This included clinic workload and time-flow analyses conducted largely by clinic staff; facility checklists; and self-administered questionnaires completed by all staff, from gardeners and drivers to clinicians. Intensive workshops were held to help providers examine their own attitudes and behaviors and to understand how gender, race, and socioeconomic conditions affect clients, providers, and health care provision. The process was an eye-opening opportunity for workers and supervisors to reflect on clinic operations and provider–client interactions and on how these might be improved.

While all levels of personnel reacted positively to the project, it remains unclear whether their increased awareness and understanding of extant problems resulted in changes in practice. The limited documentation available provides reason for optimism: One clinic that participated in a time-flow and workload analysis documented measurable improvements in services. Waiting times decreased significantly; the proportion of staff time spent on direct patient care increased from 16 to 43 percent; and the average daily client load increased by 173 percent, with no increase in numbers of staff.

Several essential lessons are highlighted by the examples from India, China, and South Africa. First, words are clearly powerful tools. There are many reasons for the uneven implementation of the post-target approach in India—but lack of change in terminology is one possible cause of confusion. As a bureaucracy undergoes change, it is important to develop new nomenclature corresponding to the change. As noted above, the Chinese did this by changing the term "permit" to "service certificate"; however, in this case substantive change appears to be less far-reaching than the change in nomenclature would imply. Conversely, in India, service-delivery goals developed by health workers, based in large part on community needs assessments, are still known as "targets." The continued use of this term may undermine the intent of the policy change, which is to reorient the family planning program from a demographic agenda toward a concern with women's own fertility goals and other reproductive health issues.

A cornerstone of the South Africa project—and a need clearly delineated in the examples from China and India—is overcoming long-standing, internalized scripts for provider–client exchanges. Clients often do not expect high-quality care, are deferential to providers, and expect providers to give them correct "answers" rather than exercise their own freedom to choose between contraceptive or service options. Health care workers are still trained to believe that they "know better" than clients. In the South Africa project, participatory exercises that help workers discern these patterns and devise new approaches continue to be used to overcome these tendencies.[2]

Ingrained behavior, beliefs, and communication patterns are evident among clients as well. Many women in China have come to believe that the IUD and sterilization are always the best contraceptive options regardless of their particular circumstances. Clients in India have also internalized the priorities of the old family planning program. Women did not seem to notice the availability of a broader range of reproductive health services or a reduction of pressure to be sterilized, despite evidence that these changes had taken place. On the other hand, women in India do appear to be using a broader range of reproductive health services, and women in both India and China have shifted perceptibly away from reliance on sterilization.[3]

Finally, the three chapters in Part I reveal that the test of new policy is how it is reflected in the provider–client exchange. Improving this exchange requires changing the nature of interactions between staff and supervisors and attending to all the processes (e.g., clinic protocols and worker reward systems) that may perpetuate bad practice even when policy changes. Improving the provider–client exchange must be at the heart of any effort to institute client-centered services and must be tackled from the perspective of both the provider and the client.

Part II: Reorienting Programs to Meet the Needs of Clients and Health Workers

The two chapters in Part II explore what can be done to reorient providers to a new service-delivery paradigm, give them new protocols, and support them in their new roles. The two examples are found in Southeast Asia and East Africa, but the service-delivery challenges they concern are commonplace.

In Chapter 5 Jain and colleagues describe a simple analytic tool designed to assist community outreach workers in the Philippines to understand their clients' needs. Rather than start with the assumption that all women of reproductive age need to use contraception, the tool helps workers to elicit information about—and to respect—women's reproductive intentions and desires. Women who are pregnant, who want to become pregnant, or who want to delay or cease childbearing are all given appropriate information and services. For example, pregnant women are told about the importance and availability of antenatal care, and when and where they should go for immunization and postpartum services. Asking women about their needs contrasts starkly with the previous approach, in which workers told clients what they thought clients needed to know about contraception, with little or no input from the clients themselves.

Chapter 6 describes an EngenderHealth project in Tanzania. Dohlie and colleagues recount the efforts of staff and supervisors in a government hospital to improve the quality of family planning services by implementing a quality improvement process called COPE® (Client-Oriented Provider-Efficient). In this process, staff assess themselves using written guides that address issues ranging from clients' rights to privacy to providers' needs for facilitative supervision. Another instrument—the QMT (Quality Measuring Tool)—was used to help supervisors and staff quantify their progress in improving service quality over time. Improvements in infection-prevention procedures, informed consent protocols, and client privacy were among the many changes that staff were able to realize in response to ongoing self-assessment. These changes took place in the hospital over time and illustrate the ongoing, iterative process that represents genuine quality improvement.

These two projects, along with the South African project described in Chapter 4, changed the way in which staff worked by appealing to their desire to do good work and by offering clear, practical guidelines for doing so. They operationalized the principle of reorienting services toward meeting clients' needs and away from simply providing contraceptives. In all three of these cases, participatory research and training enlisted clinic staff as a central constituency, allowing them to identify with clients by learning that they themselves, in their capacity as health workers, have needs for training, information, supplies, equipment, and effective supervision. Just as clients have rights to services of acceptable quality, health care providers have rights to a humane and supportive work environment.[4]

The Philippines and Tanzania cases highlight the value of documenting and monitoring the process of service transformation. Participatory processes rewarded staff for identifying problems and for gathering information to question the status quo. In both cases, changes were or are being made to improve the tools used, based on shortcomings identified during implementation. For example, Jain and colleagues found a need, not anticipated by project staff at the start, to help health workers provide women desiring to get pregnant, and those using natural family planning methods, with accurate information on the fertility cycle. The COPE and QMT tools used in the Tanzania project enabled staff to continually revise and carry out plans for service improvement.[5]

Part III: Addressing Sexuality, Gender, and Partners in Services

The ICPD agenda highlighted the role of social factors that facilitate or impede women's attainment of reproductive rights and health. Service providers cannot effectively care for clients without grappling with factors related to women's sexual partnerships and social context. In providing reproductive health care, providers come face to face with inequities in gender relations; norms that inhibit women from discussing sexual matters and that condone male promiscuity; and substantial numbers of women facing coercive sexual relations.

In developing these case studies, we were directed to many programs that claimed to talk about sex, but we found relatively few that really grappled with core issues of sexuality and even fewer that dealt with power in sexual interactions. The first three case studies presented in Part III explicitly acknowledge clients as sexual beings in relationships. The final two offer specific suggestions for involving clients' partners.

In Chapter 7 Shepard describes the institutional change process undertaken by Profamilia in Colombia to incorporate sexual health services into its nationwide family planning program. As is often the case, program staff needed as much assistance as clients in dealing with social norms and biases regarding sexuality and gender. Profamilia instituted participatory training methods that helped counselors to explore their own sexuality, pleasure in relationships, and the connections between their professional and personal experiences. A counselor's manual, developed by the counselors themselves, provides guidance on the types of sexual health issues to address with clients with different needs and backgrounds. The manual includes readings on such topics as human sexual response, self-esteem, and safer sex. The Profamilia program contributed to a qualitative leap in the quality and breadth of sexual and reproductive health counseling at the association's clinics.

In Chapter 8 Esiet and Whitaker describe the efforts of the NGO Action Health to provide sexual and reproductive health information and services to adolescents in Lagos, Nigeria. They portray the evolution of a gender-neutral, school-based program focused on abstinence into a gender-sensitive program with increasingly comprehensive sexuality education. In this case, it took time to recognize the need for and develop separate approaches for girls and boys. For example, in their sessions with girls, Action Health staff now discuss female-controlled and female-initiated contraceptive methods and strategies for getting males to wear condoms. In their discussions with boys, staff aim to help them recognize their responsibility to themselves and to their partners, including greater willingness to use condoms. Action Health also lobbied at the national level for comprehensive, gender-sensitive sexuality education.

In Chapter 9 Abdel-Tawab and colleagues demonstrate the feasibility and acceptability of sexuality counseling in the conservative cultural context of Egypt. Family planning service providers from selected government clinics participated in a three-day training session on sexuality that included discussions of providers' biases and judgments with regard to sexuality, human sexual response, solutions to sexual problems, and spousal communication. This was the least intensive of the sexuality counseling interventions documented in this volume; yet, even in this setting, and following only a short period of training, participating providers were more likely to discuss issues related to sexuality with their clients. In addition, a positive association between sexuality counseling and barrier method use was suggested. Moreover, Egyptian women sought and valued discussion of issues related to sexuality.

These three programs demonstrate that people across lines of culture, geography, age, and gender are eager and willing to discuss their sexual concerns, experiences, and needs.[6] They also demonstrate that sexuality counseling is not specifically the purview of small, women-centered NGOs. Such efforts can be effectively undertaken in a number of settings by a variety of providers, from innovative NGOs to government-run family planning clinics, and in more and less conservative settings. Both the Profamilia and Action Health cases highlight the need for in-depth work with providers to help them overcome their reticence and biases and to give them the tools and confidence they need to discuss sexuality with clients.[7] The Egypt project, which involved a single, relatively short training intervention, found, not surprisingly, that providers' technical competence, while much improved, was limited. Change in the area of sexuality counseling requires intensive, ongoing work with providers; a one-time training is unlikely to be sufficient.

In their efforts to address sexual relations and sexuality, all three programs confronted deeply rooted issues of gender and power. Esiet and Whitaker document how Action Health came to recognize the centrality of gender in its work with adolescent girls and boys. The Profamilia effort revealed that despite multiple, mutually reinforcing, institution-wide changes, some gender biases remained entrenched, as illustrated by the fact that some counselors focused on sexual coercion—not sexual pleasure—with women and on sexual pleasure—not sexual coercion—with men. Similarly, Abdel-Tawab and colleagues found that while trained providers were more likely to speak about sexuality with their clients, they were unlikely to challenge gender norms—for example, women were still expected to be ready for sex when men wanted it. In addition, no providers questioned the practice of female genital cutting (FGC), despite efforts during the training to counter such norms.

The final two chapters in Part III explore how reproductive health services might engage clients' partners. Clinic-based interventions to improve women's sexual and reproductive health are likely to have limited effects unless they consider the context in which women live, including their relations with partners and men's predominant power in sexual matters. Chapters 10 and 11 describe efforts to involve the partners of women receiving postabortion and postpartum care.

In Chapter 10 Abdel-Tawab and colleagues describe efforts in Egypt to improve women's recovery following miscarriages and induced abortions by increasing men's support of their wives during the postabortion period. In separate counseling sessions, men were informed about the need to ensure that their wives get adequate rest, warning signs of complications, women's return to fertility, contraception, the cause of miscarriage (when relevant), and sources for referral care. The project demonstrated effects on several levels, including more emotional, tangible, and family planning support for wives among counseled husbands; better physical recovery among women who received strong emotional support from their husbands; and significantly increased use of contraception among women who received high levels of family planning support from their husbands.

In Chapter 11 Molzan Turan and colleagues describe a project in Istanbul, Turkey to include men in care related to their wives' pregnancy, delivery, and postpartum recovery. Preliminary studies had indicated that many women did not use available postpartum care or modern methods of contraception, although they wanted to. An intervention was designed to stimulate partner communication on reproductive health topics through a combination of counseling services, educational materials, and a postpartum counseling telephone hotline. Among other outcomes, the investigators found that women whose husbands participated in the intervention had higher rates of contraceptive use.

These two cases indicate that many men are interested in supporting their partners' reproductive health, even in conservative settings. In both projects women expressed a desire for men's support and satisfaction with the support they received, while men expressed a desire to be involved and satisfaction with the opportunity to become involved.

Any effort to involve women's partners must place priority on women's needs. Given the disparity in power between men and women in rural Egypt, as well as sensitivities around abortion, the Egypt project took extra care to protect women's confidentiality and rights. For example, project staff asked a woman's permission to speak with her husband before approaching him, and ensured that all women were counseled individually and separately from their husbands. These safeguards are key and exemplary.

Despite the clear protocols that placed women at the center of attention, some doctors in the Egypt case thought it was more important for men than for women to receive information about recovery following miscarriage or induced abortion. In urban Turkey, where gender norms are less conservative than in rural Egypt, there was still evidence that gender dynamics required attention. Women there were less likely to attend group counseling sessions when these were for couples rather than for women only. These examples indicate that men's participation in women's reproductive health care should not be mandated. Men's inclusion may inadvertently prevent some women from getting the information they need to make decisions about their own health.[8]

Part IV: Addressing Neglected Reproductive Health Concerns

Perhaps the most widely discussed element of the ICPD agenda has been the charge to expand narrowly conceived family planning services to include neglected aspects of reproductive health care. Women have a range of pressing reproductive health concerns, including infertility, unwanted pregnancy and the complications of abortion, cervical and other gynecologic cancers, HIV/AIDS, postpartum care, emergency contraception, symptoms of menopause, obstetric fistulas, genital or uterine prolapse, and FGC. Some of these subjects are discussed elsewhere in this book.[9] Part IV focuses on efforts to incorporate specific services for postabortion care, reproductive tract infections, and gender violence, and examines a comprehensive, integrated, hospital-based reproductive health program. These cases illustrate the complexities involved in broadening a program's vision beyond customary contraceptive service delivery.

In Chapter 12 Shittu and colleagues recount the integration of compartmentalized, hospital-based family planning, gynecologic, and obstetric services into a center that brought these disparate elements together.[10] The hospital, Ahmadu Bello University Teaching Hospital in Zaria, Nigeria, also adopted the innovative strategy of using weekly rotations of paired obstetrician/gynecologists, one of whom is specially trained in integrated reproductive health service delivery, as an efficient way to expand the pool of capable medical personnel available to the center. Under the new arrangement, all clients, regardless of the reason for their visit, are informed of and appropriately referred for other reproductive health services, including Pap smears, RTI screening, and family planning. With the availability of integrated services, the hospital has seen a significant increase in its caseload of clients seeking specific reproductive health services—a near doubling of the number of new RTI patients, individual reproductive health consultations, and contraceptive users. In this case, as in others, the reinvention of reproductive health care did not require substantial additional resources. Rather, it required creativity, political will, and persistence to overcome entrenched patterns of service organization.

In Chapter 13 Langer and colleagues describe an experiment to improve the quality of postabortion care in a public hospital in Oaxaca, Mexico.[11] Baseline research painted an abysmal picture: Women were treated rudely, had no privacy, waited more than 13 hours (on average) before receiving treatment, and rarely received information about their recovery, including warning signs of complications. Among women who received postabortion contraceptive services, there were troubling signs of rights violations—for example, some women who reported not having had an IUD inserted or a tubal ligation performed did, in fact, have these procedures noted in their clinical charts, suggesting that they were performed without the woman's knowledge or consent.

Langer and colleagues involved hospital staff at all levels in reviewing these findings and initiated intensive work on interpersonal relations, technical skills training (including manual vacuum aspiration), and postabortion family planning counseling. The authors report significant improvements, including decreased waiting time, more respectful and compassionate communication with women, more clients receiving information regarding their recovery, more and better counseling on family planning, and a doubling of contraceptive use. As the authors note, there is still room for improvement: Half of the women still did not receive any information about postabortion care; pain management remained a particular concern; and counseling messages did not explicitly consider the needs of women who might have miscarried and might be eager to conceive again in the near future.[12]

While women's advocacy groups have worked for more than two decades to call attention to the abuse of women, the full magnitude of this problem is only now being recognized in the reproductive health field. Abuse by an intimate partner is one of the most common forms of violence against women. In 50 population-based surveys from around the world, between 10 percent and more than 50 percent of women reported having been abused by an intimate male partner (Heise, Ellsberg, and Gottemoeller 1999). Violence between intimate partners is a matter of concern because of its direct physical and emotional consequences for women—for example, injuries and increased risk of infection and unwanted pregnancy as a result of forced sex. Violence can increase women's risk of STIs, including HIV, because it affects their ability to negotiate the terms of their sexual relationships, including condom use. It also has been linked to adverse pregnancy outcomes and appears to increase risk for chronic pelvic pain (Heise, Ellsberg, and Gottemoeller 1999). Finally, the threat of violence also affects women's reproductive health. Fear of a negative reaction from a partner prevents many women from asserting themselves in relationships, protecting themselves from pregnancy or infection, and seeking health care.

In Chapter 14 Guedes and colleagues describes the efforts of PLAFAM (the International Planned Parenthood Federation affiliate in Venezuela) to screen for gender violence among its clients and to support women who had experienced abuse.[13] In addition to training staff and hiring psychologists, PLAFAM developed a directory of organizations providing services to victims of violence. To change the climate of public perception, PLAFAM developed posters, booklets, and bookmarks emphasizing that violence is common, but unacceptable, and informing victims where they can go for help. Under the new screening protocol, 38 percent of new clients were identified as victims of violence in the home.

PLAFAM paid unusually close attention to developing effective referral strategies. Many programs "refer" patients, but referral protocols are often vague and thus not particularly helpful. This chapter, as well as Chapter 21, describes referral systems that work because they were developed based on a careful assessment that identified relevant services and gauged their quality, and because they involve explicit referral relationships between organizations.

Concluding Part IV are two chapters that explore the challenge of managing RTIs in the context of family planning and general reproductive health service delivery. In Chapter 15 Coggins and Heimburger describe a creative and seminal experiment to overcome some of the challenges of RTI diagnosis in Mexico. This experiment tested whether women who were provided adequate information and a choice of contraceptive methods were better able than clinicians to decide whether they were appropriate IUD candidates. Its findings testify to the value of empowering clients with information and choice. Women were informed of the advantages and disadvantages of condoms, pills, and IUDs, including whether these methods protect against STIs. They were also informed that any existing STI should be treated before an IUD is inserted, that many STIs are asymptomatic in women, and that if a woman and/or her partner has sexual relations with other people and does not use condoms, the woman is at risk of infection. The results were striking: 52 percent of infected women who were given the information they needed to assess their own risks chose not to use the IUD. By comparison, only 5 percent of infected women whose risk was assessed by physicians were screened out of IUD use; and several women who indicated a preference for pills and condoms were nevertheless given an IUD by the doctor with whom they had consulted.

In light of the prevalence and gravity of HIV and other STIs, providing women with information about the relationship between sexual behavior and infection risk, and about the properties of specific contraceptives, should be a basic component of all family planning programs. Providers must also be trained to heed women's perspectives and to view a woman's right to choose and act on that choice as inalienable.

Most of the chapters in this volume describe the complexities of applying an existing technology in a manner that is more client centered and gender sensitive. In the case of RTI management, however, there are serious deficiencies in the technologies themselves, particularly in low-resource settings. In Chapter 16 Haberland and colleagues examine some of these problematic issues and potential solutions, drawing particularly on two insightful intervention studies, one in Zimbabwe and the other in Vietnam. The authors outline the scope and consequences of RTIs and the characteristics and shortcomings of prevention and diagnostic strategies. Findings from the research in Zimbabwe and Vietnam illustrate the complexities of diagnosis, but also point to viable options in some contexts. For example, given recent evidence that some endogenous RTIs may be associated with increased HIV transmission, an amplified focus that includes these infections, as well as the STIs that have typically received more attention, appears warranted.[14] The research in both countries confirms the poor results of previous validation studies of syndromic algorithms for managing cervical infection.[15] On a positive note, the Vietnam study found promise in the use of microscopy and other tests for vaginal infections, although this approach would be limited to settings where the equipment and expertise are available.[16] Finally, the chapter outlines some of the steps that family planning and general reproductive health services in virtually all settings can take to help clients prevent RTIs of all types.

Part V: Working with Communities and Women to Improve Reproductive Health and Rights

The previous parts of this volume dealt with changes at the policy level and attempts to improve services. These efforts can go only so far without addressing the social norms that perpetuate restrictive gender roles, tolerate or even foster abuse between partners, encourage unsafe sexual behavior, and limit women's power in intimate relationships and in interactions with health care providers. The chapters in Part V address three questions: How can communities be engaged in efforts to improve reproductive and sexual health? How can we work with communities to address the links between women's power and their reproductive health? How can we mobilize communities to end violence against women and girls?

Improving the quality of services and making them more responsive to women's needs requires some degree of community change. Clients' low expectations and passivity, the historical paternalism of the medical profession, and limited community engagement in the design of most health programs have curtailed the efficacy of service reform.

The first three chapters in Part V document activities that empower clients to challenge the health care status quo and to demand more as consumers. In Chapter 17 Campbell and Lambey recount the transformation of the Belize Family Life Association (BFLA) from a clinic-based program founded on contraceptive service delivery to one that facilitates community discussions on a broad range of reproductive health concerns and responds to the needs identified by community members. The intervention resulted in several clinic-level changes, including the addition of private STI counseling and a part-time psychiatric nurse-counselor. It also increased the intensity and strength of links between the community of clients and BFLA's clinical services, yielding a 30 percent increase in the number of clients. Equally important, there is now increased willingness in the community to talk about and address sensitive subjects. Participants have developed action plans to address community-level concerns, including plans to hold special sessions for men on domestic violence and to help families care for individuals living with HIV/AIDS.

In Chapter 18 Shepard documents the efforts of Consorcio Mujer, a consortium of feminist NGOs in Peru, to address both the demand and supply sides of the health service delivery system. The premise of this work is that women armed with a sense of agency and knowledge of their rights can become a significant force in health care reform. Following documentation and dissemination of quality-of-care deficiencies and violations of clients' rights, Consorcio Mujer offered separate training workshops to clients and providers, in which they explored these issues, reviewed the results of related research conducted in participating clinics, and modeled new provider–client interactions. Through facilitated discussions, both providers and clients developed concrete proposals to address the clients' rights and quality-of-care concerns identified in particular clinics. Providers and clients then came together to negotiate changes in service design that would, for example, ensure more respectful treatment, decrease waiting time, and increase privacy.

In Chapter 19 Díaz and colleagues describe a broad experiment to improve the quality and quantity of reproductive health services provided by the municipal health sector in Santa Barbara d'Oeste, Brazil. An intensive participatory process was initiated to involve providers, their supervisors, municipal authorities, community members, and researchers in a guiding executive committee. The committee reviewed diagnostic research revealing substantial barriers to access, deficiencies in quality, and inefficient use of medical personnel. For example, a complex and ineffective appointment scheduling system obliged women to arrive in the middle of the night for walk-in care or to schedule an appointment. Gynecologic exams were sometimes of poor quality (e.g., providers did not consistently wash their hands or put on gloves before an exam) and client privacy was not maintained. Gynecologists spent over half their time taking Pap smears, dispensing routine contraceptives, and conducting other tasks that could be handled by appropriately trained auxiliary personnel.

The committee identified and instituted key interventions to address these problems, including training providers, shifting job responsibilities, and establishing a model reproductive health center to serve as a referral site for the rest of the municipality. The effects of these changes were measurable, including a nearly 50 percent increase in gynecologic clinic visits, expanded method choice, increased contraceptive use, increased ease of appointment scheduling, and decreased waiting times. Of particular note is the evolution of the executive committee's awareness of what constitutes community participation. Over the course of the intervention, the representation of women's groups expanded beyond relatively elite women to include more community-based women's groups. These groups identified parts of the municipality that had remained underserved, leading to the establishment of an additional reproductive health center serving these marginalized areas.

The first three studies in Part V document mechanisms for involving community members in the development and improvement of reproductive health services offered by NGOs, government clinics, and a municipal system. As the next two chapters illustrate, the prospects for fundamental change are enhanced by the creation of safe spaces for women in which they can identify and play a role in addressing their own priority concerns.

In Chapter 20 Rogow and Wood describe Movimiento Manuela Ramos's USAID-financed ReproSalud project in Peru, which created women's solidarity groups as a key first step to improving reproductive health. In weeklong diagnostic exercises, groups of women learned about their bodies, did exercises to enhance their self-esteem and communication skills, and explored gender relations and human rights. Through these steps, women discovered and prioritized their concerns. To the surprise of project staff, RTIs surfaced as women's top priority. In response, an RTI prevalence survey was undertaken, the results of which were then used as an advocacy tool with local health authorities. At the same time, women engaged in intensive training to learn about the symptoms, causes, prevention, and treatment of RTIs. In light of women's difficulty in negotiating safe sex and seeking reproductive health care, the training addressed partner communication and negotiation skills, emphasizing women's right to say no to unwanted sex, to be safe from abuse, and to have control over their fertility. As the project proceeded, women increasingly requested that men and boys be included in reproductive health education activities. Workshops for men and boys were organized, with special emphasis on masculinity, violence, and communication.

In Chapter 21 Arens and colleagues describe their work in rural Nepal, where the organization World Neighbors linked reproductive health with social development. The authors describe the transformation of a program that compartmentalized health and development activities and provided limited reproductive health care into one that recognized women's self-defined reproductive health needs and their social context, and developed an integrated response. Clinical capacity was expanded and improved, and women's savings and credit groups were established and supported.

These two processes had a synergistic effect, increasing both the use of reproductive health services and women's sense of unity and power. Trained staff helped savings and credit group members to explore their reproductive health concerns, along with underlying biological and social factors. As the groups gained cohesion, women began to effect changes in their families and communities—for example, by sending their daughters to school, encouraging other women to do so, and confronting men about the detrimental effects of gambling. Effects on service use were measurable, with an overall 83 percent increase in visits for reproductive health care. Visits for RTI/STI management increased 70 percent; visits for uterine prolapse increased 50 percent; the number of clients presenting with urinary tract infection increased 600 percent; and antenatal care visits increased 63 percent.

The programs in Peru and Nepal both began with group formation. ReproSalud tapped local women's groups, such as mothers' clubs; World Neighbors worked with women's savings and credit groups. Both programs used participatory methods of problem identification that allowed women to articulate and prioritize their most pressing concerns. Both created safe spaces where women could discuss their concerns about relations with partners, fertility, livelihood opportunities, and health services. Expressing themselves in a group offers women practical support from their peers and the means to envision alternatives founded on a newly created base of organized females. The group mechanism also helps women develop tangible skills and create assets, whether in the form of health information or business skills.

Chapters 20 and 21 also suggest lessons for involving men without diminishing women's autonomy. The sequencing of activities is critical: Once women have gained a better understanding of their own needs and a sense of solidarity with other women they can identify their need to involve their partners in family planning and reproductive health care. In both the Peru and Nepal cases, working with women on social, economic, and health issues came first. Partner involvement was an essential next step for wider community change.

The final two case studies in this volume document an incremental process of revolution: programmatic efforts to change how entire communities regard women and to replace norms and rituals that perpetuate violence against women and girls.

In Chapter 22 Michau and colleagues describe the innovative work of Jijenge! in Mwanza, Tanzania, detailing an effort to redefine gender violence as a public matter to be discussed and challenged rather than a private matter that falls outside the purview of public discourse. Reinforcing messages were conveyed through different media and venues, including community theater, murals, radio programs, and booklet clubs. Storybooks were developed that included both women's and men's perspectives. For example, female characters in these books offer their views on how violence affects them and express their belief that they have a right to be safe in their homes. Nonviolent male characters talk with abusive male characters, offering suggestions on how to deal more appropriately with anger, the consequences of violence for women and children, and different ways of relating to their partners. To intervene in the cycle of violence, watch groups were formed to offer assistance to women in distress. In addition, workshops were organized specifically for men, with the objective of changing their behavior and attitudes regarding violence between intimate partners. While the project did not undertake a quantitative evaluation, anecdotal evidence and qualitative research findings indicate that it has had positive effects. Community members are more likely to discuss, question, and intervene against violence, and attitudes and behaviors are beginning to change.

In Chapter 23 Mohamud and colleagues document the collaboration in Kenya between Maendeleo Ya Wanawake Organization and the Program for Appropriate Technology in Health (PATH) to eradicate FGC. The authors describe how the project evolved from a focus on the health consequences of FGC to an emphasis on gender-based power and women's rights. They also detail community efforts to develop and offer an alternative rite of passage for girls and young women.

Early activities, which advocated abolishing FGC because of its negative effects on women's health, did not lead to substantial behavior change because they did not address community belief systems around sexual health, sexuality, gender, and power. Seeking to correct this, the project developed a new set of messages and strategies based on these issues. An alternative rite of passage was devised that maintained the celebratory and positive learning and coming-of-age aspects of the FGC rituals without compromising girls' bodily integrity. By December 2001 5,500 girls had experienced the alternative rite of passage without circumcision, or 20 percent of the total population of girls ages 10–19 in the target districts. A project evaluation found a significant decline in the overall prevalence of FGC, from 90 percent of women and girls ages 14–60 before the project was launched to 82 percent in 1999. The percentage of women favoring the discontinuation of the practice rose from 37 to 53 percent over the same period.

Working at the community level to change fundamental norms concerning women's sexual and reproductive health and rights requires intensive inputs. The case studies presented in Chapters 22 and 23 suggest that this change is not straightforward, but they also demonstrate that community norms and male behaviors harmful to women and girls are not immutable.

• • •

The successes and challenges documented in this volume offer many ideas and much encouragement to those engaged in efforts to realize the ICPD agenda. These efforts remain works in progress. Certainly, much remains to be done; but many creative activities in many places are taking the Cairo vision out of the realm of theory and into the realm of practice. This is the ground-level arena of real change in women's lives.

Notes

1 Recent press reports indicate that in at least one state in India, incentives and high-pressure tactics to meet contraceptive targets, especially for sterilization, continue (Dugger 2001).

2 The chapters in Part II of this book describe in greater detail efforts to reorient and support providers as they assume new roles.

3 Chapters in subsequent parts of the book discuss programs that empower women to articulate their needs and/or demand more of their service providers. See especially Chapters 17, 18, 20, and 21.

4 Efforts to reorient health care providers are also discussed elsewhere in this book. Chapter 18 describes a project to empower women to demand more of health services and to enhance providers' understanding of and respect for users' rights. Similarly, Chapter 13 describes an effort to improve providers' interpersonal skills and respect for women's choice and fully informed consent in the context of postabortion care.

5 Chapter 14, which describes a project to screen for gender violence in family planning clinics, also documents refinements to project tools as staff learned what worked and did not work in provider–client interactions.

6 See Chapter 14 for further documentation of clients' willingness and desire to discuss the sensitive topic of gender violence.

7 Chapter 17 also documents multiple, reinforcing workshops with providers as part of the Belize Family Life Association's approach to helping them consider sexuality and gender in their work.

8 Other chapters in this book also explore how to involve men without diminishing women's autonomy. See especially Chapters 20 and 21.

9 Chapters in other parts of the book cover expanded reproductive health services or address a neglected aspect of reproductive health. See, for example, Chapters 5, 10, and 21 (infertility); 9 and 23 (female genital cutting); 10 (postabortion care); 11 (postpartum care); 20 (RTIs); and 21 (prolapse, abortion).

10 See Chapter 19 for another example of creating a specialized reproductive health center, in this case within a municipal health system in Brazil.

11 See Chapter 10 for information on a postabortion care project that aimed to increase men's involvement in women's recovery following abortion.

12 An innovative way of addressing women's need for induced abortion is found in Chapter 21, which describes an effort to ensure access to safe menstrual regulation services. Staff assessed the competence of menstrual regulation providers in Kathmandu (where menstrual regulation is legal) and instituted an explicit and careful referral system for women in geographically remote areas who were seeking to terminate an early-stage pregnancy.

13 For information on gender violence projects in nonclinic settings, see Chapters 22 and 23.

14 Endogenous RTIs result from an overgrowth of organisms normally present in the reproductive tract and include yeast infection (such as candidiasis) and bacterial vaginosis.

15 Syndromic algorithms are flow charts that guide the clinician through a series of decisions that lead to a conclusion about the presence or absence of infection.

16 Vaginal infections include bacterial vaginosis, candidiasis, and trichomoniasis. Cervical infections include chlamydia and gonorrhea.

References

Dugger, Celia. 2001. "Relying on hard and soft sells, India pushes sterilization," *The New York Times*, 22 June.

Heise, Lori, Mary Ellsberg, and Megan Gottemoeller. 1999. "Ending violence against women," *Population Reports*, series L, no. 11.

United Nations. 1995. "Programme of Action of the International Conference on Population and Development, Cairo, Egypt, 5–13 September 1994," in *Report of the International Conference on Population and Development*, UNDoc.A/CONF.171/13/Rev.1. New York: United Nations.

PART I
MOVING NATIONAL HEALTH
AND FAMILY PLANNING SYSTEMS
TOWARD A CLIENT CENTER

paragraph 7.12, Programme of Action
The principle of informed free choice is essential to the long-term success of family-planning programmes. Any form of coercion has no part to play. . . . Demographic goals, while legitimately the subject of government development strategies, should not be imposed on family-planning providers in the form of targets or quotas for the recruitment of clients.

How can services be reoriented following revolutionary policy changes?

2

Dismantling India's Contraceptive Target System: An Overview and Three Case Studies

Nirmala Murthy, Lakshmi Ramachandar,
Pertti Pelto, and Akhila Vasan

From the 1940s to the 1990s, India's family planning program was narrowly focused on control of rapid population growth and characterized by a preoccupation with contraceptive targets—numbers of women to be recruited annually for sterilization and other methods. Following the 1994 International Conference on Population and Development (ICPD) in Cairo, the government of India officially renounced its contraceptive target system and adopted an ICPD-inspired approach to population policy and family planning. This new approach placed a premium on meeting women's needs for reproductive and child health services and promoting quality of care. It also decentralized the program planning process, transferring this responsibility to service providers at the local level.

A major shift in the population policy and family planning program of a country the size of India demands our serious attention. This chapter examines the dynamics of this shift at the level of service delivery, as embodied in the Community Needs Assessment (CNA) approach and the Reproductive and Child Health (RCH) program.

Our findings are based largely on field-level observations and interviews conducted with female health workers in 1997 and 1999. The perspective of these workers is particularly valuable because they are on the frontlines of service delivery, interacting directly with women in the community. Moreover, they have played and will continue to play a central role in planning and implementing the CNA/RCH initiative at the local level. We also spoke with other health care providers, district health officials, and women in the community in order to gain their perspectives.

THE CONTRACEPTIVE TARGET SYSTEM

In the early 1960s, the government of India established contraceptive targets in an effort to reduce fertility rates as quickly as possible. The highest targets were set for sterilization, followed by those for the intrauterine device (IUD). Each state was required to recruit a certain number of "contraceptive acceptors" each year. Responsibility for meeting these targets was delegated downward until it fell largely upon female health workers. Their job was to "motivate"—that is, persuade, pressure, or otherwise induce—set numbers of women to adopt permanent and temporary contraceptive methods. Workers were required to meet annual, monthly, weekly, and, in some cases, daily targets for different methods (Bandarage 1997).

Meeting the government's contraceptive targets—notably for sterilization—became a top priority of India's Ministry of Health and Family Welfare. Health workers were instructed to visit each village in their assigned area once a week, go to the homes of potential sterilization candidates, and motivate them to be sterilized. They were required to maintain registers of those to whom they had provided family planning services and to submit regular reports to the government. In monthly "performance review meetings" with their supervisors, workers were asked to report on their progress—particularly with respect to their sterilization targets. Common queries were: What was your sterilization target? How many sterilization cases did you get this month? How many cases are you going to get next month?

Health workers had other responsibilities, of course. They were supposed to conduct weekly clinics in which they were to provide immunizations, perform antenatal checkups, treat minor ailments, and distribute condoms and contraceptive pills; they were also expected to attend deliveries when called. But striving to meet their sterilization targets took up most of the workers' time and energy, leaving other aspects of reproductive and child health care relatively neglected (Visaria 1999).

The contraceptive target system operated differently from state to state and even within states, as the upcoming case studies illustrate. A 1994 study found that in Tamil Nadu, 94 percent of health workers experienced "high pressure" to meet contraceptive targets, while in Karnataka 40 percent of workers reported "high pressure" (Verma and Roy 1999). In some districts the system was particularly oppressive, as described below in the case of Coimbatore.[1]

Incentives and Disincentives: A Scheme Based on Distrust and Disrespect

The target system exposed Indian officials' dim view of low-level workers and women. In their view, rural village women and health workers could not be trusted to make the right choices without pressure and financial incentives. To this end, the government set contraceptive targets artificially high to put maximum pressure on its family planning foot soldiers. Health workers report that their assigned targets were much higher than the number of women in their communities who wanted to practice contraception. To illustrate this point, one worker showed a researcher her "Eligible Couples Register,"[2] in which the names of most women were marked by a red triangle, indicating that they had been sterilized. "Even when I show this to my supervisors they refuse to listen," the worker reported. "I have very few women left to accept any method. But the supervisors insist I should 'somehow' meet the target."

To spur workers to meet their targets and to induce women to accept contraception, the government promoted an incentive/disincentive scheme—a system of rewards and punishments. This scheme reflected the government's priorities: Sterilization was of paramount importance; temporary contraceptive methods were a secondary concern. Thus, workers were paid 50 rupees for every woman they motivated to be sterilized, but were not paid anything for the women they recruited for IUDs, oral contraceptives, or condoms. Women were generally given 160 rupees for being sterilized, but were given little or no incentive money for accepting a temporary method. Workers in some parts of India were also promised other rewards for exceeding their sterilization targets, such as desirable postings.

These incentives were coupled with strong disincentives to fall short of the government's targets: Workers who did so risked being punished in various ways. The monthly performance review was the primary arena in which this punishment was meted out. According to observations by Ramachandar and Pelto and other reports, supervisors would insult, berate, and humiliate workers who failed to meet their targets and would threaten to—and sometimes would—withhold their pay, deny them raises, fine them, demote them, or transfer them to undesirable work areas. These disincentives were effective. As one worker explained, "We were all being questioned regarding the target versus our achievement. If we showed nil in the achievement column, we were suspended from our job. Hence we did not want to have this black mark on our personal records."

Workers fearful of punishment employed various strategies to meet their targets. In some settings they spent as much as half of their time—and some of their own money—locating sterilization candidates, motivating them to undergo the procedure, accompanying them to the site of the operation, and providing support to their families. One worker reported, "Sometimes I spend three days on just one case. If there is no vehicle, I have to take her by bus and spend from my pocket."

Not surprisingly, many women came to distrust health workers, believing that they were more concerned with meeting their sterilization targets than with meeting women's needs. One woman complained, "They are interested only in the operation. Before the operation they promise us all kinds of help, but after the operation they don't care whether we are dead or alive." Another lamented, "The sister here told me to take the IUD. I took it but my husband doesn't like it. I tell her to remove it but she refuses. She says I must keep it for two years. My husband is threatening to throw me out. What can I do now?" Health workers were well aware that women in their communities distrusted them. As one observed, "Older women do not even allow us to examine their young daughters-in-law when they are pregnant. They are scared we will push family planning on them." Women's distrust often extended to the entire health care system. Even those who wished to practice contraception sometimes stayed away.

Competition, Corruption, and Coercion

The pressure on health workers to achieve their targets spawned intense competition for sterilization cases. Workers had to compete not only among themselves but often also with others charged with procuring cases. Competitors included other health care personnel and workers in other governmental departments—notably, in some areas, the Revenue Department.

Revenue workers had an advantage over health workers in that they could offer women extra material incentives to be sterilized, such as consumer goods, food, and loans. One health worker reported, "Revenue Department officials were promising clients that they would help them to procure loans from the bank and special loans from the IRDP [Integrated Rural Development Programme] and other financial institutions."

In this competitive environment, health workers tried to secure sterilization cases whenever, wherever, and however they could. Some would scavenge for cases outside of their catchment areas, in other districts, even in other states. Workers kept their eyes out for women who fit demographic profiles that made them more likely to accept sterilization. Older, high-parity women and women pregnant with their second child were prime targets. "We were very careful in following up all our clients who were pregnant for the second time," a worker reported. "Our follow-up services would start right from the inception of pregnancy. We always tried to accompany these clients to the maternity home at the time of labor pain." That way, if a client was sterilized after childbirth, the worker who brought her to the health facility could claim credit for her case.

Competition for sterilization cases gave rise to a host of unethical practices, ranging from "case stealing" to extortion and profiteering. Coercing women to "accept" sterilization was an all-too-common practice. Family planning clients were often treated like black-market commodities to be coveted, traded, bargained for, and brokered. Some "case brokers" were health workers with surplus cases beyond their quotas; others were entrepreneurs outside the health care system. These included *ayahs* (nurses' helpers) in the subdistrict and district hospitals, employees in local government offices, workers in the Tamil Nadu school lunch program, workers in other governmental sectors, and community members. One health worker reported, "Some of my cases were silently grabbed by revenue officials. I had to pay 200–300 rupees to those brokers to return my cases." Another worker described similar dirty dealings:

> When I found out that one of my clients had gone to a government facility for childbirth, I had to rush there immediately in order to follow up the case. The hospital staff person had claimed my case in order to collect the 50 rupees. Just for the sake of 50 rupees, anybody would grab our cases and claim to have motivated them. We needed the cases to reach our quotas, so we had to pay 100–200 rupees to get back a stolen case. It was like a business transaction. To get credit for a case, my name had to be written boldly on the motivation form, and the form had to be signed by the surgeon. If somebody else's name was on the form, it would look as if I had not achieved my monthly target.

Workers desperate to procure sterilization cases sometimes deliberately misled women in order to convince them to undergo the procedure. One worker confessed, "We tell them, 'Big doctors are coming from the city to perform the operations. It will be done using modern methods, so there will be no cutting open and women can go home within a day.'" Another admitted, "We don't tell them about the possible side effects because it will scare them even more."

Workers who came up short of their targets would sometimes pad their performance figures by listing nonexistent contraceptive acceptors in their registers.[3] Health officers also inflated their achievements at times, especially in states with strong reward-and-punishment systems. However, when "poor-performing" states failed to meet their targets, the national government often increased the pressure on "better-performing" states by raising *their* targets—thereby increasing the pressure on those states to inflate their achievements. This cyclical pattern of data inflation is thought to have skewed contraceptive acceptance rates upward during the target era.

Compromised Quality of Care and Violations of Women's Rights

Throughout the target era, women were sterilized en masse at government-sponsored "sterilization camps." These were not permanent sites but rather daylong medical marathons conducted at health facilities by teams of gynecologists and other personnel. Hundreds of thousands of Indian women were sterilized at these camps during the target era.[4]

Government media campaigns drew many women to sterilization camps by advertising the cash rewards awaiting those who underwent the procedure. Often, more women arrived at the camps than the space or staff could accommodate. One anesthetist observed, "The Revenue Department unnecessarily created undue demand for sterilization. . . . In the planning process, adequacy of space was not assessed."

Long waiting periods, unmanageable crowds, poor postoperative care, and shortages of vehicles to transport patients were common. The pressure to sterilize large numbers of women lowered the quality of care. Doctors were often prevented from providing competent care by the conditions under which they were forced to work. One surgeon described such conditions at a particularly large, overcrowded camp:

In one of the camps nearly 400 clients were registered. We were operating continuously in a congested theater. There was no breathing space or room for movement. We could not complete all the cases even though we worked until midnight. Some women were totally frustrated and left. The revenue officials who had motivated and brought those women complained to the district collector that we had refused to operate. After doing all this donkey's work, can you imagine that our director issued memos to all of us asking for an explanation as to why we did not operate!

The quality of care that women and children received in their communities was also compromised by the government's focus on sterilization. Health workers would visit those homes where there was a "case to be motivated," not necessarily homes where there was a sick child or a woman at high risk of pregnancy complications. Antenatal care was intermittent, deliveries were rarely attended, and other health services were neglected. One worker observed, "I was not able to give any health education to my women. There was no scope for any component other than sterilization."

The contraceptive target system undermined women's rights as well as their health. Their rights to reproductive self-determination, safe family planning services, and fully informed, voluntary consent were all sacrificed to further the government's demographic agenda.

Distrust and disrespect, worker intimidation, competition and corruption, compromised quality of care, and rights violations were the conditions fostered by the contraceptive target system. As problems proliferated, it became increasingly clear that, in the words of a health worker from Coimbatore, "It was a mad, insane world during the target era."

Some Demographic Success, but at a High Price

India's target-oriented family planning program did contribute to a fall in total fertility rates from nearly six children per woman in the early 1960s to around 3.5 in the early 1990s. The many strands of "modernization" and economic development in Indian society made a substantial, independent contribution to this decline, however, by reducing wanted fertility and increasing voluntary contraceptive use, including widespread acceptance of sterilization. In other words, an unknown but likely significant proportion of the decline in fertility would have occurred without the targets in place. The target system carried a high cost: It led to serious neglect of other aspects of health care, alienation and abuse of clients, demoralizing pressure on health workers, and, ultimately, widespread public opposition to the government. The increasingly coercive aspects of the program, particularly those concerning male sterilization, are widely considered to be a factor in the defeat of Indira Gandhi's government in 1977.

As the 1990s progressed, population experts increasingly criticized the demographic "logic" underlying the contraceptive target system. They pointed out that the system's disproportionate attention to older, high-parity women left the family planning needs of younger, low-parity couples largely unmet—although the childbearing choices of these couples would have a significant impact on India's demographic future. The strongest censure of the target system came from within India. Women's health activists were the most forceful and relentless critics of the system, declaring it a "violation of human rights . . . showing no respect to women" (Ramachandran 1996).

INDIA'S NEW APPROACH TO
POPULATION POLICY AND FAMILY PLANNING

In addition to the rising tide of internal and external opposition, several other factors persuaded the Indian government to jettison its official population policy and family planning program. These included the growing international consensus that protecting human rights must be the first-order concern of all population and development policies and programs—a position codified in the ICPD Programme of Action.

Another persuasive factor was the emergence of promising new approaches to population policy and family planning. Beginning in the early 1990s, research in India and elsewhere was yielding evidence that meeting women's reproductive and maternal/child health needs and offering them more choice in family planning methods had demographic payoffs. Experimental reproductive and maternal/child health programs in India reported substantial reductions in fertility (Measham and Heaver 1996; V. Ramasundaram 1995).

A third factor was mounting evidence that unwanted fertility could be decreased substantially in India without targets. The 1992–93 National Family Health Survey (1995) revealed that some 20 percent of women of reproductive age had an unmet need for family planning. India's fertility rate could be reduced substantially by fulfilling this unmet need—no targets would be needed.

This combination of factors convinced the Indian government, beginning in the early 1990s, to test alternatives to its contraceptive target system. It began by experimentally eliminating targets and scaling-up maternal/child health services in selected districts in all major states. The demographic results of this experiment were mixed. In some states, including Tamil Nadu, the new approach did not reduce contraceptive use; in other states it resulted in a 10–50 percent decline in contraceptive prevalence, but it also led to improvements in maternal/child health care (Khan and Townsend 1999). As noted above, because the previous contraceptive prevalence data were suspect owing to widespread data inflation under the target system, it is possible that there was little or no decline in actual prevalence.

The idea of removing the targets did not sit well with many health officials and supervisors. Supervisors complained of loss of control over health workers in the absence of the targets they used to judge performance. State health officials informed national policymakers that workers interpreted "target-free" as meaning "work-free"—based on the assumption that workers would not work unless they were under pressure to do so.

Despite this resistance, the government continued to reform its population policy and family planning program. Nearly two years after the ICPD, it formally abolished the contraceptive target system nationwide and adopted a decentralized, client-centered approach to reproductive and child health care.[5] In doing so, the government placed India at the vanguard of developing countries that were acting on the recommendations of the ICPD Programme of Action. The government hoped that its new policy and programmatic agenda would redress some of the problems created by the target system; it also hoped that the new approach would promote further declines in fertility. But first a framework for the new approach had to be designed and implemented.

Framework for the New Approach

Drawing on field experiments conducted in various states, the government adopted a framework for its new agenda that rested on two policies: (1) family planning services would be offered in the context of broad reproductive and child health services; and (2) program planning would be undertaken at the local level based on an assessment of women's needs for services. This framework took the form of two national initiatives: the Community Needs Assessment (CNA) approach and the Reproductive and Child Health (RCH) program.

In keeping with its intent to decentralize the planning process, the government offered only general guidelines for conducting community needs assessments and gave states the responsibility to work out the practical details of how to implement them. The general understanding was that health workers would conduct CNAs and then create plans to meet the service needs they identified. Workers would consult with their supervisors while developing their workplans and, in a radical departure from centrally defined targets, supervisors would then use the workers' plans to evaluate job performance.

The Reproductive and Child Health program would provide the health services that women (and children) needed, including antenatal care, safe delivery, and immunization, and would reorient contraceptive service provision in a client-oriented manner.[6] While increasing contraceptive use was a programmatic goal, meeting women's needs for a range of health services and improving quality of care were top priorities. How the program would be implemented was, again, a matter to be worked out at the local level.

The CNA and RCH initiatives were not, however, target-free. Indeed, health workers acquired *more* targets under the new approach—targets related to numerous reproductive and child health services, as well as targets for specific contraceptive methods. The difference was that—at least in theory—these targets were to be set by the workers themselves rather than by distant government bureaucrats. Workers would view their targets as performance goals that they would strive to meet not because they felt pressure to do so but because they were committed to the goal of meeting women's health care needs. In these respects, the CNA/RCH targets would be a breed apart from those of the old target system.

The government's CNA/RCH initiatives raised great hopes and serious concerns among researchers, activists, policymakers, and program managers. Would workers and supervisors establish greater or less trust following the redistribution of their roles and responsibilities? Would women's actual needs for contraception prove to be far less than the government was banking on? Would women's needs for other reproductive health services overwhelm the health care system? Would program management become simpler or more unwieldy? Would the decentralization of program planning produce too much variation in program implementation? And, finally, would the initiative simply confirm that a target is a target is a target?

We turn now to case studies documenting different aspects of the transition to the new approach to family planning.

CASE STUDY #1: DHARWAD DISTRICT, KARNATAKA

Dharwad is the largest district in the state of Karnataka, with a population exceeding 3.5 million. One in eight residents belongs to a socially and economically disadvantaged group. The literacy rate is 71 percent for males and 45 percent for females (Government of India 1991). Although the population is predominantly rural (65 percent), the national highway and several main train lines run through the district.

Most primary health care in Dharwad is provided through 85 primary health centers (PHCs), each of which has a catchment area of about 30,000, and affiliated subcenters. Through this network of facilities, the district implements national health programs, including maternal/child health care and family planning. Dharwad has been considered one of the better-performing districts in the area of family planning.

As in many districts of India, Dharwad's PHCs suffer serious deficiencies. Most report inadequate supplies of basic medicines,[7] one-fourth lack proper equipment, and one-fourth have unfilled slots for physicians. In addition, half of the subcenters have unfilled slots for male health workers. As a result, many people do not get the health care they need. For example, only 25 percent of women receive antenatal care, and less than half of all children receive required immunizations (Murthy and Vasan 1999).

During the target era, health workers in Dharwad experienced significant pressure to meet their contraceptive targets. As in other parts of the country, they focused primarily on promoting family planning services, with an emphasis on sterilization. They more often visited homes where there was a "case to be motivated for family planning" than homes where there was a pregnant woman or child. In addition, they spent an average of more than one week each month maintaining 18 required registers.

This case study, based on research conducted by Murthy and Vasan in 1995–97, describes the implementation of a community needs assessment in Dharwad. Researchers from the Foundation for Research in Health Systems analyzed the workplans prepared by 90 of the district's 450 female health workers, who represented 15 of the district's 85 PHCs.[8] Investigators also interviewed 15 PHC doctors, state and district health officers, 20–25 health workers, and 50–60 women in the community.

Resistance to Implementing the Community Needs Assessment

District health officers were initially skeptical about the feasibility and usefulness of the CNA exercise. As one officer put it:

> Each year we receive planning guidelines from the health directorate. The guidelines indicate the targets to be achieved and the size of the budget. We develop our plans accordingly. Most of the budget is already committed to salaries and medicines. Less than 10 percent of the budget is for district-specific schemes. So what difference will the community needs assessment make?

District officers complained that the CNA approach did not provide any financial flexibility, that the government had not delegated any administrative powers to them, and that it diminished their role in program planning. They were also concerned that the CNA/RCH initiative involved only female health workers, who were already overworked.

Assessing the Need for Reproductive and Child Health Services

Despite district officers' reservations, state officials decided to implement the CNA in Dharwad, since this was now the policy of the government of India. In collaboration with the Foundation for Research in Health Systems, the state family welfare officer developed guidelines for the CNA, which would assess the need for 15 family planning and maternal/child health services (see Box 1). The need for services that were not currently available—including pregnancy termination and management of reproductive tract infections (RTIs)—would not be evaluated at this stage.

A Four-Step Process

The district's family welfare officer structured the CNA as a four-step process: (1) determining "area requirements" based on state-set performance norms and local demographic data; (2) assessing women's felt needs; (3) determining service needs based on women's felt needs and the area's demographic profile; and (4) developing a workplan. Worksheets were provided to guide health workers through the process.

The state-set performance norms on which area requirements were to be based included a mix of levels of service provision considered feasible and levels considered desirable. For most services the norms were higher than previous performance. For example, pregnancy registration had been at 81 percent; the norm was set at 100 percent. A few norms were set at levels close to or lower than previous performance norms because of practical considerations. For example, institutional deliveries had been at 31 percent; the norm was set at 33 percent.

In order to assess women's felt need for services, health workers administered 15 questions[9] (based on the maternal/child health and family planning services outlined in Box 1) to a sample of 50 area women of reproductive age whose youngest child was below age 3.[10] For example, women were asked whether they felt a need for antenatal care during pregnancy; "yes" indicated their felt need for this service. Service needs were then calculated based on the sample's felt needs and the demographic profile of the catchment area. If 70 percent of women surveyed in a subcenter area said that they preferred to deliver their babies in hospitals, then the need for institutional delivery was determined to be 70 percent of the anticipated number of pregnancies in the subcenter area.

Workers then outlined their annual plans for service delivery. They were instructed to aim to meet service needs according to women's felt needs, but only if

---

Box 1. Maternal/child health and family planning service goals in Dharwad District

1. Antenatal registration of all pregnant women
2. Early registration (before 16 weeks) of as many pregnant women as possible for antenatal care
3. Referral of women at high risk of pregnancy complications
4. Treatment of severely anemic pregnant women
5. Two tetanus injections for pregnant women
6. At least three health checkups during pregnancy
7. Institutional delivery of babies
8. Home deliveries attended by a trained midwife
9. Weighing of newborns
10. Referral of high-risk newborns for medical examination
11. Child immunization (BCG, DPT, polio, measles)
12. At least five vitamin A doses for children under age 3
13. Oral rehydration therapy for children with diarrhea
14. Medical treatment of children with acute respiratory infection (ARI)
15. Provision of contraceptives to women who need them

---

these were higher than the area requirement figures developed around the state norm, which were to be regarded as minimum performance levels. Following the hypothetical example of institutional deliveries, workers would thus set their planned performance somewhere between the area requirement (33 percent) and the estimated felt need (70 percent).

Training Personnel to Carry Out the CNA

The district health officer (who oversees the work of various health program officers) was responsible for implementing the CNA. The family welfare officer (responsible for family planning) oversaw the training of all personnel after he had been trained at state headquarters. All health administrators and supervisors in the district attended one-day workshops that covered the rationale for the new approach; workplan development; quality of care; the equal importance of all RCH services; and evaluation of workers' performance based on achievement of goals in all service areas, not just recruitment of contraceptive acceptors.

During these workshops, female supervisors expressed concern that the new approach would increase the workload of female health workers. When asked why only female workers were to participate, the district health officer reportedly assured female supervisors that male workers would help. Female supervisors doubted this. As one explained, "It will be very difficult to get any work out of them [male workers] on a voluntary basis. They refuse to function as multipurpose workers. They have stopped collecting sputum from TB cases [because they did not get risk allowance, that is, monetary compensation for doing work that is hazardous to their health]. We are only pushing female workers to take on more and more work." (One district officer did try to involve male health workers in the CNA process, but doing so, indeed, proved to be problematic. Male workers—who traditionally focus on malaria and tuberculosis screening and follow-up—viewed reproductive and child health as female workers' domain.)

Heated exchanges between trainers and participants reportedly occurred in many CNA training workshops. At some, PHC staff argued that if they were expected to meet people's needs, their own needs and problems—such as staff vacancies and over-work—would have to be addressed first. District officers did not encourage discussion of these problems, possibly because they had no solutions. Despite these difficulties, however, all participants ultimately agreed to go forward with the CNA.

The next step was to train health workers to carry out the CNA. Training sessions, which consisted of two days of lectures interspersed with data collection, were held at all 85 PHCs. In the classroom, each of the four steps of the CNA process was explained in detail. Workers learned how to conduct surveys, ask survey questions, and record data on the worksheets provided. They practiced filling out these worksheets using data from a hypothetical subcenter. Following this training, the workers went to their subcenter areas and spent about three days collecting needs assessment data from 50 women. Their supervisors helped them compile the data and complete the remaining worksheets.

Most workers were able to estimate area requirements easily because doing so entailed a straightforward computation based on the number of women of reproductive age and the number of anticipated pregnancies and live births in a specified population. Workers had more difficulty grasping the concept of felt need and how this might differ from service-seeking behavior. Some workers converted felt-need questions into questions that assessed actual practice—and vice versa. For example, the question "Do you feel the need to register for antenatal care?" was sometimes converted to "Did you register for antenatal care?"

Calculating Needs and Setting Goals for Service Delivery: Tinkering with Calculations

For most of the 15 services, area requirement and needs assessment figures were fairly consistent. In the case of child immunization, for example, performance norms dictated 100 percent coverage, and 90 percent of women felt a need for this service. On the other hand, while 41 percent of recently delivered women expressed a need for delaying the next pregnancy, the area requirement for birth spacing based on the state-set norm was 55 percent. Workers had been asked to assume that "need for spacing" could be converted into acceptance of temporary methods; this was unlikely, however, given that only 0.2 percent of married women reported using spacing methods. Interestingly, 54 percent of women expressed a need for sterilization services, but the area requirement was only 45 percent.

Workers' self-assigned performance goals for family planning were often higher than their contraceptive targets had been and tended to be more closely aligned with area requirements than with women's expressed needs. When workers were told that they could set goals that reflected women's felt needs, many responded that it was better to anticipate what their supervisors wanted (i.e., meet area requirements). Despite trainers' attempts to overcome the tendency of workers to word the felt-need questions in a manner that would generate data showing high levels of need, this tendency may have persisted during the surveys. Some workers apparently feared that their supervisors would accuse them of not having performed their health education work well enough if levels of felt need for services were low. District officers suspected the opposite: that workers would intentionally underreport women's felt need for services so as to set lower performance goals for themselves.

To counteract this alleged misconduct, officers instructed workers to calculate service needs by applying felt-need figures to population data from the 1991 census rather than population figures from the workers' annual enumeration, which they distrusted.[11] To account for the increase in population since 1991, they instructed workers to multiply the village population of 1991 by 1.9. Officers believed that these calculations would force workers to increase their performance goals. Ironically, the older census data—even when multiplied by 1.9—yielded a lower population than the workers themselves had enumerated the previous year.

PHC staff were frustrated that they had been instructed to develop plans for areas in which there were no health workers to implement them. District officers claimed these instructions had come from above. One PHC physician commented that this hardly constituted decentralized planning: "Why are you calling it decentralized approach when we only have to follow the district's instructions?"

State or district health officers sometimes lowered performance goals in keeping with the perceived capacity of the health care system. For example, the expected number of diarrhea cases and women's felt need for oral rehydration salts (ORS) were four times higher than the number of ORS packets available. Similarly, women's felt need for treatment for acute respiratory infection (ARI) was calculated to be five times higher than the number of ARI cases treated at PHCs the previous year. Knowing that ORS supplies would remain erratic and that many individuals would seek ARI treatment from private doctors, the officers lowered their performance goals for these two services.

For similar reasons, state health officers intervened in the way performance goals were set by setting lower norms in the area of obstetric care. While 68 percent of women preferred a hospital delivery to delivery at home, the officers doubted the district's capacity to meet this need; hence they set the area requirement for institutional delivery services at 33 percent. The officers justified this by asserting (in contradiction to the data) that most women preferred home deliveries and that this preference was not likely to change for some time. The officers also set low area requirements for early antenatal care and for referrals of woman at high risk of pregnancy complications.

At the end of this planning exercise, the district officers told PHC staff that the plans they had prepared were now their "targets" for the year. At the end of the year, their performance would be evaluated against these new targets.

The Effects of the CNA

Effect on health workers. In the year after the CNA was completed, health workers achieved over 90 percent of their performance goals. Under the old system, they had generally achieved 80–85 percent of their targets. This improvement in job performance occurred even though they received no additional resources. Furthermore, workers reported that they did not feel pressured by their supervisors to achieve family planning targets, nor were they as likely to be threatened with punishment for failing to do so.

Health workers' job performance improved even though their overall workload increased—just as they had feared. They now had performance goals for 15 services rather than targets for contraceptive methods only; moreover, as noted earlier, their contraceptive targets were in some cases slightly higher than before. Workers made an effort to assign more or less equal importance to all 15 goals. One worker commented, "I have more work now than before. Earlier I could meet my family planning targets. Then nobody would ask me any more questions. Now it is different."

While CNA program-planning responsibilities added to health workers' workload, the responsibilities also increased their sense of pride and personal investment in their work. Workers eagerly displayed their service-delivery plans on subcenter walls. One pointed to her plan and stated proudly, "These are now our targets. We know how to calculate them."

As health workers talked less about family planning and more about maternal/child health, they gained a more positive image in their communities. One worker commented, "Earlier we felt that we were beggars, begging women to come for an operation. Women behaved as if they were doing us a favor. Now I don't feel that way. I feel that I give them the services they need." Another remarked, "I am not doing only family planning. That is why it is easy for me to work in the community." A third observed, "We are better accepted in the community. People do not avoid us."

Workers were more comfortable with their self-assigned sterilization goals than they had been with the sterilization targets assigned to them under the old system. This was true even in subcenter areas where workers' sterilization goals were as high as or higher than their old targets. One worker commented, "Earlier all of us were asked to recruit two sterilization cases per month. That meant our annual target was 24. Now my plan shows 25 women need sterilization this year—but it's okay."

The new system brought about a change in the structure and atmosphere of monthly performance review meetings. Workers no longer complained to their supervisors that their targets were unrealistic. Meetings no longer focused exclusively on contraceptive targets. Workers would report how many deliveries they had attended and how many pregnant women in their area had completed three antenatal visits, in addition to how many women had adopted contraception. The tone of review meetings improved markedly. As one worker observed, "Our work has increased, but our officers don't shout or threaten us."

Effect on clients. We spoke with women in the community to assess whether they perceived any change in the way services were provided after the target system was replaced with CNA. Some women reported that health workers called on them more frequently. Others remembered workers writing down the names of all pregnant women and telling them that it was important to go to the hospital to deliver babies. But most of the women we interviewed did not perceive much change.

We asked women whether workers spent adequate time with them, answered their questions, and provided them with information. One woman's response summed up the feelings of others: "She cannot spend much time with us. She has many houses to visit." Some women said it was not necessary for workers to visit them or to motivate them for family planning; they had wanted and obtained sterilization on their own. Overall, women did not notice any improvement in the quality of services. They did say, however, that health workers inquired about their needs, and felt that the government was concerned about the welfare of pregnant women and children. Whether or not this is a result of decentralized planning is not clear: Women had not heard about decentralized planning or about the targets being removed. While these impressions suggest that the new system did not benefit women greatly, our data show that women's use of services increased and that health workers spent more time providing a wider range of services.

Table 1. Indicators of reproductive and child health service use in Dharwad District before and after implementation of the CNA

Outcome indicator	Before[a]	After[b]
Institutional deliveries (% all deliveries)	20.0	28.0
Deliveries by midwifery-trained personnel (% all deliveries)	51.0	55.0
Complete immunization (% children 12–23 months old)	48.0	73.0
Antenatal care checkup (% pregnant women)	23.0	53.0
Contraceptive use (% women with children under age 5)	37.0	43.0

[a] Baseline survey conducted by Foundation for Research in Health Systems in September 1994.
[b] Rapid household survey in 15 PHCs conducted by Foundation for Research in Health Systems in September 1997.

As workers encouraged women to use the various services for which they had professed a need, use of those services increased (see Table 1). Use of antenatal care increased from 23 percent in 1994 (one-and-a-half years before the CNA was implemented) to 53 percent in 1997 (one-and-a-half years after CNA implementation). Child immunization increased from 48 percent to 73 percent during the same period, and institutional deliveries increased from 20 percent to 28 percent. Sterilization rates rose very slightly, and the use of temporary contraceptive methods barely increased, from 0.2 percent to 1.3 percent, despite the fact that the CNA had revealed a need for delaying the next birth roughly equal to that of stopping births altogether.

Quality-of-Care Issues

While health workers are now evaluated on their success in promoting use of a wider range of services, the quality of the services provided is not taken into account. For example, district health officers have given little attention to women's satisfaction with contraceptive methods (in terms of side effects, follow-up care, and the choice of methods workers provide). Asked why women's satisfaction with services is not considered, one health officer replied, "Because women attribute any discomfort to contraception. We cannot rely on their reports."

Summary

The CNA pilot project in Dharwad highlights the strengths and weakness of the decentralized approach. On the positive side, most health workers were able to gather CNA data and carry out computations. Helpful worksheets, assistance from trained supervisors, and workers' past exposure to sample surveys all contributed to this success.

Health workers' central role in carrying out the CNA had several benefits. Interviewing women for the needs assessment increased workers' awareness of women's perspectives on their own needs. Workers also learned that the local health care system was not capable of meeting all of women's felt needs for services, and that women did not always feel a need for potentially beneficial services. In such cases, workers were able to identify a need for health education.

Perhaps most importantly, workers developed a greater sense of personal investment in their work. They showed more commitment to the plans and performance goals they themselves established for the purpose of meeting women's needs than to the targets that had been set for them under the old system. This was true even when their self-assigned targets were equal to or greater than their old targets.

Implementing the CNA approach in Dharwad has also had some measurable benefits for women. Use of reproductive and child health services increased after the new approach was instituted. Under the new system, relations between women and health workers improved in some respects: Workers reported feeling more welcome and respected in the communities they serve, for example.

On the negative side, some health officers did not approve of the CNA process. They regarded the CNA as an academic exercise, a mere formality that did not reflect their own mandate, which they continued to feel was the achievement of contraceptive targets. As one district officer observed, "Even though workers don't have [externally imposed] targets, we continue to have them as before. We have to somehow meet those targets."

The efficacy of the new approach was constrained by staffing shortages and the increased work demands on female health workers. It was also hampered by persistent distrust between health officers and workers and between workers and the women they serve. District officers were unwilling to accept workers' calculations as accurate. Some workers doubted whether women had given them accurate and honest answers to their survey questions. For the CNA approach to succeed in the future, district officers must have a more serious commitment to the program—and to health workers.

CASE STUDY #2: KOLAR DISTRICT, KARNATAKA

The district of Kolar is approximately two hours east of Bangalore, the capital of Karnataka, to which it is linked by highways and a railroad. While not affluent, the district has an active economy and strong trade links to external markets. Modern aspirations and consumer lifestyles are prevalent. Social norms about family size have changed rapidly, with many people choosing to invest in the education and well-being of a smaller number of children.

Data were gathered in Kolar District from October to December 1999 by Ramachandar and Pelto. To learn about the effect of eliminating the target system in this district, we focused on one major *taluka* (subdistrict) with a population of around 265,000.[12]

We gathered much of our information from in-depth interviews with 23 of the 47 auxiliary nurse midwives (ANMs) in the subdistrict (ANMs function as the primary grassroots interface between the health care system and the community). We also observed five sterilization camps, which gave us opportunities to talk with clients and their family members. We conducted in-depth interviews with over 20 males (mostly husbands) in PHCs and the *taluka* hospital. We also met with the RCH officer and his staff at the district headquarters, and were provided with data on a range of RCH services.

Conditions Under the Target System

The former contraceptive target system had never been as draconian in Kolar as it had been in other districts of India. The ANMs we interviewed reported that they had few difficulties meeting their targets. While both revenue and health workers were required to recruit women for sterilization, they cooperated unusually well. ANMs reported that they had to "buy" sterilization cases, but, compared to the complex machinations necessary elsewhere, these were relatively simple transactions that mainly took place at the *taluka* hospital. ANMs in Kolar could buy cases from locales outside of their work area ("out-of-area cases") for 30–50 rupees per case. Informants also reported that ANMs swapped cases when one had more cases than she needed to meet her target while another did not have enough.

Training, Supervision, and Staffing Under the New System

The launching of the national Community Needs Assessment and Reproductive and Child Health initiatives prompted a limited programmatic response in Kolar. The district's ANMs were trained to provide a broader range of RCH services, including temporary contraceptive methods. The training, however, was brief. ANMs reported that they received very little information about such topics as HIV/AIDS.

In keeping with the spirit of the government's new RCH program, Kolar has incorporated *anganwadi* (children's daycare) workers into its community health care system. These workers play a major role in identifying pregnant women; they also attend the monthly review meetings with ANMs. This arrangement has facilitated close cooperation between ANMs and *anganwadi* workers, thereby strengthening efforts by the latter to identify pregnant women and to promote use of temporary contraceptive methods.

More Targets Under the New System

The target system has not been dismantled in Kolar. On the contrary, ANMs in this district (as elsewhere) now have more targets than they did before. These include targets for temporary contraceptive methods, antenatal care registration, treatment of diarrhea cases with oral rehydration therapy, and other RCH services. The ANMs we interviewed listed ten targets that they are now expected to meet.

As in Dharwad, the task of calculating targets was transferred from state and national officials to local health workers. In Kolar, ANMs now conduct careful household surveys to enumerate the local population and identify all couples of childbearing age. These surveys are the first step in developing targets based on state performance norms, local demographic data, and women's felt need for services using CNA, as described above in the case of Dharwad.

According to our informants, there have been several problems with the calculation of targets in Kolar. First, the computational steps outlined in the state CNA manual are reportedly complicated and result in unrealistic targets. After ANMs have completed their calculations by following these instructions, the PHC medical officer and district health administrators reportedly increase these numbers arbitrarily. In some instances they add numbers to the total (enumerated) population. One of our informants expressed her frustration with this situation:

> We spend a minimum of seven days every year to enumerate our subcenter populations. We go door to door to count the household members and get a thorough house listing. We note down new births and deaths, and accordingly we arrive at an exact population. Based on this enumerated population, we fix our targets for different activities. When they [inflate our demographic data] they say that they do not believe our counting. If they do not believe us, why do they waste our time?

Health officers reportedly also inflate the targets that ANMs have set for themselves. One ANM reported to us:

> I took courage and asked the medical officer why they are giving additional targets. He said, "Our primary health center's target has been increased and I came to know this from the Kolar district officials when I went for my monthly meeting." I asked, "Who increased the target for Kolar?" "It came from the state capital," he said.

Another ANM remarked:

> Why do we calculate and set our own targets? What is the use? Suddenly our superiors give us shocks by saying, "Add this extra number to your target." We are not supposed to know why it is given and who is giving it. If we question them, they label us "argumentative." We have to unquestioningly obey their orders.

The ANMs in Kolar still have strong fears of being punished for failing to meet their targets. They fear being denied pay increases and allowances for purchasing work uniforms and being transferred to less desirable locations. According to our observa-

Table 2. Contraceptive trends in Kolar District, 1990–2000

Year	Sterilization		IUD		Oral contraceptives (OCs)	
	No. of clients	% of mix[a]	No. of clients	% of mix[a]	No. of clients	% of mix[a]
1990–91	12,971	48.0	9,756	36.1	4,316	16.0
1991–92	15,523	49.2	11,020	34.9	5,017	15.9
1992–93	16,004	49.0	11,678	35.7	4,991	15.3
1993–94	18,735	47.1	15,008	37.7	6,052	15.2
1994–95	20,557	45.2	15,997	35.2	8,889	19.6
1995–96	19,910	42.3	18,137	38.6	8,988	19.1
1996–97	19,844	40.2	20,215	41.0	9,270	18.8
1997–98	19,468	41.3	19,092	40.5	8,608	18.2
1998–99	20,234	43.1	18,832	40.2	7,837	16.7
1999–2000[b]	16,225	43.3	13,634	36.4	7,641	20.4

[a] Defined as sterilization, IUD, OCs.
[b] To November.
Source: Based on statistics from the Bureau of Health and Family Welfare, Kolar District.

tions and the ANMs' interview responses, punishment begins with verbal abuse during monthly review meetings; such abuse appears to be routine.

A New Formula for Assigning Contraceptive Methods

The use of temporary contraceptive methods (notably the IUD) has increased in Kolar. This can be attributed to several factors: (1) the government's new endorsement of temporary methods; (2) the growing proportion of sterilization clients who voluntarily choose to undergo the procedure, thereby reducing the amount of time that ANMs must spend motivating women to be sterilized; (3) the presence and cooperation of *anganwadi* workers and community educators, who have enabled ANMs to devote more attention to providing temporary methods; and (4) the increasing acceptance of temporary contraceptive methods among people in the district. All of the health workers we interviewed commented on people's increased awareness of the need for spacing methods and the choices available. Table 2 presents data showing the increased use of IUDs and oral contraceptives. Such data are difficult to interpret. Other data have shown that use of temporary methods was already on the rise before the end of the target era; however, those numbers may be inaccurate, given the evidence that ANMs and PHC personnel may have routinely inflated their performance figures.

The ANMs in Kolar use a parity-based formula to determine which methods to offer particular women. An ANM explained, "We review the couples in our [Eligible Couples Register], study their marital status, and accordingly motivate them to use different kinds of contraception." Newly married women are given information about delaying their first pregnancy and about oral contraceptives, condoms, or IUDs, but are not "motivated" to accept a contraceptive method. Women with one child are motivated to use an IUD. Women who present with symptoms contraindicating IUD use are asked to try oral contraceptives. Women with two or more children are generally only offered the "option" of sterilization.

While the pressure on ANMs to motivate women to accept sterilization has diminished, the pressure to motivate women to use IUDs has increased. As one ANM reported:

> Our target for the copper-T has doubled now. They [PHC medical officers] have no sense, asking me to get 36 copper-T cases. Women with a single child are motivated to use the copper-T as a spacing method. How can I manage to get 36 copper-T cases, that is, women with single children? When I explain to the doctors that I do not have that many cases in my field area, they do not seem to understand.

The ANMs are instructed to screen women for symptoms that would contraindicate IUD use. If such symptoms are detected in a client, the ANM is supposed to provide her with an alternate temporary contraceptive method (usually oral contraceptives). While this benefits women to some degree, it does not benefit ANMs under pressure to meet high IUD targets. This conflict of interests is not conducive to rigorous compliance with screening guidelines. As one ANM explains:

> They have increased the IUD target and also they have given us a set of conditions before inserting IUDs. Clients should not present symptoms of white discharge. There must be no previous history of heart disease. She should not complain of giddiness. She should not suffer any physical weakness. She should not have more than one child [women with two or three children are strongly urged to go for sterilization, but in some cases are given IUDs]. Her first delivery should not have been a cesarean. She should not be diabetic. She should not have [high] blood pressure. She should not have tuberculosis or a history of it. She should not complain about bleeding. If we keep searching for IUD cases in the whole area, keeping these conditions, we would not get a single case.

Inadequate Attention to Reproductive Health Care Needs

With their work week stretched to the limit and their attention still focused primarily on meeting their contraceptive targets, ANMs in Kolar simply have no mandate or time to address broader reproductive health concerns. As a result, they pay relatively little attention to RTIs/STIs (including HIV/AIDS). ANMs receive some training on this topic, but they rarely put it to use. They are supposed to visit schools occasionally to talk about health issues, but this activity is infrequent and involves limited contact with students.

Haphazard Record Keeping

Record keeping appears to be haphazard. We often saw ANMs jotting data on miscellaneous slips of paper and in small notebooks. It appears that they only update their records and registers once a month, in time for their monthly review meeting.

The ANMs we spoke with complained vehemently that the state government has not given them registers for record keeping. As one noted:

> The government has not supplied us with the registers. They are busy giving extra work and are always questioning our work. Where should we record all our work? For two years we have not received registers. We cannot buy 20 registers at our own expense.

Summary

Under the former target system in Kolar, there were few targets and the environment in which ANMs worked to meet them was relatively relaxed. Under the new system, health care personnel have been trained to provide a range of reproductive health services, temporary methods of contraception have gained ground, and ANMs are collaborating with *anganwadi* workers. However, the target system is alive and well in Kolar. Indeed, the commendable shift in emphasis toward a broader range of reproductive health concerns and a wider array of contraceptive methods has only increased the number of targets that ANMs are required to meet. In addition, district and state administrators have not abandoned the idea that health workers must be pressured to do their work in response to quantitative performance demands from above. Pressure on ANMs to meet their targets, if anything, has increased. One ANM explained:

> The government says that there are no targets, but there are. The medical officer dictates his terms to me. He says, "You have to get these many tubectomies and IUDs. Somehow you have to meet these targets." They talk in the same authoritarian tone and style. They say, "I don't know how you are going to get the cases but getting cases is your problem, not my problem."

CASE STUDY #3: COIMBATORE DISTRICT, TAMIL NADU

Coimbatore is one of the wealthier districts in the state of Tamil Nadu. Fertility rates have fallen sharply in the state, as they have in much of southern India. Indeed, Tamil Nadu has achieved its goal of reducing fertility to the replacement level.

The 70 PHCs that serve Coimbatore's 3.6 million residents are better funded than those in many rural districts; nevertheless, Coimbatore still suffers shortages of medical supplies, equipment, and other resources (including water).[13]

This case study is based on 60 interviews with health care providers and observations at health facilities, all conducted in 1997 by Ramachandar and Pelto. Half of the interviews were with visiting health nurses (VHNs) and half were with other health care personnel, including physicians, nurses, and statisticians. Although the interviews took place several years after the demise of the contraceptive target system, respondents—who were selected to represent Coimbatore's main subregions—were eager to talk about that system.

Harsh Conditions Under the Target System

The contraceptive target system was particularly harsh in Coimbatore, as it was throughout Tamil Nadu. Responsibility for meeting sterilization targets was assigned to the district revenue, health, education, and rural development departments, which competed fiercely for sterilization cases.

VHNs in Coimbatore hunted far and wide for sterilization cases. Stealing, brokering, and trading cases were common practice. One VHN reported, "Just to get one case I have gone all the way to Mettupalyam or Pollachi *taluka* hospitals, away from my own operational area. I had to go that far just because my area case was cleverly grabbed by someone and taken to the *taluka* hospital."

Workers in all departments would lure women with the promise of the 160-rupee reward that they would receive from the government for undergoing sterilization. But revenue workers would also offer women consumer goods—such as pressure cookers, table fans, saris, and water containers—as additional incentives. To advertise these incentives, the Revenue Department would place announcements in local newspapers that identified the location of sterilization camps where the goods would be available. One informant described the methods used by department workers to secure sterilization cases:

> *A revenue official of a subdistrict would go all the way to area Y to distribute pamphlets announcing that five kilos of rice would be given to women who got sterilized in area X. Then the official of area Y had to stop women from going to area X to be sterilized, so immediately he would print another pamphlet announcing that sterilization clients would get free transportation from their home to the sterilization facility in area Y and back home again. They would also get consumer goods, such as steel water containers, in addition to the government cash incentive.*

The government's 50-rupee reward for procuring a sterilization case was the primary motivation for revenue workers to comply with the contraceptive target system. The main motivation for VHNs, on the other hand, appears to have been the fear of being berated or otherwise punished for failing to meet targets.

One VHN described the stressful conditions she worked under during the target era: "Night and day I am thinking and getting worried about my target. How to achieve the target, how to get back the stolen cases, and at what cost. It was an era of nightmare."

An Early and Gradual Change in Policy

Efforts to reform the contraceptive target system began in Tamil Nadu several years before the national government officially abolished the system. Beginning in 1991–92, the government of Tamil Nadu assigned the Directorate of Health and Family Welfare sole responsibility for meeting contraceptive targets throughout the state, eliminating much of the competition for sterilization cases. To the surprise of state administrators, relieving the Revenue Department of responsibility for meeting contraceptive targets did not prevent the state from meetings its family planning goals for the year.

Tamil Nadu went on to eliminate the policy of paying workers 50 rupees for sterilization cases. This removed the main incentive for the aggressive competition over cases (S. Ramasundaram 1995). Client incentives for sterilization, which came directly from the central government, continued.

When the national government instituted the decentralized Community Needs Assessment approach to reproductive and child health program planning, VHNs in Coimbatore began to set their own targets. They were also given responsibility for maintaining the district's Eligible Couples Registers. Direct control of this register gave VHNs more power over the management of their target population and daily workloads.

Implementing the New Approach: From Training to Expanded Services

Having been relieved of the pressure to meet externally imposed sterilization targets, VHNs were able to expand the scope of their work to include provision of temporary contraceptive methods and other services. To improve the capacity of VHNs and other health care providers to meet a wider array of reproductive and child health needs, the district invested in training personnel, expanding services, and enhancing worker supervision.

In 1995 all VHNs and PHC personnel in Coimbatore attended a six-day training session to introduce them to new health concepts and skills. Participants learned about the importance of providing informed choice and good quality of care, assessing community needs, promoting participatory learning, and raising health awareness (Visaria and Visaria 1999). The district's VHNs also attended a series of training workshops over the next two years. These covered IUD insertion; general reproductive health, including signs and symptoms of gynecological problems and an introduction to HIV/AIDS; maternal/child health; identification of cataracts for treatment at "eye camps"; and identification and treatment of leprosy.

VHNs now provide a broad array of reproductive and child health services in Coimbatore. These include antenatal care, child immunization, school health camps, and expanded work on STIs and HIV/AIDS. VHNs cooperate with community nutrition workers to improve the nutritional status of pregnant women. Together with medical officers, VHNs provide health education in schools. They also conduct malaria surveillance.

All of these activities entail new record-keeping responsibilities. Our informants reported that record keeping had been quite shoddy during the target era, when data falsification was believed to be widespread. In the post-target era, accurate record keeping has taken on new importance.

Record keeping is now part of a complex information system that enables VHNs to be well informed about the communities in which they work. For example, we found that VHNs were able to provide detailed tallies of abortion cases in each of their villages, including cases they were not following themselves. The VHNs now maintain at least 20 registers, from which data are extracted and compiled at the district and state levels. The VHNs in Coimbatore are proud of and personally invested in their record-keeping responsibilities. They regularly save money from their salaries to purchase registers themselves, since they do not receive sufficient supplies from the government.

The meticulous record-keeping practices of VHNs in Coimbatore can be attributed partly to enhanced supervision, and partly to the fact that VHNs avoid harsh criticism by maintaining detailed registers. During monthly meetings in the target era, supervisors focused primarily on whether the VHNs had met their sterilization targets, offering little in the way of effective guidance or monitoring. The VHNs now meet weekly with the community health nurse and also (albeit less frequently) with the sectoral health nurse, medical officers, and district officials. These meetings sometimes involve general supervision and training, but their primary focus is review of VHNs' work progress as reflected in their registers.

The Perspective of Village Health Nurses

All of the VHNs we interviewed in Coimbatore describe conditions before and after the old target system as being dramatically different. A common reaction to the change is a profound sense of relief from the tensions of "scrambling for clients."

Nevertheless, this relief is tempered with irony. VHNs still have to meet family planning targets in Coimbatore, as they do in Dharwad and Kolar. Now, however,

Table 3. Family planning trends in Coimbatore, 1992–97

Year	Sterilization		IUD		Oral contraceptives (OCs)		Condoms	
	No. of clients	% of mix[a]	No. of clients	% of mix[a]	No. of clients	% of mix[a]	No. of clients	% of mix[a]
1992–93	23,316	46.5	10,495	20.9	5,310	10.6	11,063	22.0
1993–94	23,082	45.3	9,688	19.0	5,460	10.7	12,745	25.0
1994–95	22,804	30.6	17,220	23.1	12,251	16.4	22,308	29.9
1995–96	21,700	30.5	18,650	26.2	11,781	16.5	19,119	26.8
1996–97	22,970	36.7	19,405	31.0	8,776	14.0	11,403	18.2

[a] Defined as sterilization, IUD, OCs, condoms.
Source: Based on statistics from the Bureau of Health and Family Welfare, Coimbatore.

targets are established locally and are based on local demographic realities. In addition, the anxiety associated with meeting targets in years past has virtually evaporated.

Like their counterparts in Dharwad and Kolar, the VHNs in Coimbatore now have more work than they did previously, because of added services and increased record-keeping responsibilities. The VHNs interviewed for this study complained that they have to work extra hours during the week and on weekends to keep up with their registers.

Effects on Contraceptive Use

There have been changes in contraceptive practices in Coimbatore since the new approach to family planning was launched. For example, while the number of sterilizations per year remained nearly unchanged from 1992 to 1997, the number of IUD insertions per year doubled during that time (see Table 3). Table 3 also shows increased use of oral contraceptives and condoms beginning in 1994–95. While some of that momentum has been sustained, condom use has returned to its earlier levels.

Summary

Coimbatore's primary health centers have broadened and improved their reproductive and child health services. Health care providers at the community and PHC levels have been educated about a range of RCH issues and have been trained to deliver more such services. Unethical practices (such as coercing women to get sterilized) undertaken to meet contraceptive targets are a thing of the past.

The former target system was particularly oppressive in Coimbatore, yet this district has made great strides toward a client-centered approach to family planning.

In addition, the daily lives of health workers have improved markedly. This reflects the state's historically high investment in the health and social sectors, and the fact that Tamil Nadu's VHNs are better trained and qualified than those in most other states. As a result, the expanded RCH program was implemented more smoothly in Coimbatore. One study suggests that the experience in other districts of Tamil Nadu has been less positive (Ravindran 1999).

LESSONS LEARNED IN DHARWAD, KOLAR, AND COIMBATORE

In dismantling its long-standing contraceptive target system, the government of India had a limited objective: to make the program more client-oriented and redress some of the problems that had emerged under the old system. In addition, by revamping the system, the government hoped that India would be able to continue reducing its fertility rate. The new approach was not intended to eliminate targets or incentives altogether, but rather to modify the system in several important ways. First, through the community needs assessment, the setting of targets was to be delegated to health workers, who would assess needs in consultation with clients. Second, as part of the Reproductive and Child Health program, the number of targets was widened to include a broad array of RCH services. Third, the pressures related to meeting targets—including structured competition, psychological harassment by supervisors, and monetary incentives for workers—were to be eliminated.

Is a target still a target? As can be seen from these case studies, there are significant differences even in the experiences of three districts from two neighboring states in southern India. Coimbatore—where the former system was particularly oppressive—has made the greatest strides toward an RCH orientation and the most pronounced improvement in the daily lives of the health workers. In other settings, such as Kolar, top-down quotas for contraceptives during the target era have been replaced with, effectively, other top-down targets with concomitant pressure on workers. But a number of important lessons can be drawn from the differences—and the parallels—in the transitions of these three districts.

Quality-of-care issues are still a concern. Women in these districts are being provided with more family planning information and choice of contraceptive methods than they were in the past. Nonetheless, health workers and their superiors are still accustomed to telling women what method they should choose rather than asking women about their preferences. We see a need for more family planning counseling and contraceptive method choice, as opposed to a formulaic assignment of methods on the basis of women's parity levels or state priorities. The increased use of IUDs (especially in settings where targets for IUDs are imposed) raises serious concerns about choice, as well as whether women are being screened for active infection prior to IUD insertion and whether asepsis is being maintained.

Progress in meeting reproductive health needs beyond family planning and maternal health care has been limited. Progress is being made, though somewhat unevenly. This is attributable in part to lack of clarity in RCH program goals, as well as funding limitations and lack of trained personnel. In some areas (e.g., STI/RTI management) limited progress is in part the result of the dearth of information on cost-effective approaches appropriate to low-resource settings.[14]

The new CNA/RCH approach has increased the workload of health workers. This was the case across districts, and female health workers are most directly affected. As governments reassess their priorities for community health services, they must be sensitive to the staffing required to carry out expanded RCH programs and for a fair division of labor between male and female workers.

Implementing the CNA/RCH approach has augmented family planning outreach efforts. The new approach has made it easier for health workers to deliver family planning services. With the pressure to meet sterilization targets lifted (to a greater or lesser extent) and the programmatic focus widened to include a broader set of RCH issues, workers have gained legitimacy and greater acceptance in their communities. They now find it easier to discuss contraception with their clients. However, in settings where externally imposed targets have been reimposed (e.g., targets for IUDs in Kolar), such trust can easily be undermined.

Dismantling the contraceptive target system did not reduce contraceptive use. Instituting the new approach did not have much effect on rates of contraceptive use. In fact, sterilization rates remained about the same (or were higher) after the new approach was implemented, regardless of how it was implemented, in the three districts. The use of temporary contraceptive methods increased in all three districts after the new approach was instituted; however, this trend may have been underway nationally prior to the end of the target era.

The transition in the roles and responsibilities of health officers and supervisors—those historically responsible for achieving targets—is incomplete. The CNA/RCH approach limits health officers and supervisors to training workers and monitoring their performance in relation to workers' self-determined performance goals. Many officers appear unwilling to relinquish their authority in the absence of other avenues through which they can exercise leadership or control. Staff at all levels of the health care system need to have a stake in sustaining this new approach to family planning and reproductive health care.

Frontline health workers show greater commitment to service goals they set themselves than to targets thrust upon them from above—even if there is no numerical discrep-

ancy between the two. Most workers who were involved in setting targets and who felt protected from undue pressure to meet them reported success in meeting them and did not complain that they were unreasonable. In addition, workers who felt that they were serving community members rather than catering to government officials had a more positive view of themselves as professionals. Success in meeting performance goals was greatest where health officials abandoned the idea that health workers must be pressured to work by externally imposed, quantitative performance demands. In some settings, however, workers' own targets were summarily augmented by their superiors. Continued pressure—real or perceived—from above to meet method-specific targets demoralizes workers and can lead, at best, to circumscribed choice for women and, at worst, to coercion.

Intimidation and disrespectful treatment of health workers undermines programmatic efficacy. The denigrating attitude of many PHC medical officers and other authorities toward health workers continues to undermine the efficacy of programs in many settings. The climate of coercion, competition, and corruption that had pervaded India's contraceptive target system has not disappeared. The central complaint of workers in settings still dominated by rigid bureaucratic hierarchies is that they are treated in a patronizing, punitive, and even abusive way by their superiors. Workers in these settings report that they continue to be berated and threatened with negative sanctions when they fail to meet their targets and are not allowed to explain or defend themselves.

Clients will receive better services when personnel at all levels of the health care system work as a team united by a shared purpose: to provide high-quality health services that meet people's needs. Only when medical officers learn to trust health workers and recognize that they are a valuable source of information about local health needs will these officers become better informed and able to fulfill their own responsibilities to protect public health and well-being. Only when officers invest in ongoing and supportive training and supervision of workers will they create effective health care teams whose members carry out their tasks in a synergistic way. Only when they view community needs assessments conducted by health workers as more than perfunctory exercises can they usefully participate in finding solutions to community health problems.

And only when medical officers form collegial and respectful relationships with subordinates will they foster respectful treatment of clients by health workers: As workers are treated, so are they likely to treat clients. Even the problems of weak infrastructure and lack of sufficient funding for basic health services can be at least partially offset if the personnel providing services do their utmost to respect each other—and to respect clients' right to choose the contraceptive methods and health care services they need and prefer.

CONCLUSION

We recognize that many people regard the hierarchical structure of Indian society as highly resistant to change. But hierarchical relations within the health care system are, indeed, changing in some parts of the country. More health workers speak of medical officers who treat them with respect and dignity. Fewer feel they are at the mercy of distant bureaucrats.

Reproductive health care in India took a step forward when the national government officially retired its former population policy, declared an end to its contraceptive target system, and endorsed a new ICPD-inspired approach to family planning. The effects of this policy and programmatic shift were not felt, however, until the new approach was implemented at the grassroots level. The contrasts between the three case studies in this chapter reveal the extent to which the interpretation, implementation, and impact of national policies and programs vary at the local level. The similarities between them suggest principles and procedures that can promote further change.

We hope to have conveyed a sense of the possibilities and challenges involved in transforming a centralized, demographically driven family planning program into a decentralized, client-centered reproductive health care system. Opinions will differ as to whether any approach other than the former contraceptive target system could have been mounted in India in past decades. But now and in the future a new approach to family planning is required, one that is part of a package of reproductive health services that places a premium on quality of care, meeting clients' needs, and protecting their rights.

Acknowledgments

Lakshmi Ramachandar and Pertti Pelto gratefully acknowledge the help and support of personnel in the Departments of Health and Family Welfare in Karnataka and Tamil Nadu. We also acknowledge our large debt to the many health workers and clients who provided us with rich narratives about their experiences in the health care system. We express our thanks to the editors for their invaluable assistance in polishing the language and structure of the chapter.

Nirmala Murthy and Akhila Vasan gratefully acknowledge the support of the International Health Policy Program, which was made possible by generous funding from the Pew Charitable Trusts. We also thank Dr. G. V. Nagaraj, Program Director of the Reproductive and Child Health Program in Karnataka, and Dr. B. F. Appannanavar, District Family Welfare Officer, for their involvement in and support of our research.

Notes

1   While it is impossible to assess the target system in its entirety, there is a body of literature detailing its abuses (see, for example, Bandarage 1997 and Khan and Townsend 1999).

2   The Eligible Couples Register is a record maintained by health workers of all married couples (in which the female partner is 15–45 years old) in their assigned work area. It includes basic

information on such characteristics as age, education, number of children, age of youngest child, and contraceptive method used, if any.

3   Several studies and surveys carried out in different parts of India document this finding (see, for example, Khan and Townsend 1999).

4   While the term "camp" sometimes has negative connotations, it refers to any periodic clinical service at which a designated screening or surgical procedure is provided on a designated day, usually by specially trained personnel sent to the site. They are often held in regular clinical facilities, although others take place in makeshift, inadequate sites. The sterilization camp was an innovation of the Indian family planning program. In its early years, the program brought in expert surgeons, normally based in urban hospitals, to conduct the procedure in rural areas. Over the years the concept fell into disrepute, as too many camps were arranged with fewer and fewer resources.

5   This decentralized approach was consistent with the *panchayati raj* (elected local self-government) Act of 1993. Under this act, the national government was to transfer responsibility for planning and monitoring development programs to district levels and below.

6   India launched the RCH program in October 1997 with partial financial support from the World Bank.

7   District health officers refute this, claiming that PHC physicians use government supplies for their private practices.

8   These PHCs were chosen because the maternal health care they provided was particularly poor; the objective of the research was to demonstrate the potential impact of decentralized planning on maternal health care in this context. As such, the PHCs were not entirely representative of the district's PHCs overall.

9   The questions were: (1) Do you feel the need to register for antenatal care during pregnancy? (2) In which month of your pregnancy would you register? (3) During pregnancy did you suffer from problems for which you had to see a doctor? (4) Would you take iron and folic acid tablets during pregnancy? (5) Would you have tetanus toxoid immunization during pregnancy? (6) How many times would you go for checkups during pregnancy? (7) Where would you like to deliver: home or hospital? (8) Who would you like to conduct your delivery: trained person or relative? (9) Would you like to have your child weighed at birth? (10) Did any of your children have to be taken to a doctor soon after birth? (11) Do you feel your child should be immunized? (12) Do you think your child should receive vitamin A? (13) When your child has diarrhea, do you think you should give him/her oral rehydration salts? (14) When your child has an acute respiratory infection, do you think you should take him/her to a doctor or auxiliary nurse midwife? (15a) Do you want more children? and (15b) Would you like to delay your next child?

10   National guidelines had suggested conducting a complete household survey, which would have required health workers in Dharwad to visit about 800–900 households each.

11   Health workers in Karnataka gather data on population size and composition every April.

12   In this *taluka* there are ten PHCs, one hospital, seven primary health units, 282 *anganwadi* centers, 47 subcenters (each staffed by an auxiliary nurse midwife), three maternity centers, and one national leprosy control center.

13   The district is also served by two central hospitals, seven subdistrict (government) hospitals, and 468 subcenters staffed by visiting health nurses.

14   See Chapter 16 for more information on managing RTIs in low-resource settings.

References

Bandarage, A. 1997. *Women, Population and Global Crisis: A Political–Economic Analysis.* London: Zed Books.

Government of India. 1991. "Provisional population totals: Rural–urban distribution," series 1, paper 2. New Delhi: Registrar-General of India.

Khan, M.E. and John Townsend. 1999. "Target-free approach: Emerging evidence," in S. Pachauri (ed.), *Implementing a Reproductive Health Agenda in India: The Beginning.* New Delhi: Population Council, pp. 41–75.

Measham, Anthony R. and Richard A. Heaver. 1996. *India's Family Welfare Program: Moving to a Reproductive and Child Health Approach.* Washington, DC: World Bank.

Murthy, Nirmala and Akhila Vasan. 1999. "Improving district family welfare services: A decentralized planning model," *Journal of Health Management* 1(1): 35–53.

National Family Health Survey: MCH and Family Planning: India 1992–93. 1995. Bombay: International Institute for Population Sciences.

Ramachandran, Vimala. 1996. "NGOs in the time of globalization," *Seminar* 447(November).

Ramasundaram, S. 1995. "End of the target era," *Voices* 3(2).

Ramasundaram, Vimala. 1995. "Family welfare without targets: Tamil Nadu's experience," *HealthWatch* (Update 2): 22–24.

Ravindran, T.K. Sundari. 1999. "Rural women's experiences with family welfare services in Tamil Nadu," in M.A. Koenig and M.E. Khan (eds.), *Improving Quality of Care in India's Family Welfare Programme: The Challenge Ahead.* New York: Population Council, pp. 70–91.

Verma, Ravi K. and T.K. Roy. 1999. "Assessing the quality of family planning service providers in four Indian states," in M.A. Koenig and M.E. Khan (eds.), *Improving Quality of Care in India's Family Welfare Programme: The Challenge Ahead.* New York: Population Council, pp. 169–182.

Visaria, Leela. 1999. "The quality of reproductive health care in Gujarat: Perspectives of female health workers and their clients," in M.A. Koenig and M.E. Khan (eds.), *Improving Quality of Care in India's Family Welfare Programme: The Challenge Ahead.* New York: Population Council, pp. 143–168.

Visaria, Leela and Pravin Visaria. 1999. "Field level reflections of policy change," in S. Pachauri (ed.), *Implementing a Reproductive Health Agenda in India: The Beginning.* New Delhi: Population Council, pp. 77–111.

Contact information

Nirmala Murthy
Foundation for Research in Health Systems
6 Gurukrupa Apartment
183 Azad Society
Ahmedabad, India
telephone/fax: 91-80-672-0135
e-mail: frhs@vsnl.com

Lakshmi Ramachandar
#5 Nirmitee Terrace
South Main Road
Koregaon Park
Pune 411 001, India
telephone: 91-20-611-1530
e-mail: perttipelto@hotmail.com;
    lakshmir99@yahoo.com

3

Offering a Choice of Contraceptive Methods in Deqing County, China: Changing Practice in the Family Planning Program Since 1995

Baochang Gu, Ruth Simmons, and Diana Szatkowski

Two decades of market-oriented reform in the People's Republic of China have generated economic growth and social change, presenting both individuals and institutions with new challenges and opportunities. As people begin to experience new freedoms and average incomes increase, tolerance for the often harshly enforced population policy has lessened and requests for better family planning services and a broader range of reproductive health care have been voiced. In one survey conducted in six counties (Zhang, Gu, and Xie 1999), many women complained about the lack of follow-up in contraceptive care and indicated a need for counseling services, treatment of reproductive tract infections, and information on women's health.[1] At the same time, the 1994 International Conference on Population and Development in Cairo and the 1995 World Conference on Women in Beijing, in which China was a major participant, focused worldwide attention on client-centered models of reproductive health care.

Together these domestic and international developments prompted national-level officials of China's State Family Planning Commission (SFPC) to begin reorienting the family planning program from an exclusive focus on demographic objectives to one that is also client-centered. In 1995, Minister Peng Peiyun of the SFPC made the official call for the program's reorientation.[2] Soon after, the SFPC selected five rural counties and one urban district as pilot sites for a quality-of-care experiment (Gu 2000).[3] Personnel at the sites were encouraged to be creative in developing client-centered family planning initiatives to fit local conditions. No specific guidelines were provided. Instead, local leaders and family planning personnel were invited by the SFPC to participate in weeklong workshops during which key concepts of client-centered care and relevant changes in management practice were discussed.

We describe the experience of one of the SFPC pilot sites, Deqing County in Zhejiang Province, a fast-growing rural county that was designated one of the "hundred most prosperous counties in the country" in 1993 and 1994. Deqing is located a few hours east of Shanghai, China's most cosmopolitan city. Three-quarters of the county's population of approximately 420,000 are employed in agriculture; the average annual income for farmers in Deqing is approximately 4,098 yuan,[4] which compares favorably with provincial (3,815 yuan) and national (2,162 yuan) averages (National Bureau of Statistics 1999). In recent years the total fertility rate in Deqing has dropped as low as 1.2 children per woman, and the contraceptive prevalence rate has been as high as 93 percent.[5]

Our focus is on the county's efforts to introduce informed contraceptive choice. The data we use are derived largely from an interdisciplinary, qualitative, participatory field assessment conducted in late 1998 in the six pilot counties (Simmons, Gu, and Ward 2000).[6]

BACKGROUND

In contemporary China, centrally directed population policy and planning have defined the contours within which individual reproductive decisions are made. Population policy set a limit on the total number of children that a couple may have.[7] It also mandated that couples practice contraception, and even specified the contraceptive methods they should use—IUDs and sterilization, both of which are provider-controlled. Population plans formulated at the national, provincial, and local levels set targets consistent with the national goal of keeping the country's population below 1.4 billion by the year 2010. The plans themselves are formulated through an iterative process that involves all levels of government.

To ensure that couples comply with family planning rules and regulations, complex "planned birth management" systems have been established. While the details vary from place to place, such systems have commonly required couples to obtain written approval from the local family planning program office to carry a pregnancy to term. In order to get permission to have a child, couples have also been required to sign "family planning contracts" and to commit themselves to using particular contraceptive methods following a birth. In general, couples are expected to have an IUD inserted after the first birth and to be sterilized after the second.[8] In most of rural

China, a second child is permitted after a specified number of years as long as the first child is female and a "childbirth permit" is obtained for both births. Government leaders, program managers, and family planning workers also sign "responsibility contracts" in which they agree to meet the program's goals. Those who meet these goals receive financial rewards and community recognition. Those who fail to meet them may be reprimanded, fined, or even dismissed from their jobs.

Consistent with the program's goals and methods, evaluation of program and individual family planning worker performance has been based on quantitative indicators such as the planned birth rate,[9] the IUD acceptance rate after the first birth, and the sterilization acceptance rate after the second birth. Performing well on the basis of these measures has often meant disregarding the needs and desires of individuals and their families. As a result, relations between family planning workers and clients have often been strained.

FAMILY PLANNING IN DEQING BEFORE THE QUALITY-OF-CARE EXPERIMENT

Before the experiment, couples in Deqing were allowed to have a second child if their first child was a girl,[10] provided that they obtained a "childbirth permit" for each birth from the township family planning office. A verbal request was sufficient for the first birth, but for the second couples were required to file a written application. Couples who failed to obtain the necessary permit or who did not file an application in a timely manner were fined an amount ranging from 10 to 30 percent of their average total annual income.

As in other areas in China, contraceptive use in Deqing was mandatory and parity-driven, such that after the first birth women were required to have an IUD inserted, and after the second they or their partners were required to undergo sterilization. The program provided few viable alternatives for women who did not want to use an IUD or be sterilized, or for whom such methods were contraindicated. While a woman could, in theory, request permission to have an IUD removed, program officials and providers often discouraged them from doing so, and few authorized removals were recorded. Couples about to be married obtained a childbirth permit when they completed their marriage registration and paid an IUD deposit of 100–200 yuan. This deposit was returned when the woman had an IUD inserted after the delivery of her first child. For those who were granted permission to have a second child, a sterilization deposit of 200–500 yuan was collected when the couple received the childbirth permit authorizing a second birth. As with the IUD deposit, this fee was returned after the woman or her husband was sterilized following delivery of her second child.

Box 1. Characteristics of service delivery in the Deqing program before the experiment

- 42 percent of women said that family planning personnel made a contraceptive method choice for them.
- 50 percent of women said that they did not receive follow-up care after contraceptive adoption.
- 63 percent of women said that what they needed most was contraceptive counseling and treatment for gynecological problems.

Source: Based on a September 1995 survey of 697 married women of reproductive age conducted by the Deqing County Family Planning Commission (Zhang, Gu, and Xie 1999).

This "one rule for all" policy of contraceptive adoption was further reinforced by the mode of program and provider evaluation, which, as in the rest of China, was based largely on such indicators as the planned birth rate, the IUD acceptance rate after the first birth, and the sterilization acceptance rate after the second birth. Judged on this basis, Deqing performed well relative to national and provincial averages. Contraceptive prevalence rates were high, and both out-of-plan births and contraceptive failure rates were relatively low. Because all aspects of the program were directed toward these goals, contraceptive options were largely limited to provider-controlled methods. Other reproductive health care concerns, such as STI management and infertility treatment, received little attention.

This single-minded focus on controlling societal fertility meant that the needs and desires of individual clients were often neglected. Clients complained of family planning workers who only had an eye for the "big belly." Others said that once a family planning worker had "succeeded" in getting women to accept a given contraceptive method, that worker was seldom heard from again. Little attention was given to follow-up, and method switching was difficult, if not impossible. Results from a baseline survey (see Box 1) conducted by the Deqing County Family Planning Commission provide additional detail about the characteristics of service delivery before the introduction of the quality-of-care experiment.

Even had there been an earlier mandate to provide a broader array of reproductive health services, grassroots family planning workers lacked appropriate training and experience, and would have been ill prepared to do so. The little instruction family planning workers received focused on family planning rules and regulations and the adverse consequences of population growth. Many workers were unfamiliar with the variety of IUDs available, contraindications to their use, and their effective use-life. As one woman with two daughters, an eleven-year-old and a one-year-old, stated:

> *After the birth of my first daughter, I used an IUD. The first four years with the IUD were fine, but then I got pregnant. . . . Neither the village family planning worker nor*

I knew that the IUD was only [effective] for five to seven years. . . . The village worker did not even know what kind of IUD I had had inserted. After the [contraceptive] failure, I had an abortion, and then had another IUD inserted.

Women were aware of the workers' deficiencies and would often tease them, calling them "semidoctors" because of their limited knowledge. However, they had few alternative sources of contraceptive information. The informational materials provided for their use also focused almost exclusively on state population policy and family planning rules and regulations.

INTRODUCING GREATER CONTRACEPTIVE CHOICE

Deqing County government leaders and program managers were aware of client dissatisfaction, and once they heard about the SFPC-initiated quality-of-care experiment they expressed an interest in participating. Shortly after the first quality-of-care workshop in June 1995, county leaders decided that informed choice of contraceptive methods would be a focal point of the quality-of-care experiment in Deqing. It soon became apparent, however, that officials and leaders at various levels of the program had diverse responses to the prospect of implementing "informed choice."

County leaders had had some exposure to international debates about reproductive health and choice and supported the national initiative to reorient the program toward quality of care. Their understanding of informed choice conformed most closely to that of the project leadership in Beijing: While adherence to national birth control policy remained mandatory, people should be given greater freedom in the choice of contraceptives and be provided with information that would help them to select an appropriate method. As a county government directive stated:

Informed choice applies to married women of reproductive age who need to adopt contraception. Under the guidance of the state and with its help, they gain the necessary contraceptive knowledge, and choose a contraceptive method at their own will, one which is safe to use and effective in preventing pregnancy.

Village leaders shared the county leaders' enthusiasm for informed choice, but for different reasons. Not only were village leaders responsible for implementing family planning policies in their villages, they were also part of the community and identified with it. The stringency of family planning rules and regulations and the lack of contraceptive choice often placed them in conflict with community members. The prospect of an experiment that would allow married women to make an informed choice regarding contraceptive methods, even if it did not allow them choice about family size, would enhance their relations with village residents.

Thus, those at the top (county leaders) and those at the bottom (village leaders) welcomed reform. However, those in the middle tier (township leaders) initially resisted the proposed changes because they feared losing the financial and status rewards associated with achieving demographic objectives and disliked the prospect of the increased workload associated with quality-of-care innovations. The director of the Deqing County Family Planning Commission aptly characterized the situation as "hot at two ends, but cold in the middle." For township leaders, informed choice implied fewer sterilizations and more out-of-plan and high-parity births. As one leader lamented:

> *We've achieved a lot in population control, and we are afraid that fertility will go up under the new approach. If we introduce informed choice of contraceptives and give up the deposits [for accepting the IUD and sterilization], women will no longer accept such effective contraceptive methods.*

With the township leaders' concerns on their minds, county leaders decided to proceed cautiously and introduce informed contraceptive choice in a single village before attempting to implement it on a countywide or even townshipwide basis. In December 1995, Huanqiao Village of Xiashe Township was selected as the site for the trial, and an ad hoc task force[11] was appointed to undertake the experiment. After two weeks of preparation, including orientation meetings for task force members, development of pamphlets on informed choice, and preparation of contraceptive method samples for display, the task force was dispatched to the village.

The task force identified 37 married women of reproductive age who, on the basis of their childbearing status, might need to choose a contraceptive within the next year. Among them were women who had recently given birth, newlyweds who were either pregnant with their first child or planning to become pregnant, and women who had either experienced a contraceptive failure or were dissatisfied with their current method.

The Huanqiao Village family planning worker then visited the 37 women and told them that they had been selected to participate in a village experiment on informed choice and that they should attend a workshop at which they would receive information about their contraceptive options. At the workshop, the women were told that they no longer needed to follow the rules requiring that they use an IUD after their first birth and undergo sterilization after their second; instead, after being counseled they could make their own choice from among five available methods: IUDs, oral contraceptive pills, condoms, Norplant® implants, and sterilization. At the same time, the monetary deposits the women had paid to ensure they would accept a specific contraceptive method were returned. The return of the money helped to underscore the message that it would be up to women and couples to decide which method to use.

Following this general introduction, the task force members split up into four groups to provide the women with individual counseling. During the counseling sessions, women were given detailed information about the way the five available methods function, how they are used, and their advantages, disadvantages, possible side effects, and contraindications. Women with one child, who might be seeking to conceive again after a period of spacing, were introduced to all five methods; IUDs and, to a lesser degree, pills and condoms, were given special recommendation. Women with two children, who were viewed as being at the end of their childbearing, were also oriented to all five methods, but with longer-acting and/or permanent methods given special recommendation. Thus even though women's choices were broadened, marking a fundamental departure from the "one rule for all" policy, a bias for long-acting methods clearly prevailed. The women were told that no contraceptive method is failure-free, but that follow-up care after contraceptive adoption would help to reduce the chance of failure and would provide an opportunity to switch to another method should the first one be unsatisfactory.

Equipped with this information, each of the 37 women was asked which contraceptive method she would like to choose. Sixteen of the 37 opted for IUDs, 20 chose sterilization, and one decided to use oral contraceptives. This last case illustrates the potential significance of the introduction of informed choice for women who previously experienced extreme side effects with the IUD: The woman who switched to oral contraception was 32 years old. She had used three IUDs, each of which had resulted in a failure and three subsequent abortions. Even though she experienced these failures as well as severe side effects with each IUD, she had not been allowed to switch to another method.

Service provision occurred at a later date, thus giving women the opportunity to think things over and discuss matters with their partners. Some women, such as those who had recently given birth, selected a method shortly after the workshop. Others, such as those who were trying to become pregnant, selected a method after they had conceived and given birth.

All but three of the 37 women did, in the end, select the contraceptive method they had chosen at the workshop. The other three had initially opted for sterilization but decided, after having a physical examination at the clinic, to choose an IUD instead because of their health status. This would have been much less likely under the old system. Moreover, three of the 19 women who eventually selected an IUD already had two children. Under the "one rule for all" policy they would have had no choice but to undergo sterilization.

Local officials were pleased with the fact that all of the 37 women participating in the experiment picked highly effective methods, and that all but one chose long-acting ones. They viewed these results as proof that clients would make "responsible" choices when given more influence over their method choice. Conversations with local officials also made it clear that they were increasingly convinced that fertility preferences had changed and that most couples were satisfied with having the allowed number of children. Thus they felt there would be no demographic risk associated with adopting the informed choice approach and reasoned that other women in Deqing would, given the opportunity, make similarly responsible choices.

Analysis of these results helped to persuade skeptics, especially those at the township level, to rally behind the experiment and support the gradual introduction of informed choice to four additional townships (Sanqiao, Shilling, Xiashe, and Zhongguan) in 1996. Encouraged by the progress of the experiment in these four townships and at the request of the 16 remaining townships, the county government expanded informed choice to all 21 townships in Deqing County in 1997.

ADDITIONAL STEPS TAKEN TO SUPPORT GREATER CONTRACEPTIVE CHOICE

A variety of steps have been taken to support the introduction of informed choice in Deqing County, including training family planning workers, developing guidelines for counseling and follow-up care, developing information, education, and communication (IEC) materials for clients and providers, introducing reforms in the "birth management system," and revising the monitoring and evaluation system. Key changes in these areas are outlined below.

Special efforts have been made to upgrade and maintain providers' skills. While most of the training has focused on the technical aspects of service delivery, some attention has also been paid to the interpersonal aspects of service provision—including counseling and communication skills. In 1997, the Deqing County Family Planning Commission conducted counseling training for providers throughout the county, using a curriculum developed for the UNFPA-supported Counseling Training Project.[12] This project made extensive use of role-playing exercises to enhance empathy with the client. For example, providers were asked to play-act a situation in which a village family planning worker approaches a woman of childbearing age with an infant in her arms. What should the worker's first words be? Trainees gave several different answers, which were then discussed by the group. Participants said that they liked the new training approach. In addition to providing training, the family planning commission developed guidelines for communication and counseling skills for providers (see Box 2).

Box 2. Provider guidelines for client counseling and communication

- Make an effort to understand people's values.
- Pay attention to language, offer friendly greetings, provide praise and encouragement, and communicate in a way that is easy to understand.
- Be aware of nonverbal communication; improve observation and listening skills.
- Use auxiliary materials: anatomical models, illustrated brochures and pamphlets, and so forth.
- Master the knowledge to carry out contraceptive consultations.

Source: Deqing County Family Planning Commission 1997.

Developing a system of client-centered follow-up visits has also been key to Deqing County's efforts to institute informed choice. In the past, follow-up was motivated by demographic objectives and therefore limited to frequent ultrasound examinations for IUD users to ensure that the device was still in place. From a quality-of-care perspective, these examinations represented unnecessary medical care. Although women using IUDs are still required to receive two ultrasounds per year, follow-up services now extend to all methods and emphasize women's needs. The follow-up schedule is based on data provided by the management information system at the township level, and visits are carried out mainly by village family planning workers. Women who are experiencing problems with their method are encouraged to go to the township service station. They are now more likely to be allowed to switch methods than they were in the past, although unless there are medical contraindications providers continue to encourage women not to switch away from the IUD. Ensuring that IUDs are replaced when their period of efficacy has expired is now part of follow-up care.

Postoperative follow-up visits for induced abortion and sterilization are carried out by township service providers. The newly developed follow-up medical guidelines for tubal ligation clients are outlined in Box 3.

The Deqing County Family Planning Commission also developed written materials to improve providers' and clients' reproductive health knowledge. Providers now have the illustrated "Guide to Quality of Care in Grassroots Family Planning," which includes protocols for informed choice, record keeping, and service provision, as well as information on and samples of various contraceptive methods. After counseling, women are given IEC pamphlets that they may keep and review with their partners. The 2–3-page pamphlets provide information on reproductive health and service availability. Pamphlets developed for clients at different stages of their lives include "Please Choose the Contraceptive Method Most Appropriate for You," "Wish You Happiness in Your New Marriage," "Wish You Have a Healthy and Bright Child,"

Box 3. Provider guidelines for follow-up after tubal ligation

First follow-up visit

1. Schedule: 3–7 days after discharge
2. Check: (1) fever, (2) site of incision, (3) irregular vaginal bleeding, (4) gastrointestinal symptoms, (5) abdominal swelling, and (6) urinary problems

If any of these problems are present, refer to the clinic or hospital.

Second follow-up visit

1. Schedule: 3 months after the procedure
2. Check: (1) general (blood pressure, pulse, skin color, "spirits"), (2) menstruation (duration, quantity, pain), (3) incision (lump, new growth), (4) abdominal pain

If any of these problems are present, refer to the clinic or hospital.

Source: Deqing County Family Planning Commission 1997.

"Children Are the Future of Our Motherland," "Cherish Your Time to Be Young," and "Menopause: A Splendid Period of Life." While the newly developed materials contain a great deal of biomedical information related to reproductive physiology and contraceptive use and convey, in general, a new approach, some of the specifics remain rooted in the old system. For example, the pamphlet "Please Choose the Contraceptive Method Most Appropriate for You" still adheres to the old norm that women should use the IUD after the first birth and sterilization after the second (see Box 4).

Important changes have also been made in the birth management system—the complex array of rules and regulations that govern childbearing. First, the county leadership decided, with the endorsement of the Provincial Family Planning Commission, to abolish township- and village-level birth quotas. Individual couples, however, are allowed to have only the number of children stipulated by the local family planning regulations. Second, the childbirth permit was replaced with a "childbearing service certificate." This certificate, while retaining the childbearing management function of the permit, provides a checklist of the reproductive health services to which clients are entitled, as well as those they have already received. Third, monetary deposits guaranteeing later use of either IUDs or sterilization are no longer required.

As a result of these changes in the birth management system, married couples in Deqing County can now decide for themselves, without prior approval, when to have their first birth. The first birth is considered an "in-plan birth" (that is, one approved under childbirth management regulations) as long as both husband and wife are eight months above the minimum legal age for marriage at the time of delivery and have obtained the service certificate, which is usually delivered to the couple by the village

---

Box 4. Excerpts from the pamphlet entitled "Please Choose the Contraceptive Method Most Appropriate for You"

(1) Contraceptive choices for newlyweds

If you don't plan to have a child right away it's best to use the following contraceptive methods:

(i) Condoms

If a condom breaks, you may use emergency contraception.

(ii) Contraceptive pills

Suitable for couples who don't plan to have a child for 1–2 years after marriage. A minority of users experience nausea, vomiting, breakthrough bleeding, and other side effects. If you do, don't stop taking the pills. These side effects will go away by themselves after 1 or 2 months.[a] If you want to become pregnant, you should wait 6 months after stopping the pill before trying to conceive. Switch to condoms during this period.

(2) Contraceptive choices for couples with one child

Right after the birth of the first child, contraceptive measures should be taken. Because pill use affects the secretion of milk and infant development, pills are not suitable for lactating women. During the first 42 days after delivery you may use condoms. After that you should have an IUD inserted. The convenience and reliability of the IUD makes it an ideal choice for the woman with one child. Those for whom the IUD is not suitable can use pills, injectables, and other methods.

(3) Contraceptive choices for couples with two children

According to current family planning policy, you cannot have more than two children. Therefore, you should adopt either male or female sterilization to achieve permanent contraception. It is safe, simple to use, and reliable.

[a] This advice may not be accurate.
Source: Deqing County Family Planning Commission 1997.

---

family planning worker after the woman becomes pregnant. Couples are thus freed from the psychological and practical burden of having to go through an application process. This constitutes a significant departure from past practice.

Improvements have also been made in the monitoring and evaluation system, especially with regard to the indicators used to assess program and provider performance. In 1996, with the approval of the Provincial Family Planning Commission, method-specific targets, such as the rate of acceptance of the IUD after the first birth and of sterilization after the second birth, were eliminated. At the same time, two new quality-of-care indicators, the client satisfaction rate and the informed choice participation rate, were introduced.[13] Information on client satisfaction is derived from rotating monthly village interviews. Women who have received services in the villages are asked to rate both the attitude and technical skills of the service provider and the clinic environment and facilities on a four-point scale, ranging from satisfied to very dissatisfied.[14] This information is used to calculate the client satisfaction rate for each township. The informed choice participation rate indicates whether women who selected a contraceptive method during the period had received information on a range of methods and had been given the opportunity to make their own choice from among them.

The Deqing County Family Planning Commission set goals for these new rates: 85 percent or above for client satisfaction (85 percent of clients should be "satisfied" or "relatively satisfied" with the care that they receive) and 90 percent or above for informed choice participation. Still, demographically oriented indicators such as the planned birth rate and contraceptive prevalence rate remain an important part of program evaluation. County goals are 98 percent or above for the planned birth rate, 90 percent or above for the contraceptive prevalence rate, and 1.8 percent or below for the unwanted pregnancy rate.

PROGRESS AND CHALLENGES

As of September 1998, 14,339 couples in 21 townships in Deqing County had participated in the informed choice experiment. In order to carry out the experiment, a significant number of changes were made in the county's family planning program in a relatively short time. Contraceptive options for women at different stages of their reproductive lives were made more readily available; providers were trained to offer clients information to facilitate contraceptive decisionmaking; new IEC and training materials were developed for both clients and providers; birth management rules and regulations were revised and simplified; and information on client satisfaction and participation in informed choice was added to the monitoring and evaluation system.

The statistical data on contraceptive method mix is shown in Table 1. As can be seen, the percentage of contraceptive users who underwent sterilization has declined since the experiment was initiated. In 1994, some 43 percent of contraceptive users were recorded as having undergone a sterilization procedure; by the end of 1999, this figure had decreased to around 36 percent, owing largely to an increase in IUD use, which rose from 46 percent in 1994 to 51 percent in 1999. In addition, the percentage of contraceptive users using condoms more than doubled (from 3.8 percent in 1994 to 8.8 percent in 1999). According to the director of the Deqing County Family Planning Commission, this rise is attributable in part to an increase in condom use among couples who want to delay their first birth.

The stories clients tell about their contraceptive experiences before and after the Deqing experiment provide a more intimate view of the meaning of informed choice.

Table 1. Contraceptive method mix in Deqing County, 1994–99

Method	1994	1995	1996	1997	1998	1999
Vasectomy (%)	0.2	0.2	0.2	0.2	0.2	0.2
Tubal ligation (%)	43.3	41.9	40.9	39.2	37.6	35.8
IUDs (%)	45.7	47.1	49.1	49.5	50.0	50.8
Pills (%)	6.3	5.5	4.7	4.5	4.5	4.1
Condoms (%)	3.8	4.4	4.7	6.1	7.5	8.8
Suppositories (%)	0.2	0.1	0.2	0.2	0.2	0.2
Other (%)	0.5	0.8	0.2	0.3	0.2	0.1
Contraceptive prevalence rate (%)	92.5	92.6	92.1	93.0	92.8	92.8

Source: Deqing County Family Planning Commission.

A woman with a twelve-year-old daughter and a five-year-old son discussed her contraceptive history:

> After the birth of my first child [which took place before the introduction of informed choice], I had an IUD inserted. After the birth of the second child [after the introduction of informed choice], I was too weak to have an IUD inserted, so my husband used condoms until I was strong enough to have an IUD inserted. Later [after receiving information about various contraceptive options], I chose sterilization. But after a physical examination, the doctor said that I was not a good candidate for sterilization. If this had happened before informed choice, I would have had to undergo sterilization irrespective of my health status.

Another woman described her experience:

> After the birth of my first child, I adopted an IUD. I thought the IUD was the most convenient [method], and I wanted to use it. But once I had the IUD, I always felt dizzy and didn't feel like eating much. I then had the IUD taken out. After a few months, I had a new IUD inserted. I did this three times [taking the IUD out and later inserting a new one] and had two abortions. After informed choice was introduced in 1995, I switched to [oral contraceptive] pills. I have not had any bad reactions since.

Providers also note the contrast between the way things were and the way they are now. In the words of one provider:

> In the past people resented the "IUD after the first child and sterilization after the second" rule, which made program implementation difficult. Now, even though our workload has increased, we find the work easier and much more pleasant, and we have even become close friends with some of the clients.

The progress that has been made is, as the leaders of the project acknowledge, only a first step toward the full implementation of a client-centered program. The conceptualization and practice of informed choice in Deqing are still limited in scope. Even though there is greater freedom for a woman to choose a method, it is made clear to her that in the event of a contraceptive failure, she will not be allowed to carry the pregnancy to term. Under these circumstances many couples will feel compelled to choose a long-acting method and will view the use of short-term methods as much too risky. Providers will continue to emphasize long-acting methods for the same reasons. The fact that sterilization after the second child is no longer mandatory represents progress, but method choice remains severely constrained.

In light of these realities, it is essential that women who choose to use an IUD be assured that their choice is safe and effective. Given the fact that the Chinese program still uses IUDs that are associated with high expulsion and pregnancy rates (e.g., copper rings), many women who opt for the IUD are exposed to an unnecessarily high risk of contraceptive failure. Removing devices with high failure rates from the national program would be an important step toward providing meaningful choice.

Reproductive choice is also limited by the fact that contraceptive use continues to be mandatory for married women of reproductive age. In addition, the critical changes related to method choice are still not sufficiently well-known in the community, partly because some family planning workers do not advise women of their new rights and partly because the overall approach is still new. Although navigating the birth management system is somewhat easier than it used to be, it remains a daunting bureaucratic challenge. Women also continue to bear a disproportionate share of the contraceptive burden. Nevertheless, the changes that have been made so far constitute an explicit departure from the approach that prevailed in the past. Decisionmakers, managers, and providers have begun to acknowledge that family planning services must address people's needs and that women have a right to make their own contraceptive choices. In the Chinese context, such reorientation is indeed significant.

Acknowledgments

The authors appreciate the assistance received from the Deqing County Family Planning Commission during the assessment and subsequent data collection. We also gratefully acknowledge support from the Ford Foundation, which provided funding for the quality-of-care assessment and the analysis upon which this chapter is based. Comments from Judith Bruce, Nicole Haberland, Joan Kaufman, and Diana Measham on several versions of the chapter have been invaluable.

Notes

1   For information on early efforts to analyze quality of care in rural China see Kaufman et al. 1992 and Tu 1995.

2   The verbatim translation of the minister's statement reads as follows: "The family planning program in China must make two reorientations in both its guiding ideology and program approach, i.e., from a narrow focus on family planning alone to closely integrating it with economic and social development, and addressing population issues in a comprehensive manner; from implementing the program by primarily relying on social constraints to gradually institutionalizing a mechanism integrating interest-driven and social constraints along with coordinated comprehensive services and scientific management."

3   The Pilot Project on Quality of Care in Family Planning began as a Chinese initiative; since 1998 it has received technical assistance from an international group with representatives from the SFPC, the Ford Foundation, the Population Council, and the University of Michigan and with funding from the Ford Foundation. For a description of the Quality Project's goals and strategies, see Gu, Zhang, and Xie 1999.

4   Currently, US$1 is about 8.3 Chinese yuan/RMB (renminbi).

5   In China, the contraceptive prevalence rate is defined as the percentage of women who use contraceptives at a particular point in time among all married women of reproductive age who are required to use contraception according to local family planning regulations. The contraceptive prevalence rate thus defined can approach 100 percent. This differs from the standard definition, which is the percentage of women who use contraceptives at a particular point in time among all women of reproductive age.

6   The assessment used a methodology adapted from the strategic approach to contraceptive introduction developed by the World Health Organization. For more information on this methodology, see Simmons et al. 1997.

7   The One Child Per Couple Policy, introduced in 1979, mandated that all families, with some exceptions, have no more than one child. In practice, implementation of the policy has varied over time and from place to place.

8   While either female sterilization or male sterilization can meet the requirement for contraception, the local family planning regulations often explicitly or implicitly encourage female sterilization after the second birth.

9   The planned birth rate refers to the proportion of births that fall within local family planning regulations in a given time period, usually one year.

10 The Single-Daughter Household Policy was introduced in Zhejiang Province in the mid-1980s. According to this policy, a rural couple with an only daughter is permitted to bear a second child after a birth interval ranging from four to eight years.

11 The task force was made up of eight members: one township governor in charge of family planning; one township family planning manager; the Huanqiao Village family planning worker; two technical staff members from the county service clinic; and three staff members from the Deqing County Family Planning Commission (one deputy director; one information, education, and communication specialist; and one technical supervisor).

12 The Counseling Training Project is part of the Training of Trainers for Rural Family Planning Workers in Family Planning Technology and Interpersonal Communication and Counseling Project, carried out in China in the early 1990s by the SFPC with sponsorship from UNFPA and technical assistance from the Program for Appropriate Technology in Health (PATH).

13   The client satisfaction rate (in percent) = number of interviewed women satisfied with services/
      total number of interviewed women receiving services × 100; the informed choice participation
      rate (in percent) = number of users making informed choice/total number of new users × 100
      (Deqing County Family Planning Commission 1997).

14   To assess the township family planning office, a total of 20 women from two villages are interviewed
      each month; to assess the Deqing County Family Planning Commission, a total of 120 women
      from six villages in three townships are interviewed each month.

References

Deqing County Family Planning Commission. 1997. *Working Guides to Grassroots Family Planning
    Workers in Deqing County* (in Chinese).

Gu, Baochang. 2000. "Reorienting China's family planning program: An experiment on quality of
    care since 1995," paper presented at the annual meeting of the Population Association of America,
    Los Angeles, CA, 23–25 March.

Gu, Baochang, Erli Zhang, and Zhenming Xie. 1999. "Toward a quality of care approach: Reorienta-
    tion of the family planning programme in China," in Jay Satia, Patricia Mathews, and Aun Ting
    Lim (eds.), *Innovations: Innovative Approaches to Population Programme Management—Institu-
    tionalising Reproductive Health Programmes,* vols. 7–8. Kuala Lumpur: International Council on
    Management of Population Programmes, pp. 39–52.

Kaufman, Joan, Zhang Zhirong, Qiao Xinjian, and Zhang Yang. 1992. "The quality of family plan-
    ning services in rural China," *Studies in Family Planning* 23(2): 73–84.

National Bureau of Statistics. 1999. *China Statistical Yearbook 1999.* Beijing: China Statistics Press.

Simmons, Ruth, Baochang Gu, and Sheila Ward. 2000. "Initiating reform in the Chinese family plan-
    ning program," paper presented at the annual meeting of the Population Association of America,
    Los Angeles, CA, 23–25 March.

Simmons, Ruth, Peter Hall, Juan Díaz, Margarita Díaz, Peter Fajans, and Jay Satia. 1997. "The strate-
    gic approach to contraceptive introduction," *Studies in Family Planning* 28(2): 79–94.

Tu, Ping. 1995. "A study on the introduction of new contraceptives and improvement of service qual-
    ity in rural China" (in Chinese), *Population and Family Planning* 6: 43–48.

Zhang, Erli, Baochang Gu, and Zhenming Xie (eds.). 1999. "Assessment reports on the SFPC's first
    pilot counties/district on quality of care in family planning (1995–1998)" (in Chinese). Beijing:
    China Population Press.

Contact information

Baochang Gu
China Family Planning Association
Building 35, Shaoyaoju, Chaoyang District
Beijing 100029, China
e-mail: bagu@cpirc.org.cn

4

Transforming Reproductive Health Services in South Africa: Women's Health Advocates and Government in Partnership

Sharon Fonn and Khin San Tint

In 1994, with the whole world watching, the country of South Africa entered a new era. The same year in which the United Nations held the International Conference on Population and Development in Cairo, Nelson Mandela assumed the presidency of his country and committed the nation to a broad social transformation aimed at decreasing profound racial, social, and gender-based inequities. South Africa's apartheid era officially came to its long-awaited end.

It was clear that the legacy of apartheid would not easily be reversed. In addition to widespread poverty and discrimination, most of the black population suffered from very poor health, particularly in comparison to whites. Health statistics are alarming for much of Africa, but data from the last years of apartheid in South Africa document profound differences in health status by racial category. For example, in 1990 whites had an infant mortality rate of 7.3 deaths per 1,000 live births compared to 9.9 for Indians, 36.3 for "coloreds," and 54.7 for African blacks (Yach and Buthelezi 1995).[1] In 1989 the maternal mortality ratio was 8 per 100,000 live births for whites compared to 83 for blacks (Klugman et al. 1998).[2]

HIV/AIDS statistics are sobering. At the end of 1999, UNAIDS estimated that 20 percent of South African adults had already contracted HIV, a sizeable increase from an already high 13 percent two years previously. Estimated rates of HIV prevalence among young people ages 15–24 are significantly higher among girls than boys (22.5–27.1 percent for girls vs. 7.6–15.1 percent for boys) (Joint United Nations Programme on HIV/AIDS 2000). A recent study among family planning clients in a district of Northern Province also documented endemic reproductive tract infections (RTIs): 18 percent had trichomoniasis, 29 percent suffered from bacterial vaginosis, 12 percent had chlamydia, and 3 percent tested positive for gonorrhea (Schneider et al. 1998).

Along with a population in poor health, the new South African government inherited a health system that was sorely inadequate; the scope of available services correlated closely with the race of clients served and, therefore, inversely with need. Sixteen percent of pregnant women who gave birth in 1998 (most of whom were black) did so outside of a health care facility and without a trained provider (*South African Health Review 1999*). Postpartum care, while usually available, is often not accessible. One study of black women in an urban township found that only 53 percent of those who used antenatal care services returned for postpartum care (Xaba and Fonn 1996).

Fragmentation of reproductive health services has made access to care even more difficult. While family planning services were widespread and often available at the local level, they were typically offered by completely separate sets of providers, sometimes in different locations—the result of a vertical family planning program conceived of by the previous South African government to reduce the size of the black population (Kaufman 1997). Services for the diagnosis and treatment of sexually transmitted infections (STIs) have been limited for all South Africans, especially for women (Schneider 1995). Other vital reproductive health services, such as infertility care, cervical cancer screening, and services for menopausal women, could be found only at tertiary care centers, if at all.

To address such problems the new South African government—committed to radical change in all sectors of society and bolstered by a new constitution—instituted health-sector reform. The reform has aimed to improve access to care by creating a district-based primary health care system that provides comprehensive services, including reproductive health care, at the local level. Women's health has been a particular priority of the government. For example, soon after his inauguration, Mandela included maternal health among his "Presidential Lead Projects," committing the nation to extend free health care to all pregnant and lactating women and to children under six years of age. In 1996, the government passed the Choice on Termination of Pregnancy Act, recognizing the exclusive right of women to make decisions about their bodies and the continuation of pregnancy.

THE ROLE FOR WOMEN'S HEALTH ADVOCATES IN THE NEW SOUTH AFRICA

The national policies of the mid-1990s were visionary. Implementation of these policies, however, was hampered by a highly dysfunctional health system and a society that was built on overwhelming inequities.

In many countries, the role of the civil sector—including women's health advocates—is to act as an outside force that pressures government to change policies and practices. Indeed, under the apartheid system, many South Africans had worked to promote women's health, operating almost entirely outside the government system. However, the transition to a progressive government meant a new course for health advocates.

In 1991, with support from a coordinating committee, antiapartheid activist and anthropologist Barbara Klugman founded a nongovernmental organization to foster high-quality, gender-sensitive health care in South Africa through research, training, education, and advocacy. They called the organization the Women's Health Project (WHP), and it was based in the School of Public Health at the University of the Witwatersrand.

WHP leaders believed that implementing nationwide comprehensive primary care, including reproductive health services, would take more than the addition of a few new services. They felt that if the government was to provide any component of reproductive health care, the overall health system would need to function properly and the quality of all existing services would need to be improved. As one early WHP leader explained, "What was required was nothing short of a thorough transformation of the existing health system."

When the new government reorganized the country into nine provinces, previously fragmented administrative units of the health sector were unified.[3] WHP believed that the transition to the new provincial structures would provide an opportunity to intervene effectively. The organization launched a major initiative, in partnership with the government, called the Transformation of Reproductive Health Services Project, which was carried out from January 1996 to January 1997. The ultimate goal of the Transformation Project was to help the new provincial health systems meet sexual and reproductive health needs—including information about and services for STIs, pregnancy and birth, infertility, contraception, cancer, and menopause. But in keeping with its analysis of what the government needed in order to provide such care, the main focus of the Transformation Project was to support, facilitate, and participate in the development of properly functioning health systems.

The government chose the Transformation Project sites: three very poor, primarily rural provinces (Northern, Northern Cape, and North West), which together contain over one-fifth of the country's population. This chapter focuses on one part of the project—namely, direct collaboration with health care providers and users to analyze problems in the system, identify solutions, and train staff to implement those solutions. The project, a collaboration between a women's NGO and the public health system, would involve thousands of workers, from clinic janitors to senior health department administrators (Fonn et al. 1998a, 1998b).[4]

At the start of the intervention, the information base was inadequate. No one in the government knew the number or condition of existing clinics, nor was there information about the number of staff employed or their technical ability. The program philosophy of the past, built as it was upon apartheid ideology, was not only outdated but a prime obstacle to progress. Decades-old biases about race and gender still permeated the attitudes of many personnel.

To introduce the philosophies underlying the Transformation Project and to consolidate senior-level support for the process, a one-day gender and health orientation course was held for 26 senior-level health sector managers and political figures, including a provincial minister of health and welfare and two directors general of health (Fonn et al. 1997). Eighteen of the participants were male, and the majority were black. The workshop introduced participants to the project and helped them define some of the many determinants of health (e.g., social class) and the concept of *gender* (i.e., the social norms and values that shape the relative power, roles, responsibilities, and behavior of women and men) as distinct from *sex* (which distinguishes males and females by biological characteristics). Despite the fact that the interactive format was unusual for senior health bureaucrats, they valued the workshop. As one remarked, "The most important thing that we learned from the workshop was that women's issues can be discussed rationally, and most are within our ability to solve."

DATA COLLECTION: INVOLVING STAFF AND SERVICE USERS

Transformation Project staff devised a five-part data collection process, which they hoped would serve both as a diagnostic tool and as a way to increase providers' openness to change; as such, the data collection activities also served as interventions.[5] The data collected would assess both the scope and quality of existing services. The techniques used to gather this information included: (1) facility checklists; (2) primary care provider self-administered questionnaires; (3) interviews with key senior health managers; (4) clinic-based time-flow and workload studies; and (5) focus groups with community women. The techniques are described below.[6]

Data Collection Tool #1: Facility Checklist

At 378 primary care clinics, a nurse (or other supervisor) in charge completed a checklist assessing the physical facility, access to and quality of care, and contact with the community. Illustrative questions included:

- Is there clean running water? Is the supply reliable?
- Does the building need repairs? How serious are they?
- Is overcrowding common? Is it serious?

- What percentage of the client population can easily reach the clinic?
- How reliable is the system for stocking and purchasing drugs?
- How efficient is the system for retrieving patient files?
- How comfortable is the waiting area? Is it inside or outside?
- Do patients have aural and visual privacy?
- How effective are existing mechanisms for community input?
- Is the clinic involved in community development?
- To what extent are the following equipment and supplies available and functioning?
  - Antenatal (blood pressure, urinalysis, scale, syphilis screening tests [VDRL or Venereal Disease Research Laboratory], bottles, etc.)
  - Family planning (contraceptives, speculums, etc.)
  - Labor/delivery (sterilizing equipment, oxygen, delivery kits, drugs, transport, etc.)
  - Cervical cancer screening (duckbill speculums, specimen slides, fixatives, lamp, etc.)

Data Collection Tool #2: Universal Staff Questionnaires

Nearly 1,500 staff—including support staff such as gardeners, cleaners, volunteers, drivers, and so forth—at 378 primary care clinics completed a self-administered questionnaire. Although literacy levels varied, all levels of employees were able to respond. The questionnaires were designed to gather data on staff characteristics and the scope and quality of services.

Data collected on staff characteristics included:
- Skills and work responsibilities;
- Past participation in training and perceived training needs;
- Opinions about reproductive health service needs; and
- Awareness of related social issues (e.g., women's right to control their fertility, special needs of adolescents, causes and consequences of domestic violence, etc.).

Questions about the scope and quality of services included:
- Are reproductive health services available beyond antenatal, birth, and postpartum care?
- What is good about the clinic?
- What is bad about the clinic?

Data Collection Tool #3: Key Informant Interviews

Transformation Project staff interviewed regional and district directors as well as provincial directors of primary health care, human resource development, policy and planning, finance, and welfare. As a complement to the staff questionnaires, these interviews solicited middle and senior management views about the range and organization of existing services, supervision and monitoring practices, training needs, accessibility of services, and patients' rights.

Questions about reproductive health included:

- Nowadays people are talking about reproductive health as a new comprehensive concept. What do you think are the most important interventions to achieve good health for women?
- In an ideal situation, what services would you include in a health service that provides comprehensive reproductive health care?
- How are existing services offered? For example, are they available every day or not? Are they provided by separate providers? Are there separate queues for different services?
- How, again in the ideal situation, do you think these services should be organized from the point of view of the health care provider? From the patient's point of view?
- You have said what your *ideal* service would be. What do you think could actually be implemented in the next year? In other words, what do you think is feasible?

Questions about patients' rights included:

- People talk of rights a lot nowadays. They also talk of patients' rights. What do you think the patient has a right to?
- What do you think should be done to make it possible for patients to exercise their rights?
- If a patient is dissatisfied with the care he or she received, is there a way for him or her to voice this? Has this ever happened and, if so, how was it dealt with?

Data Collection Tool #4: Time-flow and Workload Studies

In the questionnaires and interviews, staff complained that they were too overworked and harried to be able to broaden services or expand their roles. The time-flow studies, conducted and interpreted by clinic staff themselves, helped determine whether and where efficiency gains could be made in clinic organization, and whether and how resources could be mobilized to increase the range of services. The data generated by these seemingly banal studies proved vital to fostering change.

The studies were carried out in three primary care clinics (for details, see Tint et al. 1998). Staff and patients were informed of the study intentions and asked whether they would agree to be monitored by WHP staff for three days. Information was gathered on the number of staff available to patients at any given time, the number of patients seen per day, the number and type of services provided, total patient time spent in the clinic, patient waiting time, patient time spent receiving care, patient time at each service point (e.g., at the register, with providers, with the pharmacist), allocation of staff time to different service activities (e.g., patient care, information gathering, management, cleaning), staff productive and unproductive time, and staff time spent on direct and indirect patient care.

The results were discussed in an open forum at each of the three clinics. Because the data were so readily interpretable (e.g., they showed the time taken up by each task), all levels of staff were able to see how the current system was forcing women to wait needlessly and run from one provider to another for different, but often related, health services. By considering both the capacity of providers and the needs of their clients, the studies linked the idea of high-quality care to practical possibilities for change.

Data Collection Tool #5: User Focus Groups

Transformation Project staff conducted seven focus-group discussions with users; separate groups were held in periurban and rural settings and with adult women, adolescent girls, and adolescent boys. These discussions elicited participants' opinions on the quality and scope of services offered at the local clinic. To trigger discussion about which services were most needed, the facilitator showed participants a series of cards, each containing the name of a particular kind of service (e.g., antenatal care, STI diagnosis and treatment, delivery care, cervical cancer screening, and so forth). Participants were asked whether they could think of other women's health services that were important but not listed on the cards, and these were added. The group was then asked to sort the cards into different piles according to their importance. After the most important service was chosen, the card was removed and participants were asked to identify the next most important service. This process was repeated until a list of priorities had been generated.

THE FINDINGS

The findings from these data collection exercises paint a striking picture of the state of health services in the three provinces. Problems of access to services and of quality of care emerged from both observational studies and interviews.[7]

Range of Reproductive Health Services

One of the most interesting outcomes was learning which services black women valued most. Their most common reproductive health service priorities included:

- STI treatment;
- Antenatal and obstetric care;
- Infertility testing;
- Safe abortion;
- Contraception;
- Sexuality education;
- Menopause services; and
- Cervical cancer screening and treatment.

Priorities varied by group. STI treatment, obstetric care, and safe abortion were high priorities for all groups, and safe abortion was the most important issue for adolescents. The importance placed on safe abortion was unexpected, since many people in South Africa still feel uncomfortable discussing this topic. The perceived need for cervical cancer screening was also intriguing, as there has never been an active campaign for this service in South Africa. Periurban women felt that contraception was their greatest need, while rural groups emphasized obstetric services.

Frontline managers and providers shared users' views on the need for a complete reproductive health care package, including such services as abortion and infertility testing. However, most were unable to conceptualize the organization of these individual services into a comprehensive program. Further, they knew they lacked supplies and training they needed to provide comprehensive care.

Higher-level (regional) managers tended to resist the concept of broadened services; they continued to emphasize the importance of services that were already most readily available, such as family planning and antenatal care. They noted—correctly—that broadening the scope of reproductive health care would require an overall restructuring of services.

Fragmented Services

Users complained that the clinics offered different services on different days and argued for a range of services provided at one service-delivery point (dubbed "the supermarket approach" in South Africa). Senior staff also favored a supermarket approach; however, many frontline providers, while not questioning the value of offering multiple services on one visit, contended that this would increase their workload too much. The results of the time-flow and workload studies were helpful and convincing on this point. When clinic staff reviewed these findings, they posited that responsibilities might be reallocated to facilitate a more equitable and efficient distribution of workload and an increase in the scope of services. Offering each service on a particular day did not necessarily save time. For example, when providers had to respond to a problem not "scheduled" for that day (and they were under pressure to do so because clients often could not come back), they lost significant time gathering the materials they needed. Family planning clients, for example, often had vaginal discharge, yet if STI treatment was not scheduled for that day, staff had to fetch needed equipment and supplies. In effect, while ad hoc attempts were made to offer multiple services, planning for providing them might actually have saved time and aggravation.

Waiting Time

Poor service organization also resulted in long waiting times at clinics. Observational data corroborated users' concerns: In the clinics observed, women had to wait between one and three hours to receive less than ten minutes of time with providers. One of the primary reasons behind long waiting times was the fact that, without an appointment system, most patients arrived early in the morning and then had to wait to be seen. Close to one-third of the patients were still at the clinic by early afternoon. The situation was frustrating not only for patients but also for staff, who had to work under pressure to care for the entire group. In the focus groups, users suggested that clinics offer an appointment system or a system with pre-set walk-in times.

Infrastructure and Supplies

Inadequate infrastructure and resources were also prominent concerns. Users did not believe service providers would always respond adequately in obstetric emergencies, for example. They also raised concerns about poor access to telephones and transport, as well as an undependable drug supply. Similarly, 34 percent of staff rated lack of equipment, inadequate facilities, and lack of drugs as the factors that most hindered effective job performance. Eighteen percent cited inadequate numbers of staff, and 14 percent cited transport problems as most critical.

Not surprisingly, the data generated by the facility checklists confirmed that many clinics were in need of serious repairs. Problems included poor electricity supply (a problem in 44 percent of all clinics) and inadequate or unreliable water supply (in 33 percent of clinics). These deficiencies were more than inconveniences. They impinged, often seriously, on the quality of care. Equipment could not always be sterilized and night deliveries had to be conducted in suboptimal lighting. Drug supplies were also unreliable: Oxytocin supplies (for preventing postpartum hemorrhage) were inadequate in almost two-thirds of all clinics and in 95 percent of North West Province clinics; and pethidine hydrochloride (for pain relief during labor) was not available in 90 percent of facilities.

Equipment was similarly inadequate. At least 35 percent of clinics could not test urine for infection or protein, an indicator of pre-eclampsia in pregnant women, and more than a third could not test hemoglobin levels to screen for anemia. Only one-third of the clinics had speculums, which seriously compromised access to additional reproductive health services such as cervical cancer screening. While most clinics had blood pressure monitors, many were not functional. Equipment repair was reported to take from two weeks to several months, and equipment was often lost in the system and not returned. Finally, and perhaps most importantly, reliable telephones and transport were often lacking, undermining the ability of providers to handle obstetric and other emergencies; 77 percent of clinics had no referral transport available.

Provider–Client Relationships

Women's primary concern was the provider–client relationship. Although they expressed appreciation of health workers' skills, women were critical of the way they were treated by staff. Health workers were described as rude, arrogant, unfriendly, and uncaring. In addition, women felt health workers were always rushed and responded negatively to patients who asked questions. The time-flow studies confirmed their sense of being hurried: The mean amount of time spent with family planning service providers was five and seven minutes in the Northern Cape and North West clinics, respectively. Participants in the focus groups stated that they wanted more health education and, most of all, to be treated with dignity and respect.

Supervision

The data identified another key problem: severely inadequate managerial support. Less than 50 percent of clinics reported having a visit from their appointed supervisor in the preceding six months. Within clinics, supervision was perceived not to exist, although senior clinic staff were entrusted with this responsibility. Senior health system managers themselves indicated that the few existing supervision systems were not systematically used. Moreover, many managers had not visited the clinics for which they were responsible, were not acquainted with clinic staff, and did not consider carrying out these activities a high priority.

ADDRESSING THE PROBLEMS

Health Workers for Change

The data collection exercises not only provided valuable information, they also sensitized key staff and senior managers to the idea of change, laying a foundation for reorienting providers toward a client-centered approach. This was furthered through a series of interactive workshops using the Health Workers for Change curriculum (Fonn and Xaba 1996).[8] Eight hundred twenty health workers participated in the workshops, which aimed to help providers examine their attitudes and behaviors; understand how gender inequality, race, and socioeconomic conditions affect clients, providers, and health services; and identify clinic management problems and potential solutions. The material was covered in six participatory workshops, each of which lasted about two hours and built on information presented in previous workshops.

Session 1, "Why I Am a Health Worker," helped participants examine why people become health workers and how this influences their relationships with clients. Both positive and negative factors influencing job choice were noted and their effect on the way health workers relate to clients was explored.

Session 2, "How Do Our Clients See Us?" investigated health workers' ideas about how their female clients view them and how this influences their relationship with clients. Role-plays and questionnaires developed by the health workers themselves were used to examine provider–client interactions. The majority of participants engaged in role-plays that depicted incidents highlighting poor client treatment. Health workers portrayed situations in which they were depicted as authoritative, judgmental, rude, aggressive, impatient, uncaring, unhelpful, disrespectful, and lacking in observational and listening skills. A WHP trainer described a typical role-play:

> We asked the cleaning staff to identify a situation that arises in their clinic and to prepare a role-play. They did a scene involving a woman, pregnant for the fifth time, arriving in labor. The person playing the nurse, who was tallying her monthly client statistics, did not get up from her desk. Eventually, she came to the woman, who was now lying on the floor. When she recognized her, she shouted, "Para fives must go and deliver at the hospital, not at the clinic! Why are you here?" As the nurse continued to lecture, the laboring woman said her baby was coming, and she pushed a towel out from under her dress. Finally, the nurse rushed for a delivery pack.
>
> The people watching the role-play were all nurses. They laughed, because the scene was presented in a humorous way, but then went on to talk about it. They agreed that such things happen, and they were critical of the role of the nurse. The person who played the patient said she had felt scared to come to the nurse for help. Everyone agreed that this reaction was justified, that they can be uncaring, and that this needs to change.[9]

While a few participants felt that clients saw them as resourceful and educated, the majority of providers agreed that the role-plays correctly reflected their clients' perceptions of mistreatment. They described themselves as rude, uncaring, and insensitive and acknowledged that they discriminated among clients, showing more respect to men and less to poor and illiterate women.

While many cited difficult work conditions as a factor, most agreed on the need to change their own attitudes and behaviors. They called for interpersonal skills train-

ing and suggested including the quality of the provider–client relationship as an indicator in assessing staff performance.

Session 3, "Women's Status in Society," used poems and role-plays to increase
health workers' awareness of the factors that influence the degree of control women
have over their day-to-day lives and the decisions they make about themselves and
their families. Participants discussed how these factors affect provider–client relations:

> *Because health workers are members of society, during their contact with women they
> treat them as society does. . . . If there is a male who needs attention, culturally it will
> hit you and you will attend to him first.*

While race was an issue throughout these workshops, it was in this session that
the topic surfaced most frequently. The various ways in which people discriminate—
on the basis of social status, language, race, gender, age, and literacy—were discussed.
Although participants did not always deal with the issue of race in a straightforward
manner, racial discrimination was the clear subtext of discussions about differential
treatment, attitudes, and stereotypes regarding language and culture.

Session 4, "Unmet Needs," identified women's neglected health needs and sought
to identify possible solutions. Trainers, sometimes with the help of participants, developed a story about a woman's life that reflected her social, economic, and cultural context. They then helped participants list issues that arose in the story. These included
women's limited ability to choose their partners; the risk of assault and abuse; restricted
access to education; and lack of access to needed health services, such as cervical cancer
screening, STI/HIV prevention and treatment, and emotional and substance abuse.
Participants then divided the list into issues that could be handled by the health sector
and those that required help from outside (e.g., improving education opportunities for
girls). For issues that fell within the domain of the health sector, participants grappled
with potential solutions and the resources required to put them in place.

Session 5, "Overcoming Obstacles at Work," explored health workers' job situations. Workers developed and prioritized a list of factors that impinge on their ability
to do a good job and affect their interactions with clients. The aggregated list included, in descending order of importance, inadequate equipment and supplies, autocratic and nonparticipatory management, low salaries, staff shortages, and poor
interpersonal relations among staff. Participants also discussed how each of these concerns affected their relationships with female patients. Underlying this workshop was
the belief that if health workers are expected to treat patients with respect, then health
workers need to receive respect, too.

Session 6, "Solutions," tied the sessions together and concluded with planning
activities that could be undertaken to improve quality of care. Activities that could be

conducted by participants in the clinic and those that had to be undertaken outside the clinic were discussed. For example, staff shortages could be handled by providers, who could petition for the creation of more posts and help find people to fill existing vacancies; for perceived problems with patient compliance, providers could organize a communication skills workshop.

The sessions were eye-opening. Many health workers came to a better understanding both of their clients' needs and circumstances and of their own roles and responsibilities:

> *Now I feel confident in my work environment. I actually feel in control of myself and my work.*

> *I thought [clients] did not come to the clinics through ignorance. I did not realize how rude they thought we were.*

Health workers also identified factors that would improve service use, including giving sufficient information on procedures, treating clients with care and respect, shorter waiting time, incorporating emotional and social problems of clients, and respecting clients' rights to confidentiality and privacy. Other commitments touched on the issue of discrimination, such as the need to treat illiterate people well.

An adapted version of the workshop was held with health service managers, several of whom offered positive comments:

> *It opens minds to new thinking. It makes people look into themselves and ask, "What are we doing?" You don't reorient people easily. This exercise starts the process. It then needs to be followed through with more management training.*

> *They have made a complex process seem simple. They understand that change must come from within individuals.*

> *The workshops are the most innovative management tool around.*

Gender, Power, and Health

In South Africa, as in most settings, the effect that women's low level of power has on their health status and behaviors is poorly understood by those working in the health system. Thus, WHP conducted an additional series of workshops on gender and health for 779 primary care workers. The activities allowed them to look at the influence of gender power imbalances in their own lives and link these to health and health service provision.

Participants reflected on what they had learned about managing their own lives:

> *I always came back from work to cook, even when I left work at seven in the evening. Then after the gender training, I felt that this had to change. To my surprise, my*

husband did not resist. He now cooks supper for the family some evenings, and now I have even joined a local choir because I have time to do all that. I realize that I tried to do everything because I thought that was what I was supposed to do as a woman.

LINKING THE SITES TO FOSTER A COLLECTIVE PLAN

While providers generally knew about the data collected at their own clinics, Transformation Project staff felt it was essential to pool data at the provincial level. This pooling would create a comprehensive picture of the state of services and the opinions of users and health workers, which in turn would allow providers and managers to respond in a more systematic way.

In July and August 1996, dissemination meetings were held in each of the three provinces that participated in the Transformation Project. The objective of the meetings was to use the pooled data to develop provincial action plans to improve system functioning and, consequently, reproductive health service delivery. The daylong events were attended by 60–95 people in each site, including senior managers, clinic and hospital staff, and community representatives. Each of the meetings was opened by senior representatives of the health or welfare ministry for the province (such as the director general or minister).

In order to present a composite picture of the results, the project used a method referred to as "The Train and Its Stations."[10] Each station, located in its own space in the meeting room, symbolized one of the data gathering tools or training workshops conducted by the Transformation Project. Participants were given "tickets" to guide their itinerary, so that one small group at a time would be at each station. The stations themselves were centered around a large poster summarizing the aim, methods, findings (for the entire province), and conclusions of the particular data collection exercise or training workshop. As each group arrived at a station, a facilitator presented the findings and asked questions to guide discussion.

After visiting all of the stations, each small group was asked to (1) reflect on the overall data and identify the three most important issues provincewide; and (2) develop an action plan to address these issues. The managers would then use this list of common issues to develop a unified, provincewide action plan.

In all three provinces, participants prioritized fundamental changes needed in the health system. For example, all identified revamping the supervisory system as a priority (including clarifying delineations between different levels of staff so that workers would know exactly who their supervisors were). The system used for procurement and distribution of drug supplies was also singled out as needing drastic improvement. Participants also identified improving communication—between managers and staff, staff and clients, and the clinic and the community—as a high priority. To these ends, all plans included replicating the dissemination workshop regionally. Some participants developed an action plan for training senior administrators in participatory management techniques as well as reaching more managers with the Health Workers for Change workshops. Other plans recommended using a local radio station to disseminate information on reproductive health and opening a hot line for community participation in problem-solving. Some placed emphasis on broadening the scope of existing services and recommended training for cervical cancer screening and adolescent counseling and services.

THREE YEARS LATER: LESSONS APPLIED

In the three years since the action plans were developed, there is considerable variation in the degree to which the provinces have instituted these plans and successfully transformed their services.

Many of the follow-up efforts have replicated or adapted activities undertaken during the Transformation Project. For example, Northern Province has incorporated the Health Workers for Change workshops into its ongoing in-service training program. Northern Cape Province adapted the Health Workers for Change curriculum to improve access to abortion services—one of the priority reproductive health needs identified by women during the user focus groups. North West Province, with help from WHP, sponsored two workshops aimed at reorienting managers toward improved quality of services and participatory management. Indeed, these workshops appear to have helped both senior staff and providers restructure the management process.

There are anecdotal signs that these workshops have led to changes in practice among health workers. Several health workers gave examples of changes they had made as a direct result of the workshops:

I have been taking personal responsibility for ordering equipment.

I really do confront my supervisor now.

As improvements in the system's foundations are made, the provinces are also able to make improvements in the scope and quality of services. Since the end of apartheid, a number of national-level reproductive health programs have been initiated. Notably, each province is now offering safe abortion services, upgrading its facilities for the diagnosis and treatment of STIs, and exploring—through pilot studies—how best to provide cervical cancer screening. Anecdotal evidence indicates that the acceptance of these new services is greatest when staff have been involved in the Transformation Project. For example, those who were involved with the Health Workers for Change workshops are now much more open-minded about abortion services and less judgmental of the women who seek them (Forte 1997). And while health care workers nationwide were apt to complain about having to provide cervical cancer screening, Northern Province nurses who participated in the workshops recognize the importance of this procedure and have effectively integrated it into their practice.

Unfortunately, the impact of the Transformation Project on services has not been well documented in most participating provinces. In the majority, multiple changes occurred simultaneously and synergistically (e.g., the Transformation Project and the national-level safe abortion program). Data from Northern Province, however, provide a glimpse of one site where clinic-level effects that are directly attributable to the Transformation Project have been well documented.[11]

THE CASE OF NORTHERN PROVINCE: PUTTING LESSONS LEARNED TO WORK

Northern Province had a clear goal: to offer women timely, comprehensive primary health care, including the full range of reproductive and child health services, on any day they came to a clinic. To prepare to meet this goal, the province seized on the opportunity presented by the time-flow and workload studies from the Transformation Project and applied the results to one pilot clinic in each of its seven districts.[12] We present here the results of this effort in one of those clinics.

The regional manager and clinic supervisor for the pilot clinic in Western Region had participated in the Transformation Project dissemination workshops and were eager to collaborate on the experiment. The pilot clinic served a population of 45,000 and saw 73 patients per day, on average, when the baseline time-flow and workload study was conducted. Waiting time varied depending on the service being sought. Women waited an average of 20 minutes before seeing a health worker when they presented for family planning services, but 74 minutes if they needed antenatal care. Client aggravation during their waiting time was compounded by an unsystematic process for seeing patients—even if a woman was the first to arrive, it was not certain that she would be the first (or even second or third) patient seen.

The time-flow analysis showed that only 16 percent of staff time was used for direct patient care. Thirty-eight percent of staff time was spent on "unspecified activities" (defined as non-work-related tasks done during working hours or totally nonproductive time) in addition to official breaks such as tea and lunch, which accounted for another 10–12 percent of staff time.

All clinic staff—from clinic supervisor to cleaners—were called together to discuss the baseline time-flow and workload study. WHP staff presented the findings of the analysis and facilitated discussion. During this first meeting, staff were anxious and worried about the results and were not willing to discuss the problems they faced or explore the reasons that patients waited so long and that staff time was used so inefficiently. Several other meetings, facilitated and recorded by WHP staff, were held over a period of about a year. Staff slowly became more comfortable with the issues and willing to analyze them further. Some of the problems identified included:

- Women had to see separate providers for different services. Thus a woman coming for a postpartum checkup and child immunization had to see two providers. This was neither convenient nor efficient. The brief service-focused encounters also decreased clients' ability to raise issues of concern with the provider.

- Because each patient was examined by several nurses, nurses had inadequate time to build rapport with clients.

- Workload was distributed unevenly. One professional nurse was designated for each of the primary care services, such as immunization and minor ailments. The result was that the nurse who gave immunizations finished her job early in the day, while the nurse who covered minor ailments carried most of the workload throughout the day.

- Rooms were assigned inefficiently. Each of the three consultation rooms was used for a separate service provided by a separate professional nurse. On the days that antenatal care was not offered, only two rooms were used.

- Morning prayer with patients, followed by health talks, contributed substantially to patient waiting time.

- The enrolled nurse, who did more limited work such as taking vital signs and preparing the consultation room for patients, was underutilized.

- Client files and record keeping were cumbersome. Each professional nurse had to come to the reception desk to see a patient's record, and retrieval of the record from the files was time consuming. Each nurse also had a separate register book that she maintained and used to compile monthly statistics for the head office.

- While 24-hour care was available for some services on some days of the week (e.g., delivery), in practice such services often were not available. For example, when shortages in supplies occurred (e.g., running out of linens or an interruption in the water supply) the clinic stopped providing delivery services for an unspecified period of time.

- The appearance of the clinic was dirty and depressing; as such, clients and staff found it unappealing.

- Finally, staff noted that this was the first time they had had such a frank meeting and the opportunity to collectively improve the clinic services and their work environment.

If problems in the areas of supplies and supervision were to be addressed, those who had control over these matters—that is, senior managers at both the district and provincial levels—would have to be engaged. WHP presented the baseline findings as well as the reactions and concerns of clinic staff to these senior managers. This feedback kept senior managers involved and abreast of the project and provided them with the information they needed to make changes in areas over which they alone had control (e.g., in supervisory responsibilities).

While staff had begun to suggest ways to rectify the problems outlined above, disagreements between two senior staff members hindered implementation of the changes. A pivotal point in the movement from analysis to action came after a planning meeting in March 1999, ten months after the baseline study, that included regional managers from throughout the province. Following the meeting, the regional managers gave overdue promotions to five pilot clinic staff members; this step gave three of them increased authority and enabled them to implement changes in collaboration with two other senior staff members. Decisions are now made by group consensus at staff meetings, with voting used to resolve disagreements.

The participatory process used in the time-flow and workload studies engaged staff and increased their sense of responsibility for the functioning of the clinic. When this process was coupled with improved decisionmaking and supervision, staff joined together to make the needed changes.

Ongoing monitoring and a final evaluation by WHP staff—in the form of another time-flow and workload study, among other methods—found at the 18-month follow-up that significant changes have been made.

- Clients are now seen on a first-come, first-served basis.
- Each professional nurse now provides all services, and workload is distributed evenly.
- All services—including antenatal, delivery, postpartum, family planning, STI, minor ailments, mental health, child immunization, and child health services—are now offered every day, with 24-hour delivery care.
- In an effort to increase service quality and efficiency, women who request a single service are explicitly advised of the range of services available. For example, those who come solely for family planning are seen by a professional nurse in the consulting room and given time for a full exam, discussion of methods, and consultation about any other reproductive and sexual health problems.
- The three rooms designated for specific services were converted to separate, full-service rooms. Now each patient is attended by one nurse in one consul-

tation room, regardless of the reason for her visit. Any of the nurses can use any open room (an antenatal care patient no longer has to wait for an "antenatal care room" to be free), and all three rooms are open daily.

- 24-hour delivery care is now provided consistently. Staff make sure that the equipment, supplies, and logistics necessary are available and functioning.
- Daily group health talks and morning prayer were stopped. Health education is now offered individually during clients' consultation.
- The enrolled nurse is posted at the reception desk and enters all data into one register book.
- The clinic initiated a "retained card" system whereby patients bring their patient record cards when they visit the clinic. Nurses record all information on the patient's retained card, which the patient then takes to the reception desk so that her data can be recorded in the register book.
- The clinic was scrubbed from floor to ceiling; cleaning staff felt a new sense of pride in their role.
- Regular weekly meetings of all levels of staff were instituted for decisionmaking and planning.

These last two interventions improved the appearance of the work site and encouraged far more contact across job lines—no doubt improving the efficiency and quality of services and improving staff morale.

A follow-up time-flow and workload study showed that clinic performance had improved:

- Waiting time dropped from 20–74 minutes to 1–25 minutes.
- The proportion of staff time spent on direct patient care increased to 43 percent (from 16 percent), while the proportion spent on unspecified activities decreased substantially from 38 percent to 6 percent.
- On average, daily client load increased from 73 to 200 clients per day.

Structural changes like those made by this Northern Province clinic are critical precursors to the addition of any new reproductive health services. Remarkably, these changes were brought about with no increase in staff size (in fact, the number of staff declined from 14 to 13).

CONCLUSION

While the Transformation Project was an eye-opening experience for managers, authorities, and health workers themselves, and changes have been made at the clinic level in at least some sites, many challenges remain. Often, however, it is not the failings of health workers but rather failures of the system—such as poor maintenance of facilities, inadequate supervision, and poorly functioning drug supply systems—that are major contributing factors to poor-quality care. Inadequate investment in the health sector, compounded by poor management, remains an obstacle to improved care (Ntsaluba and Pillay 1998). In addition, while the National Department of Health has initiated a ten-point plan for all nine provinces to strengthen the health system overall, a gap between policy and service delivery remains (National Department of Health, South Africa 2000). For example, while there is increasing recognition that violent and coercive relationships are a public health concern, there are as yet no nationally implemented protocols or procedures health workers can use to elicit related information from or assist clients who are in such relationships.

While problems remain, the basic premise of the Transformation Project—namely, offering a broader scope of services in the context of a functioning service-delivery system—has found operational expression. In conceptualizing the project we had argued against individual service add-ons (e.g., STI prevention, diagnosis, and treatment) on the grounds that these would not work in the long term if the health system into which they were introduced was dysfunctional. The "basic elements" we believed would need to be in place included improvements in the infrastructure (adequate buildings, equipment, and supplies), enhanced staff capacity (numbers of staff, skills in engaging with clients, and staff awareness of reproductive health and patients' rights), and reorientation of managers and staff toward client-centered, gender-sensitive care.

Such systemic change is a slow process but, we believe, is more sustainable. As South Africa's provinces continue to seek to improve the quality of their personnel, management, and physical infrastructure, they will be better able to add new reproductive health services. The Women's Health Project continues to provide the provinces with technical assistance as needed. The Northern Province Department of Health and Welfare has asked WHP to train a second group of trainers in the Health Workers for Change process, for example. Time-flow studies have been undertaken in 30 other clinics by these trained facilitators. At the end of this 30-month process, WHP conducted a workshop with all primary health care coordinators, clinic supervisors, and senior clinic staff of Northern Province to develop provincial guidelines for provision of integrated services. The initial response has been encouraging. The Primary Health Care Directorate of Northern Province is planning to formalize the guidelines into provincial regulations for primary health care. To engage the other eight provinces of South Africa, WHP will also facilitate a peer review of the Northern Province guidelines, in the hope that similar changes will be undertaken in some or all of the other provinces as well.

The Transformation Project represents a large-scale effort to reorient government health care provision, integrate reproductive health and other services at the primary-care level, and improve the gender sensitivity of care. Significant progress has been made toward integrated service provision at several sites, and the new approach is being institutionalized at the policy level in at least one province. The degree to which the care being provided is more gender-sensitive requires further evaluation. It is clear, however, that the partnership forged between women's health advocates and the new government of South Africa is having ripple effects in the provinces in which it has been active and is providing a model of responsive public-sector services for replication in other parts of the country.

Acknowledgments

We acknowledge the commitment of the staff of the Departments of Health and Welfare of the Northern Cape, North West, and Northern Provinces. We thank the Department for International Development and the United Nations Population Fund for their support of the Transformation of Reproductive Health Services Project; and the Health Systems Trust of South Africa for its support of the time-flow study.

Notes

1   Under apartheid, these were the categories into which data were classified. "Coloreds" are people of mixed race; Indians are people of South Asian heritage.

2   Since underreporting and misclassification occur more commonly in the black population, the racial disparity is likely to be greater than suggested by these data (Bradshaw, Dorrington, and Sitas 1992).

3   During apartheid, health services were independently administered and were fragmented between national, provincial, local, and homeland authorities; they were further fragmented by race, and again by curative and preventive care.

4   The project was operationally located within the Directorate of Maternal, Child, and Women's Health in the North West and Northern Cape provinces and in the Directorate of Primary Health Care in Northern Province. A provincial coordinator based in each provincial department of health was appointed to serve as the liaison with the WHP. Each of the three provincial health transformation projects was overseen by a reproductive health steering committee, and the three intervention sites were linked by a national committee chaired by the country's director of maternal, child, and women's health. The project was funded by the United Nations Population Fund and the Department for International Development.

5   Involving subjects in diagnostic and data collection exercises, often called participatory research, has been increasingly used as a means to effect change and gather data simultaneously. See, for example, the discussion of the "autodiagnóstico" process in Chapter 20 and participatory evaluation exercises described in Chapter 21.

6   See Tint et al. (1998) for additional detail on each of these tools.

7   Adapted from Fonn et al. 1998b.

8   Health Workers for Change is an internationally tested intervention to address quality of care, health system functioning, and gender inequality (Fonn and Xaba 2001; Fonn et al. 2001; Onyango-Ouma et al. 2001a, 2001b; Pittman, Blatt, and Rodriguez 2001; Vlassoff and Fonn 2001).

9   Adapted from Fonn and Xaba 1996.

10   The method is fully described in Tint et al. 1998.

11   The Integrated Services Initiative, a collaboration between WHP and the Northern Province Department of Health, was undertaken between May 1998 and October 2000 as a direct result of the Transformation Project. This project sought to assist the department in implementing policy related to integrated primary care service provision. Results from a project evaluation are forthcoming.

12   The province relied on WHP for assistance in this activity.

References

Bradshaw, Debbie, Rob E. Dorrington, and Freddy Sitas. 1992. "The level of mortality in South Africa in 1985—What does it tell us about health?" *South African Medical Journal* 82(4): 237–240.

Fonn, Sharon, Anne S. Mtonga, Hope C. Nkoloma, Grace Bantebya Kyomuhendo, Leopoldima daSilva, Ester Kazilimani, Shara Davis, and Ramata Dia. 2001. "Health providers' opinions on provider–client relations: Results of a multi-country study to test Health Workers for Change, a quality of care intervention," *Health Policy and Planning* 16(suppl 1): 19–23.

Fonn, Sharon and Makhosazana Xaba. 1996. *Health Workers for Change: A Manual to Improve Quality of Care*, TDR/GEN/95.2. Geneva: UNDP/World Bank/WHO Special Programme for Research and Training in Tropical Diseases; and Johannesburg, South Africa: Women's Health Project.

———. 2001. "Health Workers for Change: Developing the initiative," *Health Policy and Planning* 16(suppl 1): 13–18.

Fonn, Sharon, Makhosazana Xaba, Khin San Tint, Daphney Conco, and Sanjani Varkey. 1998a. "Maternal health services in South Africa," *South African Medical Journal* 88(6): 697–702.

———. 1998b. "Reproductive health services in South Africa: From rhetoric to implementation," *Reproductive Health Matters* 6(11): 22–32.

Fonn, Sharon, Makhosazana Xaba, Khin San Tint, Daphney Conco, Sanjani Varkey, Thelma Maluleke, and Barbara Klugman. 1997. "Reproductive Health Services Transformation Project: An example of mainstreaming gender in health systems development," *Innovations* 5: 15–30.

Forte, Dianne. 1997. "Evaluation of the gender and health course in phase II of the Transformation of Reproductive Health Services Project," prepared for the Women's Health Project, Johannesburg, South Africa.

Joint United Nations Programme on HIV/AIDS (UNAIDS). 2000. "Report on the global HIV/AIDS epidemic: June 2000," Geneva: UNAIDS.

Kaufman, Carol. 1997. "Reproductive control in South Africa," Policy Research Division Working Paper no. 97. New York: Population Council.

Klugman, Barbara, Marion Stevens, Alex Van den Heever, and Meryl Feder. 1998. *From Words to Action: Sexual and Reproductive Rights, Health Policies and Programming in South Africa 1994–1998*. Johannesburg: Women's Health Project, Department of Community Health, University of the Witwatersrand.

National Department of Health, South Africa. 2000. "Health sector strategic framework 1999–2004." Pretoria: National Department of Health, South Africa.

Ntsaluba, Ayanda and Yogan Pillay. 1998. "Reconstructing and developing the health system—The first 1,000 days," *South African Medical Journal* 88(1): 33–36.

Onyango-Ouma, Washington, Rose Laisser, Musiba Mbilima, Margaret Araoye, Patricia Pittman, Irene Agyepong, Mairo Zakari, Sharon Fonn, Marcel Tanner, and Carol Vlassoff. 2001a. "The impact of Health Workers for Change in seven settings: A useful management and health system development tool," *Health Policy and Planning* 16(suppl 1): 24–32.

Onyango-Ouma, Washington, Frederick W. Thiong'o, Theresa Odero, and John H. Ouma. 2001b. "The Health Workers for Change impact study in Kenya," *Health Policy and Planning* 16(suppl 1): 33–39.

Pittman, Patricia, Graciela Blatt, and Patricia Rodriguez. 2001. "An assessment of the impact of Health Workers for Change in Avellaneda, Province of Buenos Aires, Argentina," *Health Policy and Planning* 16(suppl 1): 40–46.

Schneider, Helen. 1995. "An assessment of services for the control of sexually transmitted disease in the PWV province." Johannesburg: Centre for Health Policy, Department of Community Health, University of the Witwatersrand, and National AIDS Programme, Medical Research Council.

Schneider, Helen, David J. Coetzee, H. Glenda Fehler, A. Bellingan, Y. Dangor, F. Radebe, and Ron C. Ballard. 1998. "Screening for sexually transmitted diseases in rural South African women," *Sexually Transmitted Infections* 74(suppl 1): S147–S152.

South African Health Review 1999. 1999. Durban: Health Systems Trust.

Tint, Khin San, Sanjani J. Varkey, Sharon Fonn, Makhosazana Xaba, Daphney Conco, and Barbara Klugman. 1998. *Health Systems Assessment and Planning Manual: Transforming Reproductive Health Services*. Johannesburg: Women's Health Project.

Vlassoff, Carol and Sharon Fonn. 2001. "Health Workers for Change as a health systems management and development tool: Conclusions and recommendations," *Health Policy and Planning* 16(suppl 1): 47–52.

Xaba, Makhosazana and Sharon Fonn. 1996. "Women's health," in Laetitia Rispel, Max Price, Jorge Cabral et al. (eds.), *Confronting Needs and Affordability: Guidelines for Primary Health Care Services in South Africa*. Johannesburg: Centre for Health Policy, Department of Community Health, University of the Witwatersrand.

Yach, Derek and Gcinile Buthelezi. 1995. "Health status," in *South African Health Review 1995*. Durban: Health Systems Trust and Henry J. Kaiser Family Foundation, pp. 27–52.

Contact information

Sharon Fonn, MBBCh PhD FFCH
Women's Health Project
P.O. 1038 Johannesburg 2000
South Africa
telephone: 27-011-489-9914
fax: 27-011-489-9922
e-mail: womenhp@sn.apc.org
www.sn.apc.org/whp/

PART II
REORIENTING PROGRAMS TO MEET THE NEEDS OF CLIENTS AND HEALTH WORKERS

paragraph 7.23, Programme of Action

In the coming years, all family-planning programmes must make significant efforts to improve quality of care.

principle 8, Programme of Action

. . . Reproductive health-care programmes should provide the widest range of services without any form of coercion. All couples and individuals have the basic right to decide freely and responsibly the number and spacing of their children and to have the information, education and means to do so.

How can we help providers, supervisors, and managers in the transition to a client-centered approach?

5

Learning About Clients' Needs: Family Planning Field Workers in the Philippines

Anrudh Jain, Saumya RamaRao, Marilou Costello, Marlina Lacuesta, and Napoleon Amoyen

The evolution of population policy in the Philippines reflects the country's political history. In the 1970s, the regime of Ferdinand Marcos (1969–86) provided strong support to a national program centered on fertility reduction and contraceptive distribution. Under President Corazon Aquino (1986–92), population policy was broadened beyond fertility reduction to include the status of women, maternal and child health, and other key health and social issues, such as urbanization. With this broadening came a change in the locus of responsibility for contraceptive service delivery, which shifted from the Population Commission to the Department of Health. A parallel process devolved responsibility for family planning service delivery to local government units, which took the responsibility for decisionmaking out of the hands of central bureaucrats and placed it closer to the communities being served.[1]

The administration of Fidel Ramos (1992–98) broadened policy even further, increasing its emphasis on the reproductive health agenda outlined at the International Conference on Population and Development and the Fourth World Conference on Women. Joseph Estrada's regime (1998–2001) maintained this commitment to reproductive health, although concerns about population growth and its consequences continued to be the main motivations of population policy. Further, the Department of Health continued to strengthen the family planning program with a new focus on natural family planning. Following impeachment hearings that began in late 2000, President Estrada was replaced by Gloria Macapagal-Arroyo in January 2001. The policy of this new administration is marked by a commitment to reproductive health with an additional focus on adolescent health and youth development.

Since 1997 the Department of Health has sought to operationalize the Cairo paradigm by offering family planning as a client-centered reproductive health service.

Whether or not and how this occurs locally, however, is dependent on local leadership, resources, and interests, since the devolution of power has meant that priorities, strategies to achieve these priorities, revenue collection, and budget allocation are now decided locally.

Decentralization, coupled with changing political winds and the influence of the Catholic Church,[2] has led to some confusion regarding program content and provider roles, but has also offered fertile ground for experimentation. In 1997 a project was initiated by the provincial health offices of Davao del Norte and Compostela Valley provinces in collaboration with the Ateneo de Davao University and the Population Council to further the reproductive health agenda. It introduced a model of client-centered service delivery by reorienting both clinic staff and outreach volunteers in the public-sector system. This chapter describes the process of training outreach volunteers in this new model of service delivery and the lessons learned. Work with the volunteers began in mid-1998 and continued until early 2000.

SERVICES WITHOUT CLEAR PRIORITIES

The historical shifts in program emphasis, philosophy, and responsibility described above resulted in fragmented services characterized by uneven quality and unclear priorities. These problems pervade every level of the service-delivery system, which extends from district hospitals at the top to volunteer outreach workers—known as *barangay* health workers (BHWs)—at the periphery.[3] BHWs act as the bridge between health centers and communities (they are assigned to a *barangay* health center and work under the general supervision of a midwife). They are expected to play multiple roles, including those of community organizer; educator; data-gatherer; and provider of both preventive and curative health care, ranging from dental care and first aid to child health care and malaria prevention.[4] They are also expected to offer a range of reproductive health services, including education on available contraceptive methods, prevention of sexually transmitted infections (STIs) and HIV, and antenatal and postpartum care; provide information to contraceptive users and pregnant women about potential warning signs that might require medical attention; and make referrals to health centers, rural clinics, district hospitals, and private doctors for a variety of clinical contraceptive services, management of STIs, and antenatal care (Department of Health and UNFPA 1994).

Because of the immense scope of the volunteers' work and the lack of clear instruction on priorities, reality has diverged substantially from expectations. Insufficient training has compounded the problem. According to a study of four provinces in the Philippines, 33.5 percent of the BHWs had not been trained to perform their primary outreach functions, such as conducting household visits and organizing community talks, or to function competently in key areas, including family planning (Lacuesta, Sarangani, and Amoyen 1994). BHW training often consists of a supervisor's cursory overview of the workers' role within the health system and the broad spectrum of services she is to offer, with scant attention to providing technical information on each service. Furthermore, the training has rarely focused on client needs or on creating rapport. BHWs are unable to elicit information from clients about their needs because they are not explicitly trained to do so.

The inadequacy of this training is evident from the results of the aforementioned study. BHWs who had participated in the family planning training recalled being taught about the efficacy of particular methods (97 percent) and about side effects and appropriate responses to them (90 percent). Far fewer mentioned interpersonal relations (15 percent). Almost half (45 percent) found the training to be inadequate and claimed not to have a clear understanding of how family planning methods are used or their contraindications. According to the study, BHWs spent about an equal amount of time—one to two days a week—in the clinic and in the field. Assisting midwives in the health center (64 percent), motivating clients to use family planning (40 percent), and conducting surveys to serve general administrative needs (25 percent) were the three most frequently mentioned roles they claimed to play. Far fewer viewed the tasks of disseminating information (10 percent) and resupplying pills (6 percent) as their roles (Lacuesta, Sarangani, and Amoyen 1994). Field visits in Davao del Norte also suggested that BHWs were less likely to provide any type of reproductive health care, including family planning, than to provide information on children's immunization and assist midwives with their immunization work.

It was also clear that BHWs were given little guidance as to which of their multiple tasks they needed to attend to first. Supervisors' evaluation of their reproductive health performance was based on the numbers of women they contacted or motivated to use services, rather than on the extent to which they met individual needs—reflecting the program's emphasis on such macro indicators as contraceptive prevalence and antenatal coverage.

Women who lived in the communities served by the BHWs were asked their perceptions of these volunteers and the services they offered (Lacuesta, Sarangani, and Amoyen 1994). While none of the women described BHWs in explicitly negative terms, one-third said that they were not familiar with the services BHWs offered. About half said that they had consulted with BHWs for family planning services. Only 56 percent of women who had discussed family planning with a BHW had been allowed to choose their method based on information provided on a range of available choices. Instead, BHWs tended to direct women to particular methods, as typified by the following statement: "You know, there will be scheduled ligation services provided by doctors on Saturday. Why don't you go and have yourself ligated? You already have five children and you are not getting any younger!" Researchers often overheard BHWs making such statements during field visits.

Fixed clinics exhibit parallel deficiencies in service quality, particularly with regard to contraceptive choice, information provision, and privacy. These deficiencies have been documented in a number of sites across the Philippines (Palma-Sealza 1993; Rood, Raquepo, and Ladia 1993; Zablan et al. 1998). One study of health units and lower-level *barangay* health stations (Zablan et al. 1998) found that in one-third of the observed interactions the provider encouraged one method over others during the consultation.[5] Less than 12 percent of clients were told how to use the method they left with or were informed about the method's advantages, disadvantages, and side effects. Only 22 percent of family planning clients were asked whether they had a problem or concern about a method, and 9 percent were told that they could change the method they accepted. Only 4 percent of clients discussed in any terms the nature of relations with their sexual partners, information that bears directly on the acceptability and safety of the method selected. Not surprisingly given this context, contraceptive discontinuation in the first year of use is high nationally (41 percent) (National Statistics Office, Philippines Department of Health, and Macro International 1999). Furthermore, nearly a third of the women who discontinued using their contraceptive method reported an accidental pregnancy as the cause, providing further evidence of the substantial scope for improving service quality.

BHWs thus operate within a system that is characterized by serious gaps in quality and does not provide them with the fundamental skills necessary to foster women's choice. While BHWs are seldom coercive, and the country's pronatalist societal norms are more supportive of childbearing than of contraception, many BHWs attempt to convince women to limit their fertility and often promote a particular contraceptive method—without inquiring about the client's health status, reproductive intentions, or needs.

DEFINING CLIENTS' NEEDS WITHOUT THEIR PARTICIPATION

While outreach work is one of BHWs' primary activities as originally envisioned by the Department of Health, these workers clearly have not been able to bridge the gap between clinical services and the community. In searching for a solution, the Department of Health adopted a strategy that has been widely used in other parts of the developing world: the high-risk approach. While nominally focused on an individual woman's situation, the high-risk approach is directed toward all nonusers of contraceptives "who are capable of conceiving, who are exposed to the risk of pregnancy, and who, if they were to become pregnant, would experience an elevated risk of mortality for their expected child, their living child, or themselves" (DeGraff and DeSilva 1996). It does not, however, take into account a woman's own desire to become pregnant or to prevent a pregnancy. It also ignores the needs of users who are having problems with their current method and could potentially switch contraceptives. As in other places, the high-risk approach ultimately proved to be inappropriate in the Philippines, as discussed below.

The Department of Health defined women who belonged to one or more of the following groups as being at "high risk" (Zablan et al. 1998):

1. Married women less than 20 years of age ("too young");
2. Married women over 35 years of age ("too old");
3. Married women of reproductive age with four or more previous pregnancies ("too many");
4. Women with a child younger than 15 months ("too soon");
5. Women with medical conditions such as tuberculosis, hypertension, and anemia.

Under the supervision of clinic personnel, BHWs were instructed to compile an annual survey of all married women of reproductive age. Women who were not using a contraceptive method were classified as either normal or high-risk. Each high-risk woman was then counseled on the possible complications of high-risk pregnancy and encouraged to use contraception. Because the five categories are so inclusive, over 85 percent of married women of reproductive age were classified as high-risk (Zablan et al. 1998).

Proponents of the high-risk approach argue that without such counseling these women cannot make an "informed choice" about whether or not to have another child. They further contend that it is unethical for the program not to provide this information. The approach is problematic, however. First, it uses general predictors of risk derived from rates of maternal and infant mortality and morbidity rather than relying on the client's clinical history, current health status, and reproductive intentions. Thus it has poor predictive value and identifies an enormous number of women as being at high risk who in reality are no more likely than others to have obstetric emergencies (Rooks and Winikoff 1990). Second, the high-risk approach undercuts the spirit of Cairo's client-centered philosophy. The provider elicits information about the client's childbearing history, but not her reproductive intentions. The definition of whether or not she is at risk is determined exogenously by the program, and some women with special needs are ignored. For example, a woman with a history of pregnancy complications who wants to become pregnant should not be counseled to avoid pregnancy, but given appropriate support whether her pregnancy is risky or not. Similarly, a woman who might be classified as a perfectly good candidate for pregnancy but who does not want a child should be supported in avoiding pregnancy.

Furthermore, when the provider–client exchange is centered on the high-risk approach the communication skills of the client and the provider are not developed. Accustomed to being told what to do, women rarely express their reproductive health concerns or reproductive intentions, and providers are implicitly (if not explicitly) told that women's concerns and intentions are not relevant. Thus such programs neither increase women's knowledge of reproductive health nor foster their ability to communicate their own health concerns and obtain the services they need.

In sum, while the high-risk approach appears to be an attractive strategy at first glance, it does not help workers prioritize their work or change its nature. More importantly, it obscures rather than supports women's reproductive intentions.

GUIDELINES FOR LEARNING ABOUT CLIENTS' NEEDS

The family planning roles of *barangay* health workers, as originally envisioned and selectively revised, still placed clinical or donor definitions of need over client concerns. There was no clear plan for workers' active engagement with their clientele, and little attention was paid to interpersonal communication or information exchange. An alternative was proposed that would change the operational paradigm of existing workers to one that fostered a much closer and more open relationship with clients (Jain 1996).[6] The key elements of this alternative approach included:

Eliciting information from clients. A provider must ascertain basic information about the woman's circumstances to help her select a method or provide other reproductive health services appropriate to her needs. This information ranges from the client's reproductive intentions and prior family planning experience to her contraceptive method preferences and partnership arrangements.

Involving clients in the selection of the initial method. As much as possible, the client should select or at least be involved in selecting a method appropriate to her needs and circumstances. Even if a client has a particular method in mind, it is important that the provider discuss at least one alternative. This is particularly true when a permanent method is being discussed.

Shifting providers' orientation from method to client. The provider's job should be defined not as motivating women to have small families but as helping women articulate their reproductive intentions and providing support to help them achieve those intentions. Consequently, evaluations of provider performance should be based on the ability of providers to support clients in meeting their own reproductive intentions, rather than ensuring acceptance and continued use of specific methods.

Providing adequate information to clients. There is debate over the level of information that clients should receive. Specifically, the information provided to a client may sometimes be irrelevant to her circumstances or may be so detailed that it becomes too much to absorb (Murphy and Steele 1997). At a minimum, the alternative client-centered approach to family planning posits that the provider must offer information on the following:

- Methods available and their suitability to the client's needs and circumstances (e.g., sterilization is not suitable for clients who want more children or who may not be sure about it, and intrauterine devices (IUDs) are not recommended for clients who have more than one partner or who suspect or know that their partner has multiple partners);
- How to use the method selected, its side effects, and whether or not it protects against sexually transmitted infections;
- The possibility of switching if the method is inconvenient or not suitable given a person's needs, circumstances, or health status; and
- Sources of supply, so that the client feels that s/he is in control and does not have to come back to the same source or to the same provider for resupply.

AN EXPERIMENT TO CREATE CLIENT-ORIENTED WORKERS

In search of a more client-oriented approach, the Provincial Health Office of Davao del Norte, the Social Research Office at Ateneo de Davao University, and the Population Council designed an experiment in ten municipalities of Davao del Norte and Compostela Valley provinces in collaboration with EngenderHealth (formerly AVSC International).[7] The component of the project described in this chapter trained BHWs in Panabo municipality in Davao Province and Montevista municipality in Compostela Valley Province[8] in the use of a client-service tool that focuses on helping women achieve their reproductive intentions.

In April 1998, 110 BHWs were trained in the use of a tool that would help them organize their family planning service delivery around client needs.[9] The tool was designed to help BHWs conduct individual interviews with women in the community to learn about their needs and develop a plan for working with each one of them.

The tool consisted of five questions posed to women concerning their current pregnancy status, desire for and timing of an additional child, use of contraception, and satisfaction with the method used (see Figure 1). Responses allowed BHWs to classify women as dissatisfied contraceptive users; women with unmet need for limit-

Figure 1. Scheme by which a field worker may prioritize services on the basis of a woman's answers to questions about her reproductive health needs

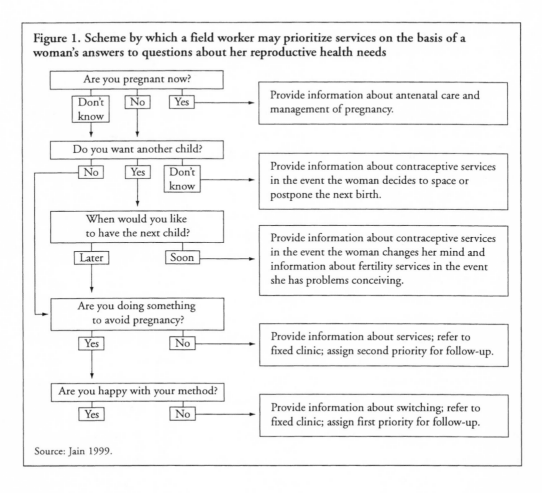

Source: Jain 1999.

ing or spacing pregnancies; women who are currently pregnant; and women who are not ready to use contraception because they are uncertain of their reproductive intentions, seek to become pregnant, or have other personal objections. The training emphasized the type of information to be provided to women according to their response and the circumstances under which they should be referred to a fixed clinic, as follows:

- Women who are pregnant are given information about managing the pregnancy safely and told when and where they should go to receive antenatal care, immunizations, and postpartum services, including family planning.
- Nonpregnant women who hope to conceive soon are given information about where to go for infertility services, if necessary, and for contraceptive services, if their intentions change.
- Nonpregnant women who do not want another child soon, are not using contraception, and would like to do so are given information on services avail-

able at the nearest clinic (e.g., injectables and the IUD) and through the BHW directly (e.g., pills and condoms).

- Nonpregnant women who do not want another child soon and who are using contraception but are not happy with the method are given information about alternatives and how they can safely switch to the method to which they are best suited.
- Nonpregnant women who are happy with their current method are resupplied if necessary and/or reminded of when and where they can obtain a resupply.
- Nonpregnant women unsure of their reproductive intentions are informed of family planning services available in the event they decide to use a contraceptive method.

The project team found that BHWs had trouble accurately classifying some women. This reflected, in part, the intransigence of their earlier approach, which emphasized increasing the numbers of contraceptive users. The project team felt that the number of unhappy or dissatisfied users identified by BHWs was too low, especially given the high national rate of contraceptive discontinuation due to side effects. Some BHWs reported that they were reluctant to record women as dissatisfied users because they feared that doing so would reflect negatively on both themselves and the clinic staff. Presumably, these BHWs had trouble getting used to the notion that listening to and meeting the client's desires were now their primary goals. Some BHWs reported they did not record dissatisfied users as such because they had provided a remedy or referral in response. In addition, given the culture of polite discourse between clients and providers, it is possible that some women were reluctant to disclose their dissatisfaction lest it reflect negatively on the providers. The project team revised the question on method satisfaction to help providers understand its purpose—both to capture the essence of the client's experience with the method and to guide their action. The first version of the question allowed only a straightforward response of satisfied or unsatisfied. It also seemed to focus on the user's perception of the method's ability to protect against pregnancy rather than the totality of her experience with the method. The revised version of the question now encompasses a range of experience from high satisfaction—indicating a sense of ease and comfort with the method—to a minimum level of satisfaction, to explicit dissatisfaction.

The project team also felt that the number of women classified as happy/satisfied was suspiciously high. By design, women who fell into the category of satisfied user were listed as requiring "no action" and did not receive follow-up visits. Also, one-third of these women reported using rhythm, withdrawal, abstinence, or lactational amenorrhea—methods that require a sound knowledge base for effective use. There was concern that even satisfied users of these methods may require more information, especially because previous studies had documented substantial inaccurate knowledge about fertility cycles and natural family planning.[10] Because natural family planning is a popular choice, and BHWs and midwives were not equipped to provide complete and accurate information, the project team gave these health workers appropriate training. Both the project team and the service providers wanted to treat these methods with the same seriousness as modern methods and felt that doing so was in keeping with the new, client-centered philosophy of care.

Women who had expressed dissatisfaction with their contraceptive method and those who wanted to cease or delay childbearing and to use contraception were referred to the fixed facility. Dissatisfied users were given blue cards, and nonusers in search of a method were given pink cards. They were instructed to hand the cards to the provider to convey the purpose of their visit and to facilitate tracking the performance of the referral system. Qualitative information from the project evaluation suggests that a number of these women took advantage of the referral opportunity; some decided to abandon the method with which they were dissatisfied in favor of natural family planning, rejecting the alternative modern methods available (i.e., condoms, pills, Depo-Provera, and the IUD). The proportion of women with referral cards who subsequently came to the health center is unclear, since it is believed that many clients neglected to bring their cards. Other experiments with referral cards report similar problems, and the project has since stopped using them.

Prioritizing Household Visits Based on Women's Needs

BHWs also developed a plan for household re-visits based on their interviews with clients. They enumerated eligible women in their areas and grouped them according to self-determined fertility status, reproductive intentions, and contraceptive use/satisfaction. Some BHWs were able to complete enumeration within two months while others needed more time because of the nature of the geographic area they covered. Those working in periurban areas with a clustering of households and a good transportation system were able to compile their lists more easily than those who had to visit far-flung households or traverse mountainous terrain with poor transportation.

A total of 6,173 currently married women of reproductive age were enumerated, and were categorized as follows:

- Pregnant (10 percent)
- Desire more children soon (4 percent)

- Not using contraception but want to cease or delay childbearing (30 percent)
- Dissatisfied users (2 percent)
- Satisfied users (32 percent)
- Satisfied users of sterilization (2 percent)
- Satisfied users of lactational amenorrhea, withdrawal, rhythm, and abstinence (20 percent)

First priority for follow-up was accorded to women who were dissatisfied with their current method and second priority to those who wanted to space or terminate childbearing but were not currently using contraception. BHWs who had a manageable number of households were able to serve all women without prioritizing their visits. BHWs who were not able to serve all the households in their area prioritized their visits and served those with lower priority during subsequent visits to the community.

While some women received relevant services or referrals during the initial visit, some BHWs mistakenly believed that the purpose of the initial visit was to elicit information and enumerate their assigned area only, and additional follow-up was required to provide any information or services clients required. BHWs learned as they went along that they could enumerate and provide information at the same time.

Implementation of the client-oriented strategy was not seamless, and many of the problems encountered are still being resolved. It became clear, for example, that the assigned areas were not clearly delineated because of uncertain or overlapping boundaries between *barangays*. As a result, some women were enumerated by two BHWs. The assigned areas were more clearly demarcated during subsequent meetings between BHWs and supervisors. In addition, despite the time provided for the enumeration and the provision of intensive technical assistance by the project team, only a few BHWs were able to list all of the married women of reproductive age from their area; while many were able to include at least 80 percent, some covered only 50 percent. According to the midwives, this shortcoming was due to the brief canvassing period and to continuing deficiencies in BHWs' skills. In addition, because BHWs are volunteers, the midwives can only encourage them to conduct their activities in a timely and competent manner. Regular meetings to check on the status of BHWs' work helped to improve their performance and was welcomed by the volunteers, who had previously received little supervisory attention, acknowledgment, or recognition. Finally, some BHWs expressed frustration at their inability to effectively address the needs reported by some women in their areas (e.g., the needs of infertile women who wanted to become pregnant).

CONCLUSION

This pilot project has demonstrated the feasibility and difficulties of reorienting outreach workers to elicit information on women's needs and develop a plan for community visits based on those needs. The *barangay* health workers' family planning role has been more clearly defined, and its outreach component now has a structure. Under the earlier scheme, some BHWs had been asked to cover households that were far from their own residence;[11] in addition, as noted above, there was some overlap between their coverage areas. After the rosters were developed, BHWs were assigned to households near or in their own neighborhoods, and the overlap between coverage areas was eliminated. Each BHW now covers a clear and manageable number of households.

Information gathered during the researchers' field visits suggested that both midwives and BHWs appreciated the value of client-based information in designing their workplans and directing their service efforts. They had originally perceived information collection to be an administrative requirement for reporting purposes; its use as a tool for managing service delivery was entirely new to them. The client-generated database also created an opportunity for midwives and BHWs to communicate more effectively with one another. It thus increased the level of communication at all levels—between supervisors and workers and between workers and their clients.

The project has provided an experiential base for defining a good outreach worker, as follows:

- Committed and concerned about the client;
- Able to engage the client and elicit service needs;
- Able to respond appropriately to these needs; and
- Able to conduct visits based on clients' needs rather than on external criteria.

By extension, a good supervisor provides appropriate support to BHWs and encourages open exchange—both on problems that have been solved and on those for which a solution is still being sought. BHWs and midwives talk about women who are referred to the clinic, with a focus on their service needs. Increased flow of information between supervisors and BHWs has meant that their work is now effectively interdependent. When a midwife learns about the needs of BHWs' clients, she is able to provide better services when these clients are referred, and can have a more productive exchange with BHWs about the clients' status; in turn, BHWs can provide better care during follow-up visits.

This project was pilot-tested in a limited area—one municipality in each of two provinces. The provincial health officer of Davao del Norte found the experiment to be innovative and useful as it built on the resources already available within the public system. He is thus using provincial government resources to expand the project provincewide, increasing the population covered from 131,000 to over 700,000. Furthermore, he has integrated an expanded version of the project's client-based record form into the provincial health program.

Using this expanded tool, BHWs also elicit information on clients' needs for tetanus toxoid immunization for women, vitamin A supplementation for children, and child immunization, in addition to family planning. Services in all these areas are prioritized based on what the BHWs learn in their exchanges with clients. All services provided by BHWs are now recorded on a newly developed client-based form, and both BHWs and midwives have been trained to use the form.

The fact that the public system in Davao del Norte was able to scale up the pilot project, expand it to include a broader range of services, and institutionalize the new approach is a notable achievement. Other projects—particularly one being undertaken by Management Sciences for Health—are also using the lessons learned from this pilot effort to improve the client orientation of family planning services. The project demonstrates that community-based health workers can be reoriented to provide services based on client needs. Further progress and sustainability hinge on commitment to a client orientation among both decisionmakers and service providers. Translating the concept of client-centered care into practice is a key post-Cairo mandate. While this pilot experiment with outreach workers in the Philippines is not without remaining challenges, it provides a simple tool to help workers learn about—and respect—the fertility needs, concerns, and uncertainties of the client.

Acknowledgments

The authors thank the provincial health officers, Dr. Agapito Hornido of Davao del Norte and Dr. Renato Basañes of Compostela Valley; the regional director of the Department of Health, Dr. Dolores Castillo, and her staff, Ms. Nelia Gumela and Mrs. Vida Acosta; and all participating municipal health officers, nurses, BHWs, and midwives.

This study was conducted under the auspices of the Impact Studies Program, which is implemented by the Population Council and funded by USAID, the Rockefeller Foundation, and the Population Council.

Notes

1   The central office of the Department of Health retains responsibility for contraceptive supplies and logistics, standard setting, and accreditation.

2   The Catholic Church is an important participant in issues related to population policy and fertility regulation in the Philippines. Differences between the government and the Church have created an environment inimical to a strong program, and changes in policy can often be traced to the Church–state relationship.

3   A *barangay* is the smallest unit of government in the Philippines.

4   An illustrated Department of Health manual exceeding 350 pages provides *barangay* health workers with information about a broad range of health issues (from malnutrition to drowning).

5   While there is no systematic bias favoring specific methods, anecdotal evidence suggests that some methods may not be offered to women depending on their age or parity.

6   A full description is available in Costello et al. 2001.

7   The project goal was to improve the quality of family planning services by training clinic providers, with an emphasis on information exchange practices; by training supervisors in supportive supervision techniques; and by training outreach volunteers. (See Chapter 6 for more information on EngenderHealth's supportive supervision strategies.)

8   Panabo municipality has a population of around 131,000; Montevista municipality has a population of around 32,000.

9   Initially, project staff trained 49 BHWs. Immediately after this training, 61 other BHWs were trained by midwives and selected BHWs who had participated in the initial training exercise.

10   Natural family planning methods, also known as fertility awareness methods, include rhythm/keeping a calendar, monitoring cervical mucus, and tracking basal body temperature.

11   This occurred whenever the households of a BHW who had stopped volunteering were distributed among those who were still in service.

References

Costello, Marilou, Marlina Lacuesta, Saumya RamaRao, and Anrudh Jain. 2001. "A client-centered approach to family planning: The Davao Project," *Studies in Family Planning* 32(4): 302–314.

DeGraff, Deborah and Victor DeSilva. 1996. "A new perspective on the definition and measurement of unmet need for contraception," *International Family Planning Perspectives* 22(4): 140–147.

Department of Health (DOH) and UNFPA. 1994. *Health Work Is Team Work! An Operations Manual for Community Volunteer Health Workers (CVHW).* Government of the Philippines: The CVHW Program, Community Health Service, DOH.

Jain, Anrudh. 1996. "Items on information exchange to be emphasized in training of providers," internal memo. New York: Population Council.

———. 1999. "Should eliminating unmet need for contraception continue to be a program priority?" *International Family Planning Perspectives* 25(suppl): S39–S43, S49.

Lacuesta, Marlina, Segundina Sarangani, and Napoleon Amoyen. 1994. "A diagnostic study of the implementation of the DOH Health Volunteer Workers Program," final report, Asia and Near East Operations Research and Technical Assistance Project. Manila: Population Council.

Murphy, Elaine and Cynthia Steele. 1997. *Client–Provider Interactions in Family Planning Services: Guidance from Research and Program Experience: Recommendations for Updating Selected Practices in Contraceptive Use,* vol. II. Chapel Hill, NC: INTRAH.

National Statistics Office (NSO), Philippines Department of Health and Macro International, Inc. (MI). 1999. *National Demographic and Health Survey 1998.* Manila: NSO and MI.

Palma-Sealza, Lita. 1993. "Quality of care and family planning dropouts in Bukidnon Province: A survey study," *Philippine Population Journal* 9(1–4): 1–11.

Rood, Steven, Marcelo Raquepo, and Mary Ann Ladia. 1993. "A diagnostic study of Department of Health training courses for family planning providers," *Philippine Population Journal* 9(1–4): 37–48.

Rooks, Judith and Beverly Winikoff. 1990. "Chapter 12: Conclusions" and "Chapter 13: Recommendations," in *A Reassessment of the Concept of Reproductive Risk in Maternity Care and Family Planning Services,* proceedings of a seminar presented by the Population Council's Robert H. Ebert Program on Critical Issues in Reproductive Health and Population, New York, 12–13 February.

Zablan, Zelda, Josefina Cabigon, Luzviminda Muego, Marilou Costello, and Chona Echavez. 1998. "Improving the quality of care in family planning/reproductive health services of selected communities of Pangasinan Province: An intervention study," final report, Asia and Near East Operations Research and Technical Assistance Project. Manila: Population Council.

Contact information

Marilou Costello
Program Associate
Population Council
Unit 802, Pacific Place
Pearl Drive
Ortigas Center
Pasig City, Metro Manila
Philippines
telephone/fax: 63-2-638-6618
e-mail: costello@pcmanila.org

Saumya RamaRao
Program Associate
Population Council
One Dag Hammarskjold Plaza
New York, NY 10017 USA
telephone: 212-339-0603
fax: 212-755-6052
e-mail: sramarao@popcouncil.org

6

Empowering Frontline Staff to Improve the Quality of Family Planning Services: A Case Study in Tanzania

Maj-Britt Dohlie, Erin Mielke, Grace Wambwa, and Anatole Rukonge

Tanzania, with a population of more than 36 million people, is the largest country in East Africa (Population Reference Bureau 2001). The government's health policy emphasizes equity in access to services as a basic human right, with a focus on delivery of primary health care. Since 1994 the government has put increasing emphasis on the importance of reproductive health within primary health care. Tanzania faces a range of reproductive health problems, including high levels of maternal mortality (770 deaths per 100,000 live births) and HIV infection (by the end of 1999 about 8 percent of 15–49-year-olds were living with HIV/AIDS) (UNAIDS/WHO 2000). In addition, inadequate access to and quality of care translate into serious gaps in meeting women's need for contraception. Despite significant improvements in lowering unmet need, in 1996 some 24 percent of married women had an unmet need for contraception to space or limit births.[1]

While family planning services were introduced in Tanzania as early as 1959, the government did not become involved in service provision until 1974. Through the late 1980s, the government's service-delivery program focused on increasing access to temporary methods, primarily oral contraceptives. Permanent and long-term methods were virtually unavailable. The majority of female sterilizations performed in Tanzanian hospitals were done in conjunction with cesarean sections, and only two hospitals were equipped to provide minilaparotomy under local anesthesia. While the intrauterine device (IUD) was formally provided as part of the government's program, its availability was limited, and it was not available in the context of postpartum care. Norplant® and vasectomy were unavailable. In 1988, with support from the U.S. Agency for International Development (USAID), the government launched a program that sought to enhance access to permanent and long-term methods. The so-called Permanent and

Long-term Methods (P&LT) program focused on the introduction of minilaparotomy under local anesthesia, no-scalpel vasectomy, Norplant, and the postpartum IUD and emphasized provision of equipment and supplies, minor renovation of operating theaters, and training.

While the program succeeded in increasing access to sterilization and the IUD, a 1993 assessment of service-delivery needs found a range of deficiencies, which varied in severity from site to site (Ministry of Health 1993).[2] Vertically structured services, inadequate supervision, and staff who lacked the knowledge, skills, and tools to improve quality were among the systemwide problems identified. Similar concerns were found in a 1992 situation analysis in Tanzania (Ministry of Health, Tanzania, and Population Council 1992): Only 66 percent of service-delivery points had access to sterilization equipment; only 28 percent of new family planning clients were asked about their reproductive intentions; and only 5 percent of new family planning clients were told about the use and side effects of their chosen method (Miller, Jones, and Horn 1998).

As a result, in 1994 the government, USAID, and the agencies that had participated in the assessment decided to expand the mandate of the P&LT program to include a more explicit focus on quality of care and a broader perspective on reproductive health. They decided to introduce a procedure that would enable supervisors and staff at all levels to continuously improve the quality of care, with an emphasis on engaging and empowering frontline staff. The belief was that strengthening and linking supervision and training would improve the delivery system within which existing reproductive health and family planning services were provided and into which new services would be introduced. The framework on which this work was based is described in Box 1.

This chapter describes the experience of a district hospital—one of the more than 120 sites now participating in the P&LT program—as it grappled with these issues. The procedure resulted not only in a gradual shift in problem-solving from central management to staff and supervisors at the service-delivery level, but in a radical shift in the hospital's approach, from no expressed focus on quality to a focus on quality that emphasizes meeting the needs of both clients and staff.

THE STORY OF ONE HOSPITAL:
SELF-ASSESSMENT AND PROBLEM-SOLVING

The hospital, located in one of the coastal regions, serves about 7,500 inpatients each year.[3] It has 213 beds and serves as a referral site for almost 800,000 people. It joined the P&LT program in 1991, when one surgeon and two counselors from the family planning clinic were trained to provide sterilization services. As mentioned previously, it was only with great difficulty that clients could gain access to sterilization in Tanza-

---

Box 1. Framework for high-quality health services

Clients have the right to:

- *Information.* Clients have a right to accurate, appropriate, understandable, and unambiguous information related to reproductive health and sexuality, and to health overall. Informational materials designed for clients need to be available in all parts of the health care facility.

- *Access to services.* Services must be affordable; available at times and places convenient to clients; and provided without inappropriate eligibility requirements, physical barriers, or social barriers, including discrimination based on gender, age, marital status, fertility, nationality or ethnicity, social class, caste, religion, or sexual orientation.

- *Informed choice.* Services must be provided based on fully informed choice, that is, a voluntary, well-considered decision that an individual makes on the basis of options, information, and understanding. The process is a continuum that begins in the community, where people get information even before coming to a facility for services. It is the provider's responsibility either to confirm, or help the client reach, an informed choice.

- *Safe services.* Safe services require skilled providers, attention to infection prevention, and appropriate and effective medical practices. This right also refers to proper use of service-delivery guidelines, quality assurance mechanisms within the facility, counseling and instructions for clients, and management of complications related to medical and surgical procedures.

- *Privacy and confidentiality.* Clients have a right to privacy and confidentiality during delivery of services, including counseling, physical examinations and other procedures, and the handling of their medical records and other personal information by staff.

- *Dignity, comfort, and expression of opinion.* All clients have the right to be treated with respect and consideration. Providers need to ensure that clients are as comfortable as possible during procedures. Clients should be encouraged to express their views freely, including on occasions when their views differ from those of service providers.

- *Continuity of care.* All clients have a right to continuity of services and supplies, follow-up, and referral.

Health care staff have a need for:

- *Facilitative supervision and management.* Health workers function best in a supportive working environment with facilitative management and supervision that motivate and enable them to perform their tasks in ways that better meet the needs of external clients.

- *Information, training, and development.* For a facility to provide high-quality reproductive health services, staff must possess and continuously acquire the knowledge, skills, and attitudes needed to provide the best services possible.

- *Supplies, equipment, and infrastructure.* In order to provide good services, health workers need reliable and sufficient supplies, equipment in working order, and adequate infrastructure.

Source: AVSC International 1999a.

---

nia at that time. By 1995 hospital staff were performing 70 minilaparotomy procedures each year, and sterilization had become a family planning option for women in the region. By 1996, 5.2 percent of women using contraception chose to undergo sterilization, up from no women in 1991–92 (see Table 1). The IUD and injectables also became available during this period. IUD use grew from 0 to 1.5 percent of women using contraceptives, and use of injectables from 0 to 35.2 percent.

Table 1. Method mix among contraceptive users in the region, 1991–92 and 1996[a]

Year	Any modern method (%)	Pills (%)	IUD (%)	Injectables (%)	Condoms (%)	Female sterilization (%)	Any traditional method (%)
1991–92	24.3	13.3	0	0	8.1	0	75.9
1996	87.9	35.2	1.5	35.2	9.4	5.2	12.0

[a] 1991–92 figures are based on married women only; 1996 figures are based on all women of reproductive age.
Source: Derived from Bureau of Statistics Planning Commission and Macro International 1993 and 1997.

While these improvements in reach and contraceptive choice are significant, the hospital recognized that it suffered from some of the service-delivery deficiencies documented nationwide in the 1993 assessment. In 1995 hospital staff at all levels introduced a procedure for continuous self-assessment to identify and solve these problems. In doing so, they used two tools that had been developed in the field through collaboration among East African institutions and EngenderHealth (formerly AVSC International).[4] These tools—the Client-Oriented Provider-Efficient tool (COPE®) and the Quality Measuring Tool (QMT)[5]—are intended to help providers improve quality of care. COPE includes tools to determine the scope and dimensions of service-delivery problems and to assist in developing solutions; it is based on the framework of clients' rights and staff needs outlined in Box 1. QMT provides a means for supervisors and staff to jointly quantify and measure improvement in quality over time.

COPE: A Guide to Site-level Problem-solving

COPE is a process of continuous quality improvement that involves site staff at all levels in assessing and improving the services they provide. With COPE, staff assess themselves using ten written guides based on the framework of clients' rights and staff needs. Seven guides focus on clients' rights to information; access to services; informed choice; safe services; privacy and confidentiality; dignity, comfort, and expression of opinion; and continuity of care. The remaining three guides focus on providers' needs for facilitative supervision and management; information, training, and development; and supplies, equipment, and infrastructure.

COPE is introduced to staff over two days by a trained external or internal facilitator. During the initial meeting, staff and supervisors define how they would want services to be provided if they themselves were clients, and what they as providers need in order to offer such services. Staff then split up into groups, each using two to three of the self-assessment guides described above. The guides provide key questions, based on clinical and service standards, that encourage staff to evaluate the way they perform their daily tasks and, in particular, the way they interact with clients. Examples of key questions include:

- During a pelvic examination, does the provider wear gloves and use a clean speculum that has been properly disinfected or sterilized?
- Do staff assess women considering the IUD for risk of reproductive tract infections (RTIs), sexually transmitted infections (STIs), and HIV by taking detailed histories and physical examinations? Are those at risk or with indications of infection tested, treated, and counseled about other contraceptive options?
- Do staff provide condoms for dual-method use?
- Do all staff (including guards, receptionists, and medical, accounting, laboratory, and pharmacy staff) treat clients with kindness, courtesy, attentiveness, and respect?

Members of one of the staff teams interview clients to solicit their opinions on the services provided. The group using the self-assessment guide on safe services also reviews records. Staff at the site can also perform a client-flow analysis as needed to measure client waiting time and use of staff time. Members of each group then discuss the results of their component of the assessment and draft an action plan to address the problems identified. The groups then meet to discuss and finalize an overall site action plan, which outlines the problems, their causes, recommendations for solutions, specification of the individuals responsible for following up on each recommendation, and the date by which each recommendation will be implemented.

The quality improvement procedure should be viewed as continuous, with COPE exercises repeated every three to six months (AVSC International 1995, 1999a). Sites that have used the tool report being able to solve the problems they identify in about 60 percent of cases (Lynam, Rabinovitz, and Shobowale 1993).

Assessing Progress Over Time: Quality Measuring Tool

The Quality Measuring Tool was developed as a simple tool with which supervisors and staff can jointly assess and quantify their progress in improving quality over time. It relies on a combination of self-assessment, verification by supervisors, and problem-solving while the supervisor is onsite. To use the tool effectively, supervisors should visit the site at least every three months. Once a year, during a supervisory visit, staff and supervisors complete the QMT by consensus. Completing the QMT requires answering questions based on the COPE self-assessment guides.

Examples of questions in the QMT related to a client's right to information include:

- Do staff explain available alternative procedures?
- Do staff explain the consequences of procedures before they undertake them?

- Do staff inform clients of contraindications or side effects of the service or family planning method they want?

Examples of questions related to a client's right to access include:

- Is the family planning clinic open at least five days per week?
- Is the family planning clinic open all day (with no interruptions for tea break or lunch)?

An example of a question related to a client's right to choice is:

- For clients who require diagnosis and treatment of RTIs (including STIs), are facilities or referrals in place to ensure that they and their sexual contacts get these services?

A positive response is worth one point, and each negative answer yields no points. According to the answers provided, staff can calculate an overall score in each category, with 100 percent indicating that all questions were answered positively. Conducting the QMT on a regular basis enables staff to measure their progress over time. The results supplement other medical monitoring data routinely collected by supervisors, and all such data are incorporated into the staff's COPE action plan for solving site-level quality problems. Currently the QMT is being revised to incorporate an even broader range of reproductive health issues.

IMPROVING QUALITY OF CARE IN THE HOSPITAL: COPE AND QMT IN PRACTICE

The hospital conducted a COPE exercise in mid-1995. As a result, a number of the problems identified were documented and resolved. This was followed in December 1995 by a more quantitative QMT assessment. The QMT served as a baseline for the site and made it possible to track the process of identifying problems, implementing solutions, and documenting results.

Problems regarding rights to access and informed choice included:

- A woman had to have her husband's consent to receive sterilization services.
- The maternity ward did not provide any contraceptive methods.
- Postpartum IUD services were not available.

Problems regarding the right to safe services included:

- The operating theater lacked emergency drugs.
- Supplies to prevent infection were inadequate in the family planning clinic, maternity ward, and operating theater; locally purchased chlorine bleach was of uneven quality.
- An inadequate supply of gloves and syringes made it necessary to ask clients to supply these items themselves.

- The family planning clinic, maternity ward, and operating theater lacked appropriate containers for safe disposal of syringes and other sharp objects.

Problems concerning the right to facilitative supervision and management included:

- No district supervisors had visited the hospital in the last six months.
- Service statistics had not been compiled recently, were not well organized, and were not displayed.
- No COPE exercises had taken place during the past six months.
- The facility had no regular forum for discussing family planning services.

EMPOWERING STAFF THROUGH
IMPROVED SUPERVISION AND TRAINING

The initial COPE exercise had made it clear that prevailing supervision and management practices were not conducive to high-quality services and that improved training was needed in a number of key areas. Rather than institute top-down measures to improve quality, the hospital decided to focus on staff needs in the belief that empowering and supporting staff would also result in a better response to clients' rights and needs.

To decentralize program supervision, a medical coordinator was hired in 1996 to work with sites in four coastal regions. The coordinator's role was to train local supervisors in facilitative supervision, which emphasizes two-way communication, coaching, mentoring, and joint problem-solving (Ben Salem and Beattie 1996). Supervisors then serve as catalysts for improving quality by facilitating better work performance, creating a positive work environment, and considering their staff to be "internal customers." The COPE procedure helped supervisors adopt this approach by encouraging teamwork among all levels of staff, providing a forum in which staff and supervisors can exchange ideas, and relying on staff experience to identify and solve problems through self-assessment.

The medical coordinator also helped supervisors respond more actively to the learning needs of staff at all levels by making quarterly visits to the site—during which the coordinator met with both supervisors and staff—and by training regional, district, and site supervisors at annual workshops. In turn, site supervisors met with staff on a weekly basis. Because this approach to staff development considers the learning needs of all staff, it better meets the needs of the entire site and is called whole-site training (Bradley, Lynam et al. 1998). As supervisors became more involved in activities designed to expand learning through skills training, orientations, and updates, they began to provide better post-training support and follow-up. Supervisors also received training in intrainstitutional outreach—or "Inreach"—a process through which staff organize orientations for other departments and wards to encourage links and referrals (Lynam, Dwyer, and Bradley 1994).

Several changes in the functioning of the facility can be attributed to the processes described above:

- The hospital established a COPE committee, and four staff members were trained in COPE facilitation. Sessions were subsequently conducted every three to six months.
- Copies of the COPE action plan were displayed. As one staff member commented, "Before, teamwork was weak; . . . now administrators and staff are working as a team. All staff feel free to express their opinions freely in department meetings."[6]
- Supervisory visits increased in frequency and length; external supervisors visited the site at least once every six months and stayed for at least one day. As one staff member said, "[Regional supervisors] come more often and really work to help us solve our problems. . . . Sometimes they spend a whole day with us, which gives us [more time] to share ideas and discuss problems. . . . It makes us feel good."[7]
- The QMT was revised to reflect additional areas for training, including how to use service statistics for decisionmaking, planning, and follow-up by external supervisors.

In sum, with COPE and the QMT, staff and supervisors assessed and participated in improving their own work, a process that motivated them to find ways to improve quality with local resources. The activities also provided a forum in which supervisors and staff could discuss and solve problems together, often for the first time. Supervisors play a critical role in setting expectations and goals, serving as role models, meeting training needs, making resources available, and linking the site to the larger system when problems cannot be solved onsite.

THE IMPACT OF STAFF EMPOWERMENT ON QUALITY OF CARE

While the new approach resulted in some immediate changes, others occurred over the long term. Between 1995 and 1998, life at the hospital changed for both clients and staff.

Right to Safe Services

Although the hospital's family planning staff had been trained in infection prevention practices and technical skills, the training was not always well understood or applied. In addition, basic infection prevention supplies often were not available. With the introduction of self-assessment, facilitative supervision, and whole-site training in 1996, the family planning clinic's efforts at improving quality became more consistent. The clinic also benefited from similar efforts elsewhere in the facility: Onsite training and orientations for all staff made it possible to extend improved infection prevention practices to the operating theater and to all wards, including the maternity and gynecology wards. All levels of staff learned appropriate procedures, and supervisors provided the necessary supplies, support, and feedback to ensure that staff were implementing improved practices. Examples of changed practices include:

- Staff posted wall charts that showed how to prevent infection.
- By calling attention to the inadequacy of drugs and supplies in the operating theater, staff succeeded in improving inventory; most emergency drugs became available (however, cupboard space became a problem when drug supplies improved).
- Staff donated cooking oil buckets to use for decontaminating equipment and linens.
- As awareness of the need for antisepsis increased, the hospital became concerned about the cost of commercially bottled chlorine bleach. As an alternative, the pharmacist began preparing a bleach solution using chlorinated lime powder.
- Staff reduced overflow at the medical waste pit by bagging some waste to take to another dumpsite. Staff also requested boots for cleaning staff who carry waste to the pit as well as for mortuary and laundry staff, and these were provided.
- Heavy-duty gloves were made available in the operating theater.

Right to Informed Choice

When the hospital joined the Permanent and Long-Term Methods program in 1991, family planning staff (including the surgeons and assistants who perform tubal ligations) received extensive training in counseling and informed choice. The informed choice procedure for permanent methods requires that information be provided on alternative methods, that the client be carefully screened, and that the client give his or her written informed consent after counseling and before the clinical procedure. Performance on these measures was imperfect. In 1995, staff found insufficient and incorrect information in a sample of 20 consent forms for tubal ligation clients. Performance improved after the introduction of self-assessment, facilitative supervision, and whole-site training. In a 1998 sample, all 20 forms were correctly completed by staff and signed by clients. Training was also expanded to other wards: Staff in the gynecology, maternity, and pediatric wards were trained by coworkers to counsel clients on family planning, to provide services, or to refer clients to the family planning clinic for services.

Right to Access to Services

- In response to staff concerns about continuing inadequate choice of long-term methods at the site, Norplant was added to the method mix in mid-1996.
- The maternity ward gradually began to offer contraception directly, beginning with IUDs and later expanding to other methods.
- Signs providing information on the location and hours of operation of the family planning clinic were posted around the hospital.
- According to national policy, the requirement for husbands' consent for tubal ligation was eliminated.
- Previously, women who arrived in search of both family planning services and health care for sick children, for example, were referred to outpatient services, which required a separate visit and a long wait. As a result of a COPE exercise, a new building was made available for family planning and maternal and child health (FP/MCH) services, and staff were able to ensure that clients' children were seen during the same visit.
- Previously, women had to go to another part of the hospital to have blood drawn. Blood samples were now taken in the FP/MCH clinic.
- Special patient visiting hours were established.

Improving the Quality of Other Reproductive Health Services

- In response to a high-level program decision regarding shortcomings in postabortion care nationwide, in 1997 two service providers at the hospital were trained in manual vacuum aspiration (MVA) and other elements of postabortion care and returned to the hospital to provide on-the-job training to coworkers in the gynecology ward.[8] Senior medical officers, all department heads, and gynecology, maternity, and MCH nurses received orientation to postabortion care and counseling, including infection prevention related to MVA.[9]
- In 1998 a nurse was hired to work with the medical coordinator to form a supervisory team, a step that signified the beginning of closer collaboration with the maternity and gynecology wards. In 1999 the nurse helped the maternity ward introduce COPE tools specifically developed for assessing maternity services (see Box 2).
- In response to the AIDS epidemic, staff have been trained in both infection prevention and STI/AIDS counseling. In three of the four QMT surveys,

---

Box 2. Applying COPE to maternity care

Applying COPE to the assessment of maternity services, staff identified the following problems for clients:
- Lack of information on nutrition;
- No signs showing when and where maternity services are offered;
- Long waiting time in the laboratory;
- No involvement of men in antenatal, delivery, and postpartum care;
- Less availability of chlorine and gloves as compared to the family planning clinic;
- No incubators and bathing supplies for babies;
- No lockers for mothers;
- Unclean toilets;
- No screens in wards;
- Congestion in wards;
- Poor interpersonal relations between staff and patients;
- Women having to deliver alone because staff are too busy; and
- Provider bias against postpartum IUD insertion.

Staff cited unmet needs of their own as well:
- Inadequate communication and quality assurance;
- No proper tracking of records;
- No job descriptions;
- Few trained counselors;
- No library/reference materials; and
- Inadequate information on current breastfeeding issues.

---

staff indicated that all family planning workers were able and willing to counsel clients about STIs and AIDS. The most recent survey indicates that additional staff require training in this area, as a result of staff turnover.[10]

Right to Privacy and Confidentiality

In one of their COPE exercises, staff identified lack of privacy for family planning clients as a problem. Initially, the family planning program had use of only one small room in the already crowded MCH clinic. When the new building became available, the staff reorganized all FP/MCH services, assigning two private rooms for family planning counseling and one for exams and IUD insertions, and ensuring that the rooms had a lock or a "Do not disturb" sign to prevent interruptions.

Community Outreach to Promote Access to and Use of Services

The communities surrounding the hospital were unaware of the range and content of services the hospital provided. Staff began working with local clinics to improve their

Rights and needs	Dec. 1995	Apr. 1997	Jan. 1998	Oct. 1998
Clients' rights				
Information (%)	50	64	69	80
Safe services (%)	35	81	90	94
Choice (%)	50	59	81	92
Access (%)	64	72	79	89
Privacy, confidentiality (%)	64	57	79	87
Dignity, comfort, expression of opinion (%)	80	85	77	91
Continuity of care (%)	40	65	69	89
Staff needs				
Supervision (%)	4	92	85	93
Information, training (%)	71	67	86	81
Supplies, equipment (%)	63	95	85	100

Table 2. Improvements in service quality, 1995–98

counseling services as well as their understanding of the hospital as a referral source for methods such as Norplant and minilaparotomy, emergency treatment of abortion complications, and other services. One staff member stated, "We are even providing training in family planning counseling and referral to most of the community-based workers serving this area. Through on-the-job training, we've been able to expand the services we provide without taking staff away from the hospital." Another commented, "Information has reached everybody, not just one person. Many women have understood the meaning of family planning. And clients are getting correct directions to family planning services from gatekeepers."

CONCLUSIONS: MEASURABLE RESULTS IN KEY AREAS

As discussed earlier, the Quality Measuring Tool provides a means of charting a site's progress over time based on staff and supervisor assessments. Results between 1995 and 1998 show progress in all ten indexes of clients' rights and staff needs (each index consists of several related indicators or questions), as early improvements were largely sustained and additional improvements were achieved over time (see Table 2).[11]

The most dramatic change recorded was in scores for supervision, which increased from 4 percent in 1995 to 93 percent in 1998 (the drop between 1997 and 1998 reflects the addition of new elements to the assessment tool). As discussed earlier, meeting staff needs by improving supervisory practices was the key to enabling staff to meet clients' needs for safe services, choice, and access to care more effectively than they had before. Scores for safe services, for example, improved from 35 percent to 94 percent between

1995 and 1998. In two areas of clients' rights, scores dropped slightly in the middle of the period assessed. In one case (dignity and comfort), this drop was due to the addition of new questions about client waiting times, which both staff and clients felt were unreasonable. By October 1998 both staff and clients felt that waiting times had improved and the score improved commensurately, reaching 91 percent. In the second case (privacy and confidentiality), the drop in the score between 1995 and 1997 occurred because auditory privacy declined in the counseling/examination room, probably because of an increase in the number of clients visiting the facility and crowding in the waiting area close to this room. Staff were able to provide more privacy for counseling and examinations when the new building became available. By 1998 the site had achieved a score of 87 percent in the privacy and confidentiality category.

Clients' Perspectives on Service Improvements

Interviews with six clients conducted at the FP/MCH clinic in April 1999 suggest that progress is being made from the perspective of clients. The interviews also pointed out areas for further improvement, particularly in the area of information provision. All six clients said they had received the services they came for. However, only one said she had heard a health talk, and several said they would like to receive more information on family planning and other issues related to reproductive health. Most said they appreciated not having to leave the FP/MCH clinic to have blood drawn. Several commented that the hospital was cleaner than in the previous year, and another expressed approval of the new visiting hours.

An earlier set of interviews with 16 gynecology ward patients in 1997 found that all had received family planning information during their visit. These clients also made suggestions for service improvements. Eight said information on family planning "should reach villages" or should "reach more people." Thirteen said services in the ward were good, "even better than in other hospitals," but one said providers should be "closer to patients" and drugs should be more available. One recommended that the hospital set up a shop to sell commodities that are not available in the wards.

The Cost of Quality

While some would argue that quality improvement is too expensive, in a health-care setting poor quality is costly—in both financial and health terms. For example, if equipment is improperly sterilized, staff and clients can get infections that require treatment, additional staff time, and medications and other supplies.

The main program-level costs of this initiative were for supervision and training, and the emphasis has been on approaches to quality improvement that are sustainable. Most of the improvements were made using the hospital's existing resources: Staff trained one another in new skills and techniques and donated buckets for infection prevention, and hospital managers reorganized the flow of services. Because the QMT assessments were integrated with site-level supervisory activities, information on the costs of the evaluation is not available.[12]

REMAINING CHALLENGES

Although this hospital and other sites in Tanzania have significantly improved quality using relatively simple self-assessment tools and more effective approaches to supervision and training, many challenges remain (Bradley, Wambwa et al. 1998; Bradley et al. 2000). These include continuing to improve both access to and the quality of existing services, as well as adding new reproductive health services. For example, when the QMT was used in 1998, the site had yet to offer Pap smears for cervical cancer screening or vasectomy services for men, both of which had been identified as deficiencies in the constellation of services. While such deficiencies can always be identified, their solutions are not always within reach. The government does not have the resources to implement all needed interventions at one time.

Another challenge faced by the program—at this hospital and elsewhere—is the high attrition rate of technical staff as a result of transfers, rotations, and, more importantly, deaths (Riwa et al. 2000), including deaths from AIDS. The loss in human resources highlights the critical importance of sustainable, continuous capacity building, as well as the urgent need to institute effective HIV/AIDS prevention programs.[13] The effects of attrition could be minimized by training more clinical officers and nurses in the provision of clinical reproductive health services (e.g., training nurses to insert and remove Norplant and training clinical officers to conduct minilaparotomies and no-scalpel vasectomies).

Quality improvement requires considerable capacity building in terms of skills improvement, change in staff attitudes, and better systems overall. One systemwide constraint is the insufficient supply of chlorine to prevent infection. Currently, chlorine is not included on the essential drugs list, and it is not consistently available for purchase at reduced rates through the medical stores department. Even the chlorinated lime powder used by the pharmacist to make a cheaper bleach solution onsite is not consistently available through this department. These deficiencies are under review by the Ministry of Health, which also plans to develop national infection prevention guidelines and standards (Riwa et al. 2000). Ongoing commitment to continuous quality improvement at the site, combined with increasing support from the top, will help ensure that these deficiencies are gradually overcome.

Acknowledgments

This chapter could not have been written without the involvement and commitment of managers and staff at all levels in the Ministry of Health, at the Tanzania Family Planning Association, and at the hospital described here. Support for the Permanent and Long-term Methods program described in this chapter was provided by USAID.

Notes

1   Except where noted, the information in this section is drawn from Bureau of Statistics Planning Commission and Macro International 1993 and 1997.

2   The assessment team included representatives of the Tanzania Ministry of Health, the Tanzania Family Planning Association, USAID, USAID's Family Planning Service Expansion and Technical Support project, Intrah, and EngenderHealth (formerly AVSC International).

3   The authors and the Tanzania Ministry of Health have agreed to keep the site name confidential.

4   See Dohlie et al. 1999 for details on this package of tools.

5   QMT was formerly known as the Quality Improvement Quotient (QIQ) (AVSC International 1995). Revised documentation of the QMT is forthcoming (EngenderHealth 2002).

6   This statement was made by a hospital staff member at the Annual Facilitative Supervision Workshop in Arusha, June 1998.

7   This quotation and the others cited in following pages are from a 1997 site visit report by Erin Mielke.

8   The three elements of postabortion care are: (1) emergency treatment for complications of spontaneous or induced abortion; (2) effective postabortion family planning counseling and services; and (3) effective links between emergency treatment services and comprehensive reproductive health services (Achwal et al. 1999).

9   In response to the success of the pilot project at this site, the Ministry of Health has expanded postabortion care services to 28 additional sites.

10 To help meet the needs of sites like this, EngenderHealth recently produced a set of STI/HIV prevention quick-reference cards for health care providers for use in counseling clients seeking family planning, antenatal care, and general health care (AVSC International 2000).

11 As described earlier, a score of 100 percent implies that all questions contributing to the index were answered positively.

12 Cost elements included staff time for a research specialist to develop the evaluation tool, pilot-testing and adapting the tool as part of a one-week annual supervision workshop for medical coordinators, and local travel costs to the sites to conduct the evaluation (one day per assessment, per site). Site-level data were analyzed on the day the evaluation was conducted. Staff time was also allocated to analyze the information across sites.

13 AIDS is the leading cause of death among adults in Tanzania. Donor support for the Ministry of Health aims to increase use of FP/MCH and HIV/AIDS prevention measures, improve the policy environment for HIV/AIDS, and increase the availability of quality services (including condom availability, peer education and youth activities, voluntary counseling and testing, and home-based care, among others). A severe shortage of drugs to treat STIs is one of the constraints to these efforts (USAID/Tanzania 2001).

References

Achwal, Isaac, Andrew Kilonzo, Erasmus Malekela, Manisha Mehta, Elizabeth M'Mbando, Dawson Mrosso, Anatole Rukonge, Grace Wambwa, and Meck Wikedzi. 1999. "Final evaluation: Improving postabortion care in three Tanzanian hospitals," internal final report. New York: AVSC International.

AVSC International. 1995. *COPE: Client-Oriented, Provider-Efficient Services.* New York: AVSC International.

———. 1999a. *COPE Self-Assessment Guides for Reproductive Health Services.* New York: AVSC International.

———. 1999b. *Facilitative Supervision Handbook.* New York: AVSC International.

———. 2000. *STI/HIV Prevention Quick-reference Cards for Health Care Providers: What Every Client Should Know.* New York: AVSC International.

Ben Salem, Beverly and Karen J. Beattie. 1996. "Facilitative supervision: A vital link in quality reproductive health service delivery," AVSC Working Paper no. 10. New York: AVSC International.

Bradley, Janet, Pamela Fenney Lynam, Joseph C. Dwyer, and Grace E. Wambwa. 1998. "Whole-site training: A new approach to the organization of training," AVSC Working Paper no. 11. New York: AVSC International.

Bradley, Janet, Erin Mielke, Grace Wambwa, Joseph Mashafi, and Manase Nasania. 2000. "Family planning services in Tanzania: Results from a project to improve quality, 1996–1999," internal report. New York: AVSC International.

Bradley, Janet, Grace Wambwa, Karen Beattie, and Joseph Dwyer. 1998. "Quality of care in family planning services: An assessment of change in Tanzania 1995/6 to 1996/7," internal report. New York: AVSC International.

Bureau of Statistics Planning Commission and Macro International. 1993. *Tanzania Demographic and Health Survey 1991/1992.* Columbia, MD: Macro International, Inc.

———. 1997. *Tanzania Demographic and Health Survey 1996.* Calverton, MD: Macro International, Inc.

Dohlie, Maj-Britt, Erin Mielke, Feddis K. Mumba, Grace E. Wambwa, Anatole Rukonge, and Wilfred Mongo. 1999. "Using practical quality improvement approaches and tools in reproductive health services in East Africa," *The Joint Commission Journal on Quality Improvement* 25(11): 574–587.

EngenderHealth. 2002. "The quality measuring tool for reproductive health services: A manual for using the quality measuring tool for managers, supervisors, and providers." New York: EngenderHealth. Forthcoming.

Lynam, Pamela F., Joseph C. Dwyer, and Janet Bradley. 1994. "Inreach: Reaching potential family planning clients within health institutions," AVSC Working Paper no. 5. New York: AVSC International.

Lynam, Pamela, Leslie McNeil Rabinovitz, and Mofoluke Shobowale. 1993. "Using self-assessment to improve the quality of family planning clinic services," *Studies in Family Planning* 24(4): 252–260.

Miller, Kate, Heidi Jones, and Marjorie C. Horn. 1998. "Indicators of readiness and quality: Basic findings," in Kate Miller, Robert Miller, Ian Askew, Marjorie C. Horn, and Lewis Ndhlovu (eds.), *Clinic-Based Family Planning and Reproductive Health Services in Africa: Findings from Situation Analysis Studies.* New York: Population Council, pp. 29–85.

Ministry of Health. 1993. "Tanzania assessment: Program for permanent and long-term contraception," report. Nairobi, Kenya: AVSC International.

Ministry of Health, Tanzania, and Population Council. 1992. "Tanzania: The family planning situation analysis study," report. Nairobi, Kenya: Population Council.

Population Reference Bureau. 2001. *2001 World Population Data Sheet of the Population Reference Bureau: Demographic Data and Estimates for the Countries and Regions of the World*, book edition. Washington, DC: Population Reference Bureau.

Riwa, Peter, Rhodes Mwaikambo, Anatole Rukonge, Isaac Achwal, and Carol Camlin. 2000. "A report on the review of long-term and permanent contraceptive methods and quality improvement program in Tanzania," prepared for the Ministry of Health, Reproductive and Child Health Section.

UNAIDS/WHO. 2000. "United Republic of Tanzania: Epidemiological fact sheet on HIV/AIDS and sexually transmitted infections." Geneva: WHO.

USAID/Tanzania. 2001. "Supporting an accelerated response to HIV/AIDS in Tanzania," presentation to the Reproductive Health and Child Health Section/USAID Performance Improvement Work Planning Meeting, Dar es Salaam, Tanzania, February.

Contact information

Erin Mielke
Program Manager, Quality Improvement
EngenderHealth
440 Ninth Avenue
New York, NY 10001 USA
telephone: 212-561-8061
fax: 212-561-8067
Info@engenderhealth.org

Grace Wambwa
Program Manager
EngenderHealth
1st Floor
PO Box 57964
ABC Place
Waiyaki Way
Nairobi, Kenya
telephone: 254-2-444-922
Engenderhealthkenya@engenderhealth.org

PART III
ADDRESSING SEXUALITY, GENDER, AND PARTNERS IN SERVICES

paragraph 7.36, Programme of Action

The objectives are: (a) To promote adequate development of responsible sexuality, permitting relations of equity and mutual respect between the genders and contributing to improving the quality of life of individuals; (b) To ensure that women and men have access to the information, education and services needed to achieve good sexual health and exercise their reproductive rights and responsibilities.

paragraph 7.41, Programme of Action

. . . information and services should be made available to adolescents to help them understand their sexuality and protect them from unwanted pregnancies, sexually transmitted diseases and subsequent risk of infertility.

How can reproductive health programs bring sexuality and gender into their services?

---

paragraph 4.27, Programme of Action

Special efforts should be made to emphasize men's shared responsibility and promote their active involvement in responsible parenthood, sexual and reproductive behaviour, including family planning; prenatal, maternal and child health; prevention of sexually transmitted diseases, including HIV; prevention of unwanted and high-risk pregnancies. . . .

How can reproductive health services engage the partners of their clients?

7

"When I Talk About Sexuality, I Use Myself as an Example": Sexuality Counseling and Family Planning in Colombia

Bonnie Shepard

For a long time, it was a joke in the reproductive health field that most family planning services operated as though contraceptive use had nothing to do with sex. Evidence from around the world has brought to light how profoundly the power dynamics in sexual relations restrict women's use and choice of contraceptive methods, or force them to use methods secretively. The onset of the HIV/AIDS epidemic and rising consciousness about sexually transmitted infections (STIs) and reproductive tract infections (RTIs) have provided additional and urgent reasons to put promotion of sexual health on the agenda of all family planning agencies.

This increasing awareness has led to specific operational challenges. How can personnel at all levels be trained to address sexual health in ways that are respectful of diverse service users when the surrounding culture inculcates lack of respect? How can they deal with gender-based power dynamics that determine women's ability to protect themselves from STIs, sexual coercion, or violence? This case study of institutional change describes how one family planning organization—Profamilia in Colombia—confronted these challenges and expanded its mission and services by adopting a sexual and reproductive health approach.[1]

THE EVOLUTION OF PROFAMILIA

As a family planning organization, Profamilia is an often-cited success story. Founded in 1965 by Fernando Tamayo as a nonprofit, nongovernmental organization, Profamilia is Colombia's International Planned Parenthood Federation (IPPF) affiliate, one of the largest in IPPF's worldwide network. With 35 clinics in 31 cities and almost three-quarters of a million client visits each year, Profamilia is a major service provider in Colombia, delivering approximately 60 percent of all family planning services in the country.[2]

Although Profamilia originally focused exclusively on contraceptive delivery, in 1967 it began to diversify. It expanded its services, first by providing Pap smears and, later, gynecologic services and some pediatric and general medical care. By the mid-1980s, Profamilia had broadened its mandate beyond women's medical services, and over the next ten years (1985–94) it gradually launched an impressive range of new services. First the agency opened men's clinics in Bogotá and Medellín; while vasectomy provision was perhaps the driving force for opening these clinics, many men came for treatment of STIs and urologic problems. Next, it began to provide legal services for women and opened youth centers. Profamilia continued to expand its sexual and reproductive health services by conducting a workshop for clinic directors on gender issues and reproductive rights, undertaking an AIDS prevention campaign, and establishing an advisory office for issues related to sexual and reproductive rights and gender. In 1995, María Isabel Plata, a cofounder of Profamilia's legal services for women and a lawyer internationally recognized for her work on women's rights, became Profamilia's executive director.

In the midst of this expansion, foreign donors, most notably the U.S. Agency for International Development (USAID), began withdrawing support from Colombia. In 1995 the Colombian government implemented health-sector reform through Law 100. Law 100 is notable for its progressive commitment to equity and universal access in the health care system, its coverage of a range of family planning and sexual and reproductive health services, and its support for community-based health promotion. The opportunity for financial reimbursement from the government created by Law 100 induced many public and private institutions to begin offering reproductive and sexual health services. While the law's passage resulted in the loss of Profamilia's "monopoly" as the national provider of private-sector family planning and reproductive health services, it also gave the organization additional opportunities for attaining financial sustainability (Profamilia and AVSC International 1996).

TURNING CHALLENGES INTO OPPORTUNITIES

By the early 1990s, Profamilia found itself with a shrinking donor base and a deepening philosophical commitment to diversifying services. Rather than retreat in the face of uncertain finances, the organization invested further in a holistic approach to reproductive health, sexual and reproductive rights, and gender equity—programmatic steps that would resonate with the principles of the 1994 International Conference on Population and Development (ICPD) in Cairo and the 1995 World Conference on Women in Beijing. The organization opted to emphasize increased quality and diversity of services, enhance responsiveness to users' concerns and rights, and expand sexual health services beyond the confines of the male clinics. What had been a slow but steady process of diversification accelerated.

Financing the growing range of services was a daunting task. Because neither legal nor psychological services were covered by Law 100, Profamilia had to increase its fees for these services. On the other hand, many of its reproductive health services—including educational activities such as talks on violence or sexuality in the community and schools—became universally reimbursable for the first time, giving Profamilia the potential to achieve greater financial self-sufficiency in the process of implementing ICPD principles.

Plata explains the synergy generated by these strategic challenges as Profamilia adapted to the new situation:

> Diversification of services and involvement in women's rights, adolescent programs, and men's services has caused more youth, women, and men to come to Profamilia. When we give talks on these topics, it opens the doors to other institutions [with which Profamilia gains contracts]. For example, the talks on rights and self-esteem opened the door to collaboration with Family Welfare [a major government agency]. . . . Thus, implementing the principles of holistic care, gender equity, and sexual and reproductive rights prepared Profamilia for the changes brought by Law 100. . . . If we had not taken advantage of the principles approved in Cairo and Beijing, we would not have had success under Law 100. Everything acted in concert: our financial needs, the changes in the health sector, the withdrawal of USAID, and our adoption of these principles.

Indeed, Profamilia's experience has shown that far from being too costly and complicated, providing expanded sexual and reproductive health services has been financially beneficial. Because the new clinical and community education services are reimbursed through the government's health insurance scheme, incorporating the ICPD principles of sexual and reproductive health has been key to Profamilia's financial sustainability. As of December 1998, service fees and product sales covered 74 percent of Profamilia's budget, up from 35 percent in 1989.

The organization underwent a number of administrative and programmatic changes in diversifying services as part of its larger goal of incorporating sexual and reproductive health principles. This chapter highlights one important aspect of the diversification: the incorporation of sexual health into Profamilia's services, and how the organization's broader commitment to holistic approaches, gender equity, and sexual and reproductive rights enhanced promotion of sexual health. Box 1 illustrates why the commitment to sexual health must be addressed within this broader framework of institutional change.

Box 1. Sexual health: Confronting stereotypes

According to covenants of the World Health Organization and the United Nations, sexual health involves a state of comprehensive physical, emotional, and social well-being related to one's sexuality. Promoting sexual health involves much more than prevention of disease, and doing so runs up against a host of powerful cultural and political obstacles related to interpersonal relations and communication, gender, and involvement of men. While contexts vary enormously both among and within countries, recent research on sexuality shows common patterns within or across many cultures that force much sexual behavior into hiding and add tremendous complexity to the task of promoting sexual health. These include:

• Taboos on speaking about sex;
• Acceptance of male domination in heterosexual relationships;
• Double standards for men and women regarding monogamy in sexual relationships;
• Condemnation of diverse sexual practices and nonheterosexual orientations;
• Culturally imposed sanctions on the exercise of sexuality by adolescents (particularly girls), by women, and outside of marriage;
• Tendencies to blame the victims of sexual coercion and violence, especially if they are adult and female, and to excuse male perpetrators;
• Sexual stereotyping of low-income groups and ethnic minorities; and
• Norms of masculinity that emphasize sexual conquests and risk-taking.

Confronting these patterns is the central challenge for any agency developing sexual health programs. Even staff who are normally respectful, understanding, and adequate listeners may behave differently when confronted with thorny issues of sexuality and gender. Deep-seated discriminatory attitudes related to gender, class, and ethnicity, all of which tend to have sexual components, interfere with providers' ability to counsel clients adequately. Many providers suffer from sexual traumas or problems that make it difficult for them to be unbiased listeners. Providers at all levels must hone their skills at listening, responding nonjudgmentally, and demonstrating respect for all clients regardless of their age, sex, marital status, income level, or ethnic background. Perhaps the most difficult part of this process is self-criticism—providers must learn to recognize and eradicate their own unexamined discriminatory attitudes and behavior. Adding sexual health services, therefore, entails addressing these complex sociocultural issues. Efforts to incorporate sexual health services must be linked to broader efforts to humanize provider–client relations, promote clients' rights, sensitize providers to discrimination, involve men as supportive partners, and help staff deal with their own concerns.

A COMMITMENT AT THE TOP TO A FOCUS ON SEXUAL HEALTH

Although some professional and counseling staff in Colombia's large cities had received training in reproductive health and gender as early as the late 1980s, the full-scale incorporation of sexual health into Profamilia's work began in the early 1990s. In a workshop devoted to gender issues held in 1991, all clinic directors received training from feminist health leaders from other Latin American countries. By this time, Profamilia had learned—from its experiences with the men's clinic, legal services, youth programs, and AIDS campaigns—that incorporating a sexual health framework into services and into the institutional concept of quality would require a multifaceted strategy that addressed gender and rights issues and reached all levels of the organization.

Profamilia identified the following mechanisms for change within the organization:

- Training in counseling for personnel at all levels, using both in-house and outside trainers, so that the dominant cultural attitudes on sexuality and gender would not translate into judgmental approaches with users on sexual health issues.
- New pamphlets and information, education, and communication materials aimed at both men and women on STIs and AIDS, sexual and reproductive rights, sexual dysfunction, sexual violence, adolescence and sexuality, and genital and reproductive tract infections.
- New evaluation tools, including a pilot evaluation that involved gender issues[3] such as domestic and sexual violence, and indicators that included sexual health concerns.
- Quality-of-care and ethics committees, to deal with new quality and ethical issues as reproductive and sexual health services diversified.
- Ongoing internal reinforcement through informal face-to-face and written communication (e.g., encouraging doctors and midwives to invite increased male participation, and internal discussions about ethical and rights issues that staff confront in their daily work).

A FOCUS ON COUNSELING

Because Profamilia was expanding into an area so dependent on provider–client interaction, the linchpin strategy for promoting sexual health was to improve the quality of counseling. Before the initiative, the organization's counselors were responsible for talking with users about issues specific to the services they were seeking (e.g., contraception, Pap smears, and pregnancy testing) and gave talks on reproductive health topics in workplaces, schools, and other municipal locations. They needed additional training in order to be able to discuss sensitive topics related to sexuality.

Headquarters training staff interviewed both users and staff about the quality of counseling services. Although Profamilia has always had a strong commitment to high quality, comments from users and staff made it clear that there was room for improvement.

Users' comments included:

When I came here two years ago, the woman who counseled me was quite irritable.

When I had my little girl, they treated me so badly that I didn't come back.

Staff also raised concerns:

There was a tendency to treat the person as their method ("the IUD") or as their symptom ("the vaginal infection").

Sometimes a person came for a gynecologic exam and we exhausted ourselves talking about family planning. . . . When we talked about absolutely everything, sometimes the person left more confused than when she had arrived.

Men were rarely included or invited to the women's clinics, which were completely oriented toward serving female users.

People thought of Profamilia as "tube tying, tube tying, tube tying."

Profamilia's youth clinics, which had already succeeded in adopting a more client-centered, sexual health–oriented approach, helped facilitate the incorporation of sexuality into education and counseling institutionwide. Adolescents who had "graduated" to become users of the adult centers returned to their former counselors complaining about rapid and perfunctory attention. As one trainer explained, "If we can do this with young people, we can do it with adults."

Developing Staff Skills

Sexual health workshops for counselors from all Profamilia clinics were held in 1993–94, with funding from the Canadian Planned Parenthood Federation. Evaluations of these early efforts indicated that prejudices related to homosexuality and adolescent sexuality remained deeply entrenched among family planning counselors, even after the workshops. Furthermore, staff at headquarters realized that the "internal clients"—the staff—needed as much assistance on sexual health issues in their own lives as external clients did. Accordingly, the Profamilia trainers began to use more participatory methods and to provide more opportunity in workshops for personal reflection. Germán Lopez, a Profamilia senior staff member, described the need for more intensive training and guidance in this way:

The focus groups with counselors at the beginning of the project showed that former workshops to introduce counselors to the sexual health focus had not been participatory enough. There were many prejudices and stereotypes evident. . . . The discussions . . . demonstrated that . . . the counselors had disdainful and punitive attitudes toward the sexual experiences of women and adolescents [and] they did not perceive the need to incorporate sexual partners.

Furthermore, there was a growing consensus, not only at the agency but also in the field at large, that a necessary first step toward gender equity and sexual health was for women to view themselves as worthy of respect and as having rights. To achieve these goals, Profamilia recognized that it would be crucial for the counselors to boost a woman's self-confidence so that she could begin to make and implement decisions in her own interest. In 1994, with support from the Ford Foundation, Profamilia held a workshop for family planning counselors nationwide on gender issues, sexual health, and rights. As Lopez explains, "We decided to upset completely the counselors' ideas about sexuality and sexual and reproductive health, confronting their values, myths, and prejudices." However, this training would not have been sufficient to effect needed changes in practice, even when combined with other measures such as new client education materials and other incentives from management. Profamilia had to link changes in personal attitudes to the counselors' need for day-to-day guidance and reference materials. To respond to this need, Profamilia used the workshop to solicit counselors' ideas for the basic content of a reference manual. In general, the counselors responded favorably to the chance to combine exercises that encouraged their personal development with participation in the development of a manual of protocols for their own use.

Developing Counseling Tools

Entitled "How to Incorporate Sexual and Reproductive Health in Family Planning Services and Programs with a Gender Perspective," the manual offered standard protocols for providing counseling on family planning, gynecology, infertility, pregnancy testing, cervico-uterine cancer screening, and testing for RTIs and STIs, with an explicit emphasis on connections to gender issues, rights, and sexuality.[4]

Profamilia appointed a team of three staff members (two national program coordinators and the director of the Bogotá youth center) to develop the first draft of the manual. To ensure that the manual responded to counselors' needs and to give staff a sense of ownership in the manual, the team used the ideas solicited from counselors at the workshop and conducted five focus-group discussions with counselors. Staff input was complemented with information gathered through visits to sexual health programs in Peru and Chile.

The team distributed the draft manual to all counselors for review and then, in January–April 1996, ran five three-day training workshops in four cities for counselors from all Profamilia clinics so that they could be involved in refining the protocols (see Box 2 for a list of workshop exercises).

Participants found that discussion of sexual health counseling required reflecting on and questioning their own values about gender and sexuality. Their remarks affirmed that the process of developing the manual was extremely valuable:

> *The experience with the manual [workshops] was wonderful. We [the counselors] practically developed it. . . . Although we talk about the same things, there can be deficiencies in the way we counsel people. . . . It was very personal. When one arrives at an institution like this, one changes. The change begins with us as the "internal client."*

Box 2. Workshop exercises

- Review of concepts: sexual and reproductive health and gender
- Review of one's own experiences regarding sexuality
- Reading and discussion on pleasure and relationships
- Review of one's own reproductive health concerns
- Analysis of the relationship between personal experiences and work (a communications exercise)
- Review of basic elements of counseling
- Working group review of and suggestions for improving counseling protocols
- Practice in administering protocols
- Planning session on how to implement protocols in the workplace

---

And we have to change, because if we don't, then we can't change the external client either. In the workshops [however] there are still counselors who hold prejudices, and when the training ends, you don't see the changes immediately.

It was a very intensive week, very participatory, with group exercises that helped us a lot. They taught us to know ourselves better; this helps in personal life and also on the job.

Volume I of the two-volume manual includes 30 protocols organized according to key variables such as service requested, client age, prior use of family planning, whether or not pregnancy is desired, and whether or not the client is sexually active. The organization of the manual helps the counselor determine the issues that should be addressed with different types of clients. Because many topics are included in the 30 protocols, the protocols use standardized language to discuss the couple's relationship, self-care, and information on contraceptive methods. For example, all of the protocols (except the one for clients who are not sexually active) direct the counselor to address the couple's relationship and ask many of the same sorts of questions (see Box 3). The protocols having to do with a couple's relationship open up the topic of the quality of the sexual relationship. Value judgments are evident in this text, however, that might cause users with multiple partners to feel devalued and criticized by the counselor.

Almost all of the protocols include some interview questions that vary with the user's situation. Hence, the protocol for sexually active adolescents starts with questions about the coercive versus voluntary nature of sexual activity, while the protocol for adult clients seeking Pap smears begins with general questions about the couple's relationship. While the adult protocols neither explicitly prompt the counselor to probe for violent or coercive relationships nor include an invitation to involve the sexual partner in counseling, interviews with counselors suggest that in large clinics in 1998, they were doing both in practice with female clients.

Box 3. Counseling manual's standard section on couple relationships

(Excerpt from the module for a sexually active adult who is a first-time user of family planning.)

The counselor should assume that the client coming for information on contraception either plans to have sexual relations or is currently doing so.

If the client has a stable partner, find out whether the partner supports the decision to adopt a method, and in what way he or she is supporting the decision.

Ask about the level of communication with the sexual partner, the client's knowledge of the sexual life of the partner, the client's opinion of the importance of mutual fidelity, and how long the client has been in this relationship. This information is necessary for the following reasons:

• To determine risk behaviors: whether the client has sexual relations indiscriminately without using condoms or, if the client has only one partner, whether the client is confident of the partner's fidelity and has been for a long time.

• To be used as an opening to discuss condom use in addition to use of another contraceptive method, and to ascertain whether the partner would be in agreement. The counselor could suggest communication strategies to persuade the partner if he is reluctant to use a condom (see article in Volume II on safe sex).

• To emphasize the client's responsibility for caring for her or his own body and health as well as that of her or his sexual partner (see section on self-care).

Volume II of the manual gives complementary readings on key subjects, including sexuality, human sexual response, menopause, myths and prejudices about sexual relations, self-esteem, safe sex, STIs, quality of care in services, personalized counseling for women with unwanted pregnancies, and Pap smears. Written by Profamilia staff and other Latin American authors, the readings were compiled to provide relevant background information for staff on these topics and their relationship to sexuality.

Participants in the workshops were expected to return to their clinics and replicate the training with other staff involved in service provision. As can be expected, this strategy had mixed results. Some reported that high turnover among doctors made their involvement in training difficult; others, however, ran successful workshops with all levels of staff, including doctors.

PROGRESS

Sexual and reproductive health counseling has taken a huge leap forward at Profamilia. In a six-month post-training evaluation that began in late 1996, counselors reported many successes and changes in their clinics, including incorporation of the new topics into counseling, increased user satisfaction, increased use of services other than family planning, and remodeling of clinics to provide more privacy for counseling. In interviews conducted in 1998, counselors reported feeling comfortable asking a very general question, often related to whether or not a spouse was in agreement with the use of family planning or the quality of the couple's relationship, that left an opening for a conversation on relationships and sexuality.[5] Others described greater ease in discussing issues of sexuality: "When I talk about sexuality, I include myself. . . . Eight years ago it would not have been possible to talk about sexuality—now we plunge into these topics without worries or fears." Counselors also expressed confidence that they could refer users to the psychologist when faced with concerns they could not handle.

Staff psychologists have emerged as key figures in the incorporation of sexuality into Profamilia's work. As the counseling sessions began identifying a greater number of women with emotional concerns, the psychologists (who had originally been hired to work in the youth centers but had taken on some adult clients) expanded their duties. Clinic-based psychologists now regularly counsel women who are victims of domestic or sexual violence, as well as couples with infertility and sexual problems. They also serve as a mental health referral agent whenever an adult client demonstrates to a counselor or other clinician the need for more sophisticated psychological support and intervention than counselors can provide. For example, user concerns about orgasm or communication with sexual partners can usually be handled by the counselors, but a client suffering from physical abuse will be referred to a psychologist for more extensive counseling and assistance. Some psychologists also accompany those counselors who feel the need for extra support when they give community talks on sexuality.

Analysis of comments from client focus groups suggests that counseling has improved as a result of the ongoing internal examination and training.

> This time when I was in counseling, the young woman was very nice and told me that the information I had received [two years earlier] was not correct.

> I came two years ago, but now the counselors explain things much better, they are more concrete . . . and they spend more time explaining each method.

REMAINING CHALLENGES

Profamilia is justifiably proud of its progress in incorporating sexual health into its services. But change does not come without some institutional upheaval. A number of remaining challenges were identified during this case study of institutional change at Profamilia.

Persistent Ambivalence About Sexuality Counseling

The emphasis on expanded counseling generated some ambivalence at the managerial level regarding what a counselor can and should handle. Contrary to the picture painted by the counselors, one administrator felt that "women don't like us to talk about sexuality, and the gynecologists don't want to ask about it. It seems very intrusive."

However, in focus groups female users acknowledged that they lack information about self-care, STIs, and HIV/AIDS prevention, and stated that they are completely uninformed about sexual and reproductive rights, women's rights, and users' rights. Many indicated that they would be willing to stay in the counseling sessions for a longer period of time in order to gain this information. Believing that women want this information does not, however, solve the problem. As another administrator stated, "The users can become very distressed and talk so much that the counselors can't handle it" [in the time allotted for the session].

Counselors themselves worry that they lack the skills necessary to deal with situations that are difficult but not rare—for example, women experiencing sexual violence, unwanted pregnancy, and problems with gender identity and sexual response or dysfunction. As one youth center staff member commented, "Some of the situations covered in the manual are still difficult for me to deal with at times, such as rape, unwanted pregnancies, and lack of self-esteem." Executive staff recognize that for sexual and reproductive health to be definitively incorporated into counseling services, continuing staff training will always be needed owing to normal staff turnover and the lack of a psychologist in smaller clinics.

The incorporation of sexuality and gender issues into counseling at the men's clinic has also been uneven. The vasectomy service has a counselor/coordinator, and vasectomy counseling now addresses sexuality, particularly users' fears and myths about sexual pleasure and performance following the procedure. As one satisfied user reported after the counselor applied the new protocols, "I never imagined that vasectomy would raise so many issues. Now I am less worried." However, the vast majority of clients (87 percent in one study[6]) come to the men's clinic with other concerns (primarily related to urologic problems and screening for STIs), and it is unclear whether the male counselors are comfortable discussing sexual health outside the context of vasectomy counseling. None of the counselors interviewed in 1998 spontaneously referred to counseling clients who came for STI and HIV/AIDS screening, and they had little to say in response to direct questions. The clinics prominently advertised the availability of Viagra, although one counselor said that there had been little demand for it. Counselors reported that women tend to be the more talkative members of couples, and that the counselor often needed to encourage men to speak.

Gender Bias in Sexuality Counseling

The quality of counseling for male and female clients has improved, but gender bias remains. Women are asked about patterns of sexual coercion or violence on the part of their male partners, but they are not encouraged to delve into issues of their own sexual satisfaction and pleasure. Men are encouraged to discuss their concerns about pleasure and performance, but they are not asked questions that might reveal violence or sexually coercive patterns on their part. While these may be the concerns that users present, counselors may also be reinforcing gender stereotypes accepted by the culture (e.g., that a "real man" must always be ready for sex and that women should not be concerned with pleasure and satisfaction), thus shortchanging both male and female clients in important ways.

Approaching Sexual Partners Appropriately

Most counselors and clinic directors stated that a client is routinely asked to invite his or her sexual partner, and that they counsel more couples now than they did before. When working with a couple, counselors pay attention to the couple's interactions and to the rights of the person who is about to adopt a contraceptive method or undergo a medical procedure. Sometimes, however, involvement of partners can be taken too far; after the training there were a few reports of counselors who demanded rather than invited the presence of the partner, possibly pressuring the client to bring a partner when he or she did not want to. The best routine question might be, "Do you have a sexual partner you would like to invite to the next visit?" Most counselors interviewed already seemed to have incorporated this practice.

Time Constraints

Counselors also feel time pressures when sessions involve discussion of relationships and sexuality. While the average counseling session is 15–20 minutes long, sessions with clients who have a pressing problem can last up to an hour. Post-training evaluations from different sites in late 1996 found that the lack of time and personnel had become a critical issue in some clinics.

Staff responded in several ways. Counselors made it a point to inquire about a client's primary concerns at the beginning of the session so that they could focus on these points of interest and leave time at the end to broach new topics having to do with sexual and reproductive health. Difficult cases were often referred to the psychologist, and, in cases of sexual or physical violence, also to legal services. Clinic directors also began placing new information materials related to sexual and reproductive health in all waiting rooms.

In the last few years, the larger clinics have dealt with the lack of time by training all staff to deal with sexuality issues to some extent. Doing so serves multiple purposes: It provides extra capacity for dealing with clients, and it creates an environment that is more understanding of sexuality concerns and a staff that works better as a team. This strategy was facilitated by the organization's historical commitment to training staff at all levels in sexual and reproductive health. At the Cali clinic, for example, the cashiers design the monthly poster display, and an accountant had read the entire counseling manual. In all three cities there are training events that include all levels of personnel. One counselor in a male clinic commented:

> It is so important to train everybody, because when an interview turns into a lengthy one, the nurses or the receptionists have to give at least a minimal level of counseling, and they are trained to do so. Everyone here fills more than one function. The administrative staff also attends to the public. . . . Even the security guards know how to give basic information on the services we provide.

Training all staff also makes it possible for administrative staff to climb the career ladder and become counselors.

Lack of Privacy

Both executive staff and counselors highlighted lack of privacy in the physical infrastructure of some clinics as a major obstacle to offering counseling on sensitive topics such as sexuality. As noted earlier, several clinics nationwide have made remodeling the counseling space a high priority.

Evaluation

While Profamilia has conducted pilot evaluations of incorporating sexual health and gender issues into the services it provides, there is no evidence that these issues have been incorporated into the routine monitoring and evaluation of quality of care. This situation is not unique to Profamilia. It reflects one of the major challenges to providers of sexual and reproductive health services worldwide. The preoccupation with "indicators" in the donor and NGO communities in this field is indicative of the difficulty of evaluating progress on sexual health and gender issues through routinely gathered measures.

INCORPORATING SEXUAL HEALTH INTO SERVICES: A MATTER OF INSTITUTIONAL AND CULTURAL CHANGE

Profamilia's experience illustrates that transforming provider–client interaction is not a simple before-and-after story. Profamilia's executive director, María Isabel Plata, explains that incorporating sexual health into services in any institution is necessarily "both an institutional and a cultural process. It takes time." Precisely because the cultural barriers to the promotion of sexual health in most societies are numerous and deeply rooted, the process requires ongoing investment. Still, despite uneven achievements, Profamilia staff agree on the basic philosophy underlying counseling. As one staff member explained:

> *The most important aspect of learning to do individual counseling is to learn to listen to the person facing us before giving any information.*

In incorporating sexual health into its services, Profamilia had much to build on and many subsequent opportunities to reinforce the gains achieved through the early training and the development of the manual of counseling protocols. Before 1994 the organization had positioned itself to incorporate the principles of the Cairo conference through a historical commitment to quality of care and good management practices; development of superior evaluation systems; the presence of feminists in leadership positions; long-standing civic involvement in policy dialogues on sexual, reproductive, and women's rights; recognition of the importance of staff training; and a spirit of innovation.

In the four years following its initial counselor training, Profamilia adopted two main strategies to consolidate its progress, as follows:

- *Standardized incorporation of sexual health issues into education and services.* Examples include incorporating sexual health themes into its curriculum for sex education in the schools, and adding questions to the clinical record form used nationwide that relate to sexuality (pleasure and risks), violence (physical, psychological, and sexual), and negotiation between couples.

- *In-service training opportunities that focus on sexual health and gender.* Recent examples include conferences on sexuality for Bogotá clinic staff, research on adolescent sexuality supported by WHO, and an internal study group on masculinity. In 2001, Profamilia's Gender and Rights office coordinated an effort with the youth centers of the largest nine clinics to strengthen their approach to sexuality and sexual rights. The program, entitled "Constructing Bridges of Respect for Difference," involves center directors, staff, and peer educators in addressing homophobia and other prejudices.

CONCLUSION

How transferable is Profamilia's experience? Undoubtedly, several factors enhanced the sexual health initiative. Profamilia has a reputation for being well-managed and innovative, with an ability to adapt to changing circumstances, be forward-looking, and institutionalize principles of quality of care. The growing presence of women's rights advocates in leadership positions has greatly strengthened the organization's commitment to holistic approaches, gender equity, and sexual and reproductive rights. Finally, the progressive aspects of Colombia's health system reform enabled Profamilia to implement these commitments while achieving greater financial sustainability.

Although these internal and external factors served as important building blocks for the sexual health initiative, the challenges faced by Profamilia are still comparable to those faced by all other service organizations whose historical focus has been family planning.

The deep cultural roots of attitudes about sexuality demand that providers undergo a "shake-up" of their attitudes, to enable them to counsel users on sensitive sexual health issues without being judgmental or punitive. Most counseling and medical staff need to examine these issues in their own lives. The participatory education and training methods used by Profamilia stimulated both personal reflection and attitudinal change among the counselors and involved them in developing their own counseling guidelines. While such training is necessary, it is not sufficient. Profamilia uses many strategies to complement the counselor training and reference manual, including training medical and administrative staff, producing new client educational materials, developing new evaluation strategies, participating in national and municipal campaigns on AIDS, and taking out subscriptions to key journals to which staff have access. The key to having staff take institutional initiatives seriously is to promote guiding principles consistently over time through a range of synergistic strategies, rather than to rely on one-shot interventions with no follow-up.

In the process, Profamilia discovered that it must draw on skills and validation from a variety of in-house resources and community partners. The adolescent program fostered an openness to matters of sexuality that the staff had resisted earlier. This was a surprise, but an important lesson. Feminist health advocates provided information and experience that were valuable in framing the curriculum and getting a sense of women's needs. Legal services staff contributed their expertise by dealing with issues of rights and gender, such as violence against women. Psychologists, once involved, added professional credibility to the counseling sessions, made sensitive subjects discussable, and connected them to health in a formal way. There was a surprising openness among all staff, and even inexperienced staff contributed to the development of written materials and manuals. Indeed, sexuality is a subject that people at all levels need to explore more fully.

Acknowledgments

Special thanks to the staff at Profamilia for their generosity with their time, insights, and institutional information. María Isabel Plata, Patricia Ospina, Gabriel Ojeda, Germán Lopez, Ana Cristina Gonzalez, and Maria Cristina Calderón at headquarters gave me an institutional overview, while the directors and counselors at the clinics in Bogotá, Cali, Ciudad Kennedy, and Medellín provided valuable insight on how institutionwide initiatives translate into changes in services. The writing of this chapter was made possible by generous support from the Ford Foundation and the David Rockefeller Center for Latin American Studies at Harvard University.

Notes

1   This case study is based on data from a project supported by the Ford Foundation from 1994–96, and on data collected during two weeks in October 1998 during site visits to Profamilia clinics in Bogotá, Cali, Ciudad Kennedy (in the urban periphery of Bogotá), and Medellín. During these visits, I collected additional documents and interviewed key informants, including executive staff at headquarters, clinic directors, one or two counselors in male and female clinics, and psychologists from the youth centers. Given the limitations of the data and the sample, this case does not necessarily represent the situation of Profamilia services in other cities and in rural areas, nor can it approach the validity of a full evaluation.

2   Before 1995, when a new health insurance law took effect, Profamilia provided 70 percent of the country's family planning services. See Galvis 1995 for details.

3   IPPF/Western Hemisphere Region involved Profamilia and two other Latin American IPPF affiliates in a four-year effort to develop an evaluation manual that incorporates gender issues. The manual was published in English and Spanish (IPPF/WHR 2000).

4   Urology and antenatal services were not included in the protocols because of low client volume, and because most urology and antenatal clients use one of the other services included in the protocols.

5   The counselors were aware that they should have been incorporating sexual health topics into their counseling. Therefore, the interviews cannot serve as evidence of consistent behavior in counseling, but they demonstrate new internalized norms and experiences of implementing them.

6   From a 1997 quality-of-care study in the Bogotá men's clinic (Barker 1998).

References

Barker, Gary. 1998. "Cinco casos de estudio" [Five case studies], prepared for the Symposium on Participation in Sexual and Reproductive Health: New Paradigms, Oaxaca, Mexico, October. New York: IPPF/WHR and AVSC International.

Galvis, Silvia. 1995. *Se Hace Camino al Andar* [Making new paths]. Bogotá: Profamilia.

International Planned Parenthood Federation/Western Hemisphere Region (IPPF/WHR). 2000. *Manual to Evaluate Quality of Care from a Gender Perspective.* New York: IPPF/WHR.

Profamilia and AVSC International. 1996. *Profamilia y la Seguridad Social en Salud* [Profamilia and social security in the health system]. Bogotá: Profamilia.

Contact information

Bonnie Shepard
Senior Program Manager
François-Xavier Bagnoud Center
   for Health and Human Rights
Harvard School of Public Health
651 Huntington Avenue, 7th Floor
Boston, MA 02115 USA
telephone: 617-432-1008
fax: 617-432-4310
e-mail: Bonnie_Shepard@alumni.ksg.harvard.edu

María Isabel Plata
Executive Director
Susan Holland-Muter
Gender Advisory Officer
Profamilia
Calle 34 No. 14-52
Santafé de Bogotá D.C.
Colombia
telephone: 57-1-339-0900
fax: 57-1-338-3159
e-mail: genero@profamilia.org.co

8

Coming to Terms with Politics and Gender: The Evolution of an Adolescent Reproductive Health Program in Nigeria

Adenike O. Esiet and Corinne Whitaker

Nigeria, the most populous country in Africa, has a young population. Twenty percent of its estimated 123 million inhabitants are between the ages of 10 and 19, and another 30 percent are in the first decade of life. In addition to normal adolescent struggles with identity, the transition to adulthood for young Nigerians has been complicated by economic, political, and cultural turmoil. The health and education sectors have been deeply affected by years of neglect, material shortages, and corruption; job scarcity has forced hoards of young people into hawking merchandise along the crowded streets of the metropolis; and globalization, rapid urbanization, and a media-saturated environment have disrupted the traditional culture in which children become young adults.

Adolescents in Nigeria face serious reproductive health risks, many the result of cultural and parental pressures and the stark differentiation of the roles and prospects of adolescent girls and boys.[1] One set of health challenges is the result of early marriage for girls, which is often justified as a cultural imperative and undertaken at the behest of families concerned about finding suitable husbands for their daughters before they are deemed unacceptable for the marriage market (e.g., because they have conceived out of wedlock). Nigerian law specifies no minimum age of marriage, and age at marriage among females is among the lowest in the world. Further, once married, many girls have very little choice but to end their schooling and become pregnant.[2] This is particularly striking in the northeast part of the country, where girls tend to marry in mid-adolescence (median age at marriage among 25–29-year-olds was 14.9) and half become mothers by age 18.0; girls in the southwest typically delay marriage until later adolescence (median age at marriage among 25–29-year-olds was 20.5) and childbirth until after age 20 (Federal Office of Statistics [Nigeria] and IRD/Macro International 1992).

Sexual activity among unmarried adolescents is also rising and carries its own risks. According to one study of urban in-school youth, 72 percent of males and 82 percent of females have had sexual intercourse by the age of 20 (Makinwa-Adebusoye 1992). Unprotected sexual activity among unmarried girls results in a high demand for abortion, which is usually performed under unsafe conditions. A small study among adolescent females in Lagos showed that 24 percent of sexually active respondents had had at least one abortion, and less than half of these young women had had the proce- dure performed by a medical doctor (Odujinrin 1991).

Hence while all adolescents face significant sexual and reproductive health chal- lenges, the degree and nature of their risk vary substantially by gender. In particular, early pregnancy—both within and outside of marriage—is a serious risk faced exclu- sively by young females. Both unsafe abortion and early childbearing contribute to one of the highest maternal mortality ratios in the world.[3]

Girls are also at high risk of acquiring HIV. One of every 20 Nigerians is cur- rently HIV-positive. However, the rate among girls (4.4–5.9 percent) is higher than that among boys (1.7–3.4 percent) (UNAIDS 2000), which is indicative of girls' greater social and physiological vulnerability.

Both male and female adolescents have trouble gaining access to basic informa- tion about how to protect their health. In a study among adolescents in five schools in and around the city of Lagos, knowledge about HIV was uneven: 76 percent had heard of AIDS but over one-third believed that HIV infection could be spread through kissing. In two semiurban schools, one-fifth of students rejected the statement that HIV is transmitted through sexual intercourse (Oloko and Omoboye 1993). Of the 30 percent of girls 15–19 years old who attend school, 43 percent have heard of one modern contraceptive, compared to 37 percent of out-of-school girls (Population Council tabulations of 1990 Nigeria DHS data from Federal Office of Statistics [Ni- geria] and IRD/Macro International 1992).

There are strong links between girls' economic disadvantage and their reproduc- tive health. For example, it is a fairly common practice for single girls still in school to assist parents by selling goods after school to contribute toward financing their own schooling and their families' livelihoods. This activity renders them vulnerable to many pressures, and some must resort to exchanging sexual favors for cash—for example, older men buy the inexpensive food or household items the girls sell for a high price in exchange for sex. When the young girl returns home with a larger-than-expected "take," her economically distressed parents may praise her rather than question the source of the money. According to one study, this is common even among female university students, who enjoy relative economic advantage: Up to 18 percent are in relationships in which they exchange sex for favors or material rewards (Uwakwe, Mansaray, and Onwu 1994).

Traditionally, adolescents were guided through the transition to adulthood by mentoring from older community members, initiation rites, and cultural restrictions on sexual activity both inside and outside of marriage. For example, if an unmarried girl had sexual relations with a man—freely or against her will—her partner could be identified and sanctions could be imposed. Adults also shared information (albeit sometimes incorrect information) about sexuality and reproduction in "age-group associations," where girls and boys of a certain age experienced socialization rites together. Socioeconomic pressures, AIDS, and the influence of Western media have increased the need of adolescents for accurate sexual and reproductive health education; unfortunately, as Nigeria modernizes, the traditional vehicles for such education have weakened and providing such education for adolescents remains a contentious issue. Efforts to meet adolescents' needs are constantly attacked by influential individuals and groups (some religion-based, some fearful of the loss of "tradition and cultural distinction") who believe that such information will encourage adolescents to become sexually active.

Nigeria's policymakers have shaped the country's modern population agenda with attention to growth rates, but have not considered the close links between large families, early marriage, women's status (including their access to and control of resources), and poverty. Nor has there been much public discussion of adolescent sexuality and reproduction. The public schools' population education program provides only broad-based demographic information and guidelines on the government's "preferred family size." Even in anatomy lessons, teachers often fail to use the proper terminology for the vulva or penis, referring instead to "private parts." An exceptional new pamphlet on HIV produced for the public schools acknowledges that young people are sexually active but sends the message that "bad" adolescents have sex and get HIV. Most public-sector education campaigns are not specifically directed at adolescents, and health services designed especially for unmarried or recently married adolescents are almost nonexistent.

THE CREATION OF ACTION HEALTH

It was against this backdrop in 1989 that eight individuals—drawn from the fields of medicine, education, law, psychology, and journalism—created Action Health, Incorporated, a nongovernmental organization (NGO) dedicated to improving the health and upholding the rights of adolescents in Nigeria. We understood from the onset that the larger policy and cultural milieu would prove an obstacle to our work. With time we came to understand that gender issues are inseparable from other adolescent issues, and gender dynamics both within and beyond our own program would significantly hinder our efforts. This case study is the story of how Action Health has encountered and confronted these challenges.

Our fundamental premise was that adolescents themselves could best define their own needs and concerns. We initially decided to focus our efforts on secondary school students, who represent a small but rising proportion of Nigeria's total adolescent population. We reasoned that these students are potential leaders of their generation, and that changes in their attitudes and circumstances would have far-reaching effects in Nigerian society. From a practical standpoint, these adolescents are nominally under the control of the educational system, and it was our hope that this system would be the standard-bearer for a more progressive and supportive attitude toward this age group. Finally, secondary school students are much easier to find than their more numerous out-of-school counterparts.

We began by consulting secondary school students and some of the adults who were influential in their lives. The first activity carried out with the adolescents was a school-based workshop on teenage pregnancy and drug abuse, which was held in a section of Lagos close to Action Health's home office. The 150 students who participated were drawn from 33 coeducational, all-girls, and all-boys schools. Discussions began in mixed-sex groups and were followed by the submission of anonymous questions, which allowed us to deal with more sensitive (and salient) issues.

As students articulated their concerns, it became clear that some issues were more pertinent to boys and others more relevant to girls. For example, girls felt substantial pressure to have sex; as such, their questions often revolved around power in their relationships and how they could begin relationships with trustworthy men. They were also concerned about menstruation, its management, and how it related to their sexuality. They asked whether sex helps reduce menstrual cramps, whether a person could have sexual intercourse and still be considered a virgin, and whether boys "have to" have sex to be healthy. Boys were more concerned about attracting female attention, issues of sexual performance, and the functioning of the penis (e.g., whether masturbation "wastes their energy or sperm"). Both boys and girls struggled with how to keep their friends without compromising their own self-esteem or their parents' trust.

Relationships with parents were a central concern. Students actively struggled with getting their parents to listen to them and with how and when to ask parents difficult questions about sex, love, and their future. They felt that no one listened to or cared about their problems. Parents were described as leaving children to fend for themselves. Many of the students described being sent off to school with no food and no funds to get

---

Box 1. Students' communiqué on teen pregnancy

In their communiqué, the students identified a range of factors underlying teen pregnancy and drug use, along with recommended solutions. The following items are adapted from the section of the document that addressed pregnancy.

Problem	Solution
Personal	
Lack of maturity, self-discipline	Adopt principles of self-control and discipline
Peer group influence	Make good friends, positive peers
Familial	
Parents' inability to provide for children	Parents should care more for children, seek to meet their needs and have rapport
Parents' exposing their children to promiscuity through their own actions	
Unhappy and broken homes	
Parents' reluctance to discuss sexuality	Parents should discuss sexuality with children
Societal	
Availability of pornography	
Overly materialistic values	Reorient societal values, priorities, and morals
General level of poverty	Provide community youth centers, recreation facilities
Schools	
Low level of awareness	Establish peer counseling, sexuality education, symposia, and other public educational events; involve teachers' union and parent–teacher association
Sexual harassment by male teachers	Impose penalties for sexual harassment by teachers
Female students who take advantage of their femininity to secure favor from male teachers	
Male students exploiting female students	Control sexual harassment
Blues parties (dance parties where maximum body contact is encouraged)	Supervision and prohibition of these events by local authorities

---

food, and some felt that their parents didn't care if something bad happened to them. Again, gender differences emerged: Girls spoke of being blamed when they reported teachers who pressured them to have sex in exchange for a passing grade. The students asked for a "safe place" to talk with their peers and with other adults who would listen to them, stating, "Parents talk down at us," and "We'd like to know all there is to know from people as young as ourselves, because they'll tell us the truth."

The workshop participants produced a communiqué (see Box 1) that reflected many of these concerns and included a summary of their major health problems and a list of their needs. This communiqué was used to initiate discussion with other students through new clubs, existing structures, and informal student networks, and it provided a basis for additional input from other students (and eventually from parents and teachers).

We carried out a parallel set of activities with teachers, parents, parent–teacher associations, and school principals from the selected schools, along with local community leaders. Just as girls' and boys' differing perceptions and expectations were gender-related, so were those of the adults in their lives. The characteristics of a "good girl" were viewed as very different from those of a "good boy." Although the intensity varied, girls were often the focus of adult concerns. They questioned what a girl who was tardy or absent at school might be doing, whether girls and boys were distracted from learning by their emerging sexuality, whether young people were modestly enough dressed (many schools have dress codes), and the extent to which gangs of boys posed threats to girls' safety.

On the basis of these preliminary consultations, we decided to move forward with two initiatives: a school-based peer-education program and a youth center, both in central Lagos. Despite their pioneering nature, our initial aims for these projects were modest. We had little idea of the ways in which time and events would force us to redefine our approach.

THE SCHOOL-BASED PROGRAM:
PEER-LED HEALTH AND LIFE-PLANNING CLUBS

One teenager was selected from each of the original 33 public schools in the district to serve as peer educators. The peer educators—many of whom had participated in the original teenage pregnancy and drug abuse workshop—would provide information to fellow students. Action Health would provide training, ongoing support, and evaluation of this program.

The schools already had a functioning club system, so the peer educators decided to make use of this familiar structure for their work. They established health and life-planning clubs that would meet once a week to discuss and receive factual information on sexual health and development. In keeping with the requirements of the schools, however, information about preventing pregnancy had to be limited to abstinence. We brought the 33 peer educators together every three months for a peer-education forum, in which we provided them with material support, opportunities for discussion, awards, guidance on content, and assistance in formalizing the curriculum.

We simultaneously trained volunteer adult mentors—teachers and parents who would form connections with the young people and assist the clubs' efforts. Mentors were selected on the basis of students' assessments of which adults were already most responsive and sensitive to students' sexual health concerns. In addition to training the mentors, we also routinely participated in health club activities to be sure that the factual information provided was correct and to dispel prevailing myths about topics such as sexuality.

The clubs attracted wide attention at the schools. In many cases, between 80 and 200 adolescents in a school of several thousand students would participate. With a single peer educator responsible for the sexual and reproductive health enlightenment of two to three thousand students, we quickly saw the need for additional resources. With additional funding, the program began training two to six new peer educators in each school every year. We selected students who had at least one year of school left and were therefore old enough to be respected and knowledgeable but not yet at the point of graduation. As we expanded the number of peer educators, we faced more broadly the issue of selection. Initially, peer educators were chosen by school principals, presumably on the basis of academic performance and their appeal to adults. Later, as students participated in nominating peer educators, the criteria shifted toward an emphasis on an individual's flexibility, approachability, and popularity.

Having teenagers work with trained adult mentors proved an effective approach. While students felt comfortable discussing some issues among themselves, they began to seek out the adult mentors to air other problems. Some girls disclosed to the adult mentor that a teacher was pressuring them for sex; others reported incest. Teachers also offered support to girls who were being pressured to leave school. Together with Action Health staff, these teachers created small teams that, with the girls' consent, would visit those families seeking to remove their daughters from school to encourage them to reconsider.

Although the clubs were succeeding in their initial objectives, we began to sense the limits of our approach. First, we were learning that gender issues had a great deal of influence on club leadership, participation, and dynamics. The peer educators were more active in schools for girls than in those for boys. In coeducational schools, female peer educators had difficulty sustaining leadership positions; hence, these girls were the least active of all the peer educators in the program, despite the fact that there tended to be more girls than boys in the coeducational clubs.

Gender dynamics also influenced the way that students responded to the peer-led sessions. Girls tended to be willing to ask questions but were shy about acting in role-plays. Boys were less trusting of the peer educators, but they participated easily in inventing and enacting role-play scenarios. In the coeducational schools, the participants tended to be less trusting at first because they felt they might be judged as "sexually active" in front of members of the other sex; but once discussions got underway, girls participated as actively as boys.

As was true in the initial workshop, the content of students' concerns tended to be gender-specific. A common dilemma enacted by girls was how to remove themselves from a sexual situation without getting hurt or raped. As female peer educator Adeọla Olunloyo explains, "The girls themselves think girls are the weak ones, the

---

Box 2. Teaching girls how to reduce their risk of date or acquaintance rape

- Set sexual limits at the beginning of a relationship
- Go on group dates rather than going out alone with a boy
- On a date, avoid alcoholic drinks
- At a party or on a date, avoid any bottled drink that is not opened in your presence (to avoid being drugged)
- Before accepting gifts, be sure that there are no strings attached and no expectations of sexual favors; avoid accepting expensive gifts to avoid being accused of "leading him on"
- "There is no such thing as a free Coke!"

---

obedient ones." When given the role of resisting a sexual advance, many girls screamed and kicked in an attempt to get free. The peer educators emphasized the need for girls to develop and use negotiation skills, be assertive but diplomatic, and be smart as a way to be powerful. Noting that most rape in their community is perpetrated by acquaintances, they also taught girls how to reduce their risk of "date rape" (see Box 2).

Boys, on the other hand, tended to mock the abstinence message and wanted to enact scenarios in which it was already assumed that intercourse would take place. Since males are expected to want sex all the time, boys felt ridiculed if the scenario depicted a boy resisting sexual advances; since they are expected to be in control, they felt equally ridiculed in a role-play in which a girl resisted a boy's sexual advances in a way that bruised his ego.[4] According to Olunloyo, "Guys feel a girl is supposed to want sex." The boys therefore preferred to jump ahead to negotiating the use of condoms. Although condom use is technically a taboo subject, the boys wanted to role-play how to negotiate condom use without making the girl feel as though she was being accused of being a prostitute and without losing the upper hand in the relationship. They were also concerned about reduced physical sensitivity associated with condom use.

Gender issues were not the only challenge we faced. Another was related to external political realities. Young people were requesting information about contraception, safe sex practices, setting and negotiating sexual limits, power differentials in relationships, and sexual abuse. We had been clearly directed by the school authorities, however, to limit information regarding prevention of pregnancy and sexually transmitted infections (STIs) to abstinence. Topics such as contraception, treatment for STIs, and the fundamentals of sexuality were "out of bounds" for Nigerian schools. In fact, the very first sexuality education sessions intentionally concealed the sexuality component within a discussion of broader health issues, including malaria and diarrhea.

We recognized the need to provide more in-depth information on sexuality and reproductive health and on the social issues that bear on them than was possible in the schools. We also realized that there is probably no truly "gender-neutral" territory. The venue for addressing these issues in program design was the community-based youth center.

THE YOUTH CENTER: CREATING A SAFE SPACE FOR GIRLS AND BOYS

We hoped to create a safe space where any young person 10–21 years old could have a productive learning experience. Hence when we opened a youth center, we planned activities that would overcome some of the limits of the school-based program. First, we offered educational sessions on reproductive and sexual health, where young people could receive information that schools considered taboo. Second, we generally held these sessions between 2:00 and 5:00 in the afternoon, when both in-school and out-of-school young people could attend. Third, we organized gender-neutral social activities, such as board games and table tennis.

Our approach to the educational sessions evolved significantly. When we began, our approach to the presentation of material was very pedagogic, as is typical for Nigeria. In part, this style reflected our own lack of knowledge about how to effectively engage and equip youth. Over time, we began using more participatory and diverse educational approaches, including films, role-plays, games, and structured exercises such as quizzes and debates. We also organized a number of initiatives to involve young people in producing their own magazine and videos. The magazine, *Growing Up*, is published quarterly and is distributed to in-school clubs, libraries, school boards, Ministry of Education officials, and other agencies. Producing the magazine teaches adolescents marketable skills in word processing and desktop publishing, and the magazine itself addresses generic adolescent concerns (e.g., fostering better communication with parents), gender-specific issues (e.g., concerns boys have about growing up and girls' concerns about female genital cutting), and policy issues. The videos highlight the divergent experiences of boys and girls. For example, one adolescent produced a video entitled "Dimming Stars," which is the story of a girl who, after reluctantly agreeing to have sex with her longtime boyfriend, gets pregnant and is expelled from school, while the consequences to the boyfriend are negligible.

We also began formalizing our educational programs by posting a monthly schedule of topics and activities. This schedule includes a range of activities—for example, the showing of a film; a body awareness class; student-produced videos; Anonymous Questions Day; a personal empowerment skills workshop; and observation of a special day such as World AIDS Day or Women's Health Day. A library, printed materials, and one-on-one sessions with an educator—if needed—complemented the monthly schedule of activities.

As in the school-based program, we were achieving real successes but facing the inescapable and central reality of gender-based power differences. A prime example of this problem arose in addressing condom use. Girls, duly informed about contraceptives, would still explain, "I can't request for a condom to be used because my boyfriend will believe I am a loose girl." On the other hand, even boys who had never used condoms would often say that the condom is not effective and "robs you of pleasure." Another example of how gender dynamics manifested themselves was more painful for Action Health as an institution. We knew that some adult men in authority felt they could provoke and even exploit girls sexually. We came to the painful realization that this danger could exist even in our adolescent reproductive health program.[5]

From our experiences in the schools and the youth center, we learned important lessons about promoting health awareness among adolescents:

- The idea of reproductive health is inadequate unless one grapples with such issues as power in sexual relations, power between the sexes, and power between generations; we would have to challenge, in particular, the notion that men have a greater right to pleasure than do women and girls.
- Parental and adult values may themselves be antagonistic to the welfare of adolescents, especially adolescent girls.

As we learned these lessons, our program evolved in several important ways. Our educational curriculum—both in the school-based peer-education program and at the youth center—became more gender-sensitive. With girls, we began to include discussion of female-controlled or female-initiated contraceptive methods, and to emphasize strategies to encourage males to wear condoms. In discussions with boys, we sought to help them recognize their responsibility to themselves and their partners, including being more open to condom use. We also decided as an institution that, to maintain the sexual safety and acceptability of our centers for adolescent girls, we would employ only females as adult mentors. We decided that the only males we would train to join the staff were boys we identified through the peer-education clubs who seemed to internalize and demonstrate respectful attitudes toward females.

As we began addressing these gender issues, we were again confronted by harsh realities—this time external political opposition. Individuals and church groups were increasingly attacking Action Health for "sharing too much information with young people and for talking about family planning." An anonymous letter published in a national newspaper in late 1992 alleged that Action Health "corrupts" children by promoting family planning.

As a result, the Commissioner for Education banned the program from operating in any government school in Lagos State. Most parents then refused to allow their children to visit an officially discredited organization, and even the youth center was deserted. Action Health was in crisis.

THE TURNING POINT

Faced with the government shutdown, we had to reassess our program both politically and in terms of content. We followed our basic philosophy of consulting with young people. The peer educators urged us to push at the highest political level for a lifting of the ban. Parents and trustees helped us to organize meetings with influential government officials. For example, one trustee had worked in the Institute of Child Health at the Lagos University Teaching Hospital and had key contacts in the Ministry of Education. We distributed press information kits clarifying the organization's purposes and sponsorship and offered journalists the opportunity to visit the youth center, meet with the young people, and debunk the negative public perception. As frightening as the prospect of confronting the government seemed, we were determined to defend all we had achieved on behalf of young people in our country.

After three months of targeted efforts to educate local journalists, accurate and fair newspaper reports began to appear. In reaction to this turning tide, the government asked the principals of secondary schools in which we had worked to express their views of Action Health's activities. One principal after another reported that the school-based program was providing valuable information and skills that young people needed but that were not provided in the school curriculum. The government conceded that it had taken action without "looking at the merits of the case." A memorandum issued by the Lagos State Ministry of Education reinstated the school program, allowing us to resume our activities.

While this was a remarkable victory for Action Health, we were not content simply to re-establish the school-based program. Perhaps emboldened by our success in the policy arena, we decided to advocate for more meaningful adolescent sexuality education, which meant challenging the constraints on discussions of adolescent sexuality initially imposed by school administrators and communities. We wished to move beyond perfunctory public health messages on malaria and diarrhea prevention simply to give the sexuality information an acceptable "cover." One important limitation remained, however: Discussion of contraception in the classroom continued to be prohibited. We would still have to refer students in need of such information to the youth center, where we provided increasingly comprehensive information on STIs; contraception; the importance of seeking timely services for sexual abuse, incest, and menstrual irregularities; pregnancy options; and how to negotiate sexual encounters.

Of course, the more we allowed students to talk about their real health needs, the more we had to face the limits of education alone in meeting those needs. Many students were already having sexual experiences, pleasurable and consensual in some cases, unwanted and abusive in others. These young people complained that the abstinence message did not address their real needs. They wanted to know how to protect themselves more effectively, whether from pregnancy, disease, or exploitative relationships.

Our policy of offering information alone had been put to the test and had come up short. Adolescents facing sexual encounters needed negotiating skills, which we had begun to address at the youth center but not yet in school settings. Many also needed clinical services. For a time we offered referrals, but many young people did not trust the providers or lacked the courage or the funds to follow up. Further, the referral clinics did not provide the individualized education or skills-building that was needed to complement and reinforce our educational programs. Gradually, we explored a possibility that had never been part of our original vision and that would undoubtedly generate renewed public resistance: We opened a teen clinic of our own.

ESTABLISHMENT OF THE CLINIC

Action Health opened its own clinic in a small room within the youth center and offered a wide range of medical and reproductive health services and counseling. The budget ($5,000) was limited, so we hired one nurse-midwife and depended in part on time and supplies donated by board members. We also charged below-market rates and established a revolving fund for all drugs and pregnancy tests. Some clients still found it difficult to pay and were allowed to pay on very lenient credit terms. The income from the revolving fund helped to offset the impact of inflation on replenishing drug supplies. The clinic was open to any young person using the center and to participants in the school program.

Initially, most clients came for general health concerns such as skin infections or fevers. It took some time for them to trust the clinic personnel with more intimate reproductive health concerns. By treating general medical problems, we were able to attract young people and bring them back for follow-up visits that provided opportunities for discussing reproductive health issues.

To expand the reach of the clinic, we established health awareness outreach clinics in the communities surrounding the youth center. At first, we conducted only weight and blood pressure checks, along with an orientation about our reproductive health activities. The outreach clinics put clinic staff into the community and enabled them to reach many more young out-of-school girls, who tended to be married and often already had children.

Given the community's positive reception to the mobile clinics, we expanded this effort to the schools themselves, setting up rotating morning clinics in 12 schools. We provided all services on a drop-in basis; follow-up appointments were made at the center-based clinic when necessary. Staff provided a general health exam and counseling and education based on the client's sexual history. We provided pelvic exams and a range of diagnostic tests. While the schools allowed students access to the mobile clinics, they also continued to constrain the type of information we could provide. Ironically, we could test for and treat STIs, but, because we were on school premises, we could not teach students to use condoms for prevention. Pregnancy testing could be carried out, but counseling about abortion was prohibited. For this reason, we offered students the option of receiving their test results at the youth center, where we could provide more comprehensive counseling. The mobile clinics and accompanying outreach have had a significant effect on the youth center clinic's client volume. From an initial eight clients a month in 1993, over 1,300 young people came to the clinic in 2000, each visiting the clinic twice on average. These numbers continue to grow.

As noted earlier, young people's initial visits tended to be for general health concerns such as skin infections, malaria and fevers, and injuries. Today, 50 percent of young people come seeking information about and treatment for suspected reproductive tract infections; sexual abuse or violence; concerns about the effects of female genital cutting (which affects one-third of our clients); premature ejaculation; and a host of other reproductive and sexual health concerns. This suggests that some of the stigma surrounding sexual and reproductive health issues has been overcome, but meeting the expanded range of young clients' needs has also strained the counseling skills of our staff. In response, we organized specially designed training sessions for clinic staff. Clinicians now provide a broadened range of in-house diagnostic tests for reproductive tract infections, including gonorrhea, syphilis, bacterial vaginosis, trichomoniasis, candidiasis, nongonococcal urethritis, and urethritis in addition to diagnostic tests for pregnancy, genotyping for sickle cell disease or traits (to ensure proper genetic counseling before pregnancy), and malaria.

Only one-third of the clients at the clinic are young men. While this is a higher proportion than at many other clinics, we feel that reaching young males is crucial to improving all adolescents' sexual health outcomes. We are currently seeking feedback from young men regarding why they and their friends do not use the clinic. We are also exploring the possibility of holding a young men's clinic for two hours every week, using a male provider.

At this point, our program has faced and come through many challenges—most of them related either to the overwhelming centrality of gender-based power differences in adolescence or to external political sensitivities about adolescent (and particularly female) sexuality. In recent years, we have also struggled with the fact that we can reach only a tiny fraction of young people in a nation where the sheer magnitude of adolescent health needs dwarfs the combined efforts of all youth-focused NGOs. Furthermore, conservative church representatives—some of whom are clearly supported by U.S. groups—continue to target and lobby against adolescent sexual and reproductive health programs, including Action Health. Hence, we are seeking to maintain a balance between supporting the school-based peer-education program and the absolute necessity of influencing national policy on adolescent health. The final section of this case study reviews some aspects of the evolution of adolescent reproductive and sexual health policy in Nigeria.

A CHANGING NATIONAL SCENE

Our struggles were validated and our efforts reinforced by changes that followed the 1994 International Conference on Population and Development (ICPD). In 1995, Nigeria's National Adolescent Health Policy, which promoted human (adolescent) sexuality as a natural and positive part of life for both sexually active and non-sexually active youth, was adopted. This policy drew on the government's own research findings that adolescents, including secondary school students, were already sexually active, lacked information, and were taking unnecessary health risks (Federal Ministry of Health and Social Services 1994).

Since that time, national-level policy activities have become an even more important element of our work at Action Health. After ICPD, we met with long-standing allies from the NGO and government sectors to develop national guidelines for sexuality education for all age groups. These guidelines (see Box 3), prefaced by a statement from Olikoye Ransome-Kuti, a former, very popular and influential Minister of Health, helped solidify the alliances and offered a shared point of reference.

Our next goal was to develop a comprehensive national adolescent reproductive health agenda and engage those responsible for implementing the agenda. In 1998 we began educating and mobilizing a broader group of NGOs and associations, key government officials, donor agencies, groups of young people, and our colleagues in the

---

Box 3. Age-specific guidelines for sexuality education

The *Guidelines for Comprehensive Sexuality Education in Nigeria* are based on the following values: Sexuality is a natural and healthy part of living; every person is entitled to dignity and self-worth; individuals express their sexuality in varied ways; sexual relationships should never be coercive or exploitative; all sexual decisions have effects or consequences; and individuals and society benefit when children are able to discuss sexuality with their parents and/or other trusted adults.

The messages that sexuality education should cover are organized under six key topics: human development, relationships, personal skills, sexual behavior, sexual health, and society and culture. Each key concept is further delineated into subconcepts. For example, sexual behavior includes sexuality throughout life, masturbation, sexual expression with intimate partners, abstinence, human sexual response, fantasy, and sexual dysfunction. The content of messages appropriate for different developmental stages (i.e., childhood: ages 6–8; preadolescence: ages 9–12; adolescence: ages 13–17; and young adult: ages 18–24) are then outlined.

Sample messages from selected categories are outlined below:

Human development

Reproductive anatomy and physiology

- Each body part has a correct name and specific function.
- Girls and boys have body parts that, when touched, make them feel good.
- At puberty, boys begin to ejaculate and girls begin to menstruate.
- Both men and women can experience sexual pleasure throughout their lives.

Personal skills

Assertiveness

- Everyone, including children, has rights.
- Assertiveness is different from aggressiveness; aggressiveness interferes with the rights of others.
- In the past, females in our society were taught not to be assertive.
- Sometimes, people must choose between actions they believe are best and their friends' actions.
- People always have the right to refuse any person's request for any type of sexual behavior.
- Sexual partners need to communicate clearly about their needs and limits.

Sexual health

Sexual abuse

- Everyone, including children, has rights.
- It is never appropriate to force someone to engage in any kind of sexual behavior.
- People who are raped are never at fault for the rape.
- Sexual harassment (unsolicited sexual advances on a helpless or unwilling individual) can take place at school, work, home, and in the community.
- There are no social, religious, and health reasons for female genital cutting.

Note: These guidelines were developed with substantial input from the Sexuality Information and Education Council of the United States (SIECUS), which has developed flexible guidelines for sexuality education (SIECUS 1996). Source: National Guidelines Task Force 1996.

---

media. One year later, the first Nigerian National Conference on Adolescent Reproductive Health was convened by the Federal Ministry of Health and attended by representatives of the Ministries of Health, Education, and Youth and Sports, the Presidency, 100 NGOs, and over 100 young people. Action Health served as the secretariat for this historic meeting. During preparatory meetings and at the conference itself, there was some conservative political resistance to using the term "sexuality education" in the conference documents, but the language was ultimately retained. The conference and the communiqué signed by representatives of the government of Nigeria, the NGOs present, and our young adolescent guides was a dramatic affirmation of the goals to which Action Health had committed itself nine years before.

Action Health has continued to be involved in the follow-up to this conference. We recently succeeded in getting the National Council on Education to approve the integration of sexuality education into the national school curriculum. To operationalize this policy, we served on a national committee to develop a sexuality education curriculum for all Nigerian schools and explore how best to train those who will need to implement this curriculum. We developed a prototype curriculum to guide this process in collaboration with the Nigerian Educational Research and Development Council and the Federal Ministry of Education. The curriculum was formally approved by the National Council on Education in August 2001, and we have launched a process to ensure implementation at the Lagos State level, as well as to collaborate with NGOs working toward implementation in other states. Our work with girls was also highlighted in a documentary film produced by Jane Fonda and the International Women's Health Coalition for Women 2000: Gender Equality, Development and Peace for the Twenty-first Century, the five-year review of the United Nations conference in Beijing.[6]

There are other promising developments. Nigeria recently joined with almost every other country of the world in signing the U.N. Convention on the Rights of Children, which demarcates age 18 as the end of childhood. This act has facilitated much more discussion about the need to establish—and enforce—a reasonable age of legal marriage. For example, Alhaji Abubakar Alhaji, Saudana of Sokoto, a mullah in the conservative Muslim north of the country, recently indicated that he would strongly support legislation to outlaw marriage before age 18, noting that early marriage disrupts a girl's education, her job prospects, her career, and her chances for independence. Quoting the adage "If you educate a man, you educate an individual. But if you educate a woman, you educate the community, the society," he added, "So our people [in the north] have yet to realize that we cannot be educated as a community, as a society, until our women are educated" (Alhaji 2000).

This sentiment was subsequently echoed by President and Commander-in-Chief Olusegun Obasanjo, who stated that "the most important thing we can do for them is to give them education . . . it is only when girls are as educated as boys that they can be as useful in terms of development of the society." President Obasanjo further declared his support for comprehensive adolescent programs, including sexuality education, and expressed interest in learning from Action Health's experience, thereby opening the door for a new level of dialogue with the government (Obasanjo 2000).

Even as the country continues to undergo political transition, we work to sustain the political commitments made at the 1999 conference and seek adequate allocation of resources to see these commitments turned into reality. In doing so, we recall the words of one Action Health leader in describing the world in which many Nigerians grow up:

> *I experienced the deafening silence of parents who would not answer the harmless questions of an inquisitive child—simple questions about my body and my feelings— out of fear that simply talking about such issues would tempt me to "experiment."*

At the level of the individual girl or boy, the community, and the country, Action Health remains committed to overcoming such silence and to pursuing supportive, open, and meaningful dialogue. We continue to address the sexual and reproductive health issues of all adolescents, as well as to raise awareness about the fact that the term "adolescence" may mask the enormous discrepancies in power, opportunity, and risk that face girls as compared to boys. In sustaining our work, we will continue to rely on the wisdom and guidance of the young people who have come this far with us.

Acknowledgments

We thank peer educator Adeola Olunloyo for providing much of the detail on the experience of the health and life-planning clubs in different school settings. We are also grateful to the staff of the International Women's Health Coalition (IWHC) and the Population Council, and to Debbie Rogow for her research and editorial assistance. Action Health acknowledges the support of the Lagos State Ministry of Education and the principals of the schools in Somolu and Kosofe Local Education Districts in which Action Health currently operates. The programs described here receive funding from IWHC, the John D. and Catherine T. MacArthur Foundation, the Ford Foundation, and the David and Lucile Packard Foundation, among other organizations.

Notes

1   For a more complete discussion of adolescent reproductive health issues in Nigeria, see Irvin 2000, which describes gender-sensitive approaches to adolescent sexuality and provides a selected bibliography and program examples based on work supported by the International Women's Health Coalition.

2   Marriage generally signals an end to school attendance, so in-school adolescents may generally be considered nonmarried, particularly in the south. However, special vocational schools are being established for married girls in the north.

3   The maternal mortality ratio has been estimated at 800 to 1,000 deaths per 100,000 live births. The leading cause of these deaths is complications from unsafe abortion (Federal Ministry of Health and Social Services 1994).

4 Staff try to counter these deeply entrenched cultural norms, emphasizing the importance of treating girls as equals and respecting their right to say no. They also attempt to point out the exploitative nature of "sugar mommies" (adult women who offer boys food and drink in exchange for sexual attention), but boys generally say they are flattered by the attention.

5 Action Health's experience is not unique. Research into the acceptability of youth centers for girls has often found that they are ultimately dominated by men and are often places where girls experience sexual harassment rather than support for their reproductive and sexual rights and self-esteem (Erulkar and Mensch 1997; Glover, Erulkar, and Nerquaye-Tetteh 1998; Phiri and Erulkar 1997). It is disturbing that ensuring girls' rights and meeting their most pressing sexual health needs may depend on the presence of a trusted female for recourse.

6 "Generation 2000: Changing Girls' Realities" is a 15-minute documentary video featuring Action Health and two other Nigerian adolescent programs, produced by Fonda, Inc. and the International Women's Health Coalition. For more information, contact IWHC at communications@iwhc.org.

References

Alhaji, Abubakar, Saudana of Sokoto. 2000. Personal interview with Jane Fonda for the documentary "Generation 2000: Changing Girls' Realities," 9 May.

Erulkar, Annabel S. and Barbara S. Mensch. 1997. *Youth Centers in Kenya: Evaluation of the Family Planning Association of Kenya Programme*. Nairobi: Population Council.

Federal Ministry of Health and Social Services. 1994. *Nigeria Country Report for ICPD: Cairo 94*. Lagos: Federal Ministry of Health and Social Services.

Federal Office of Statistics (Nigeria) and IRD/Macro International. 1992. *Nigeria Demographic and Health Survey 1990*. Calverton, MD: Federal Office of Statistics (Nigeria) and IRD/Macro International, Inc.

Glover, Evam Kofi, Annabel S. Erulkar, and Joana Nerquaye-Tetteh. 1998. *Youth Centers in Ghana: Assessment of the Planned Parenthood Association of Ghana Programme*. Nairobi: Population Council.

Irvin, Andrea. 2000. *Taking Steps of Courage: Teaching Adolescents About Sexuality and Gender in Nigeria and Cameroun*. New York: International Women's Health Coalition.

Makinwa-Adebusoye, P. 1992. "Sexual behavior, reproductive knowledge and contraceptive use among young urban Nigerians," *International Family Planning Perspectives* 18(2): 66–70.

National Guidelines Task Force. 1996. *Guidelines for Comprehensive Sexuality Education in Nigeria*. Lagos: Action Health Incorporated and Sexuality Information and Education Council of the United States.

Obasanjo, Olusegun, President of Nigeria. 2000. Personal interview with Jane Fonda for the film "Generation 2000: Changing Girls' Realities," 9 May.

Odujinrin, O.M.T. 1991. "Sexual activity, contraceptive practice and abortion among adolescents in Lagos, Nigeria," *International Journal of Gynaecology and Obstetrics* 34(4): 361–366.

Oloko, Beatrice Adenike and A.O. Omoboye. 1993. "Sexual networking among some Lagos state adolescent Yoruba students," *Health Transition Review* 3(supplement): 151–157.

Phiri, Alford and Annabel S. Erulkar. 1997. *A Situation Analysis of the Zimbabwe National Family Planning Council's Youth Centers*. Nairobi: Population Council.

Sexuality Information and Education Council of the United States (SIECUS). 1996. *Guidelines for Comprehensive Sexuality Education* (2nd ed.). New York: SIECUS.

UNAIDS. 2000. *Report on the Global HIV/AIDS Epidemic*. Geneva: UNAIDS.

Uwakwe, Charles B.U., Abdul A. Mansaray, and Gilbert O.M. Onwu. 1994. "A psycho-educational program to motivate and foster AIDS preventive behavior among female Nigerian University students," final technical report of International Center for Research on Women, Women and AIDS Research Program (unpublished), cited in Ellen Weiss, Daniel Whelan, and Geeta Rao Gupta. 1996. *Vulnerability and Opportunity: AIDS and HIV/AIDS in the Developing World: Findings from the Women and AIDS Research Program.* Washington, DC: International Center for Research on Women.

Contact information

Adenike O. Esiet
Executive Director
Action Health Incorporated
P.O. Box 803
Yaba, Lagos
Nigeria
e-mail: ahi@linkserve.com.ng

Corinne Whitaker
Senior Program Officer for Africa
International Women's Health Coalition
24 East 21st Street, 5th Floor
New York, NY 10010 USA
e-mail: cwhitaker@iwhc.org

9

Talking About Sex in a Conservative Setting: An Experiment in Egypt

Nahla Abdel-Tawab, Laila Nawar, Hala Youssef, and Dale Huntington

Over the past decade, and increasingly since the 1994 International Conference on Population and Development, leaders in the reproductive health field have emphasized the interrelatedness of sexuality, contraceptive use, and reproductive health (Dixon-Mueller 1993; Zeidenstein and Moore 1996). Indeed, the very purpose of contraception is to allow women and men to have pleasurable sex lives without fear of unwanted pregnancy, and, in the case of condoms, sex without fear of infection. Sexual attitudes and the characteristics of sexual relationships are crucial elements in family planning method choice, influencing the client's satisfaction with the method and how effectively it will be used (Haffner and Stayton 1998). While sexuality issues are relevant to all family planning methods, the need to discuss them is greatest with methods that are coitus-dependent, such as barrier methods (Stewart 1998).

Despite studies showing that people are interested in discussing their sexual experiences, concerns, and needs, most family planning service providers avoid such topics when counseling clients, focusing instead on how the method should be used and its potential side effects. This is partly because many consider sexuality a personal matter that people are unwilling to discuss—and partly because they are not trained or supported in doing so (Moore and Helzner 1996). The difficulty of discussing sexuality may be exacerbated by cultural taboos.

While there is a need for greater attention to sexuality in family planning services worldwide, this may be particularly true in Egypt, the setting for this case study. In this conservative society, a woman's chastity is closely guarded and is considered a prime virtue. Moreover, the nearly universal practice of female circumcision—itself aimed at regulating female sexuality and thereby assuring a girl's marriageability (Helmy 1999)—may affect female sexual arousal and orgasm, potentially posing serious challenges to a couple's sexual relations.[1] At the same time, there is widespread reluctance to speak about issues of sexuality, in keeping with a general "culture of silence" about women's reproductive health issues (Khattab 1992). Indeed, a woman who discusses sexuality openly may be suspected of being too interested in sex.

Staff at the Population Council, along with Egyptian colleagues from research institutions, reproductive health nongovernmental organizations, and obstetrics/gynecology departments at university hospitals, felt that couples could benefit from greater incorporation of sexuality issues into family planning counseling. We believed that, with the assistance of a trained service provider, a woman could come to understand her own body, make more appropriate contraceptive choices, gain some measure of protection against disease, and develop strategies to improve communication with her husband; this last result could itself go a long way toward increasing sexual fulfillment and improving a woman's overall relationship with her husband. This chapter describes an effort to train Egyptian family planning service providers to address sexuality in counseling, and to learn about the feasibility, acceptability, and effects of such an initiative in a particularly conservative social setting.

CHOOSING OUR COLLABORATORS

We were eager to examine the feasibility of sexuality counseling in Egypt, but wanted to ensure that any experiment not be marginalized or considered impractical beyond the nongovernmental sector. We were also interested in putting in place partnerships and engaging the interest of key stakeholders so that, if successful, the project would have a chance of being replicated. The obvious, ideal partner was the Ministry of Health and Population (MOHP), which has the largest network of family planning clinics nationwide.

Senior MOHP staff showed an interest in the project mostly because integrating issues of sexuality into family planning services could potentially lead to improvement in the use of family planning methods (e.g., fewer discontinuations and/or less incorrect use of methods). MOHP senior staff were also interested in expanding the method mix, which was dominated by the intrauterine device (IUD) (63 percent of users) and the pill (22 percent of users) (El-Zanaty et al. 1996). Barrier methods were rarely used (less than 5 percent) (El-Zanaty et al. 1996).[2] We firmly believed that barrier methods were important methods of both contraception and disease prevention that should be available to Egyptian women. We hypothesized that greater use or effective availability was being hampered by providers' discomfort with discussing sexuality issues related to the use of these methods. We shared this rationale with the MOHP staff, and they agreed.

In 1999, the Population Council, in collaboration with the MOHP and the Clinical Services Improvement Project (CSI) and with funding from USAID, undertook an intervention to counsel family planning clients about sexuality and barrier methods in public-sector family planning clinics. We sought to find out whether family planning service providers would participate in and support training on gender and sexuality, whether family planning clients would participate in and support discussion of sexuality during family planning counseling, and whether training in sexuality would have an effect on providers' attitudes and counseling practices and on clients' attitudes toward and use of barrier methods.

The program involved providing training in gender and sexuality to physicians and nurses from three government family planning clinics, and offering them ongoing in-service technical support. Three other clinics, similar to those involved in the sexuality training in terms of number of providers per clinic, rural/urban location, socioeconomic characteristics of clientele, and provider gender, were selected to serve as controls. Providers in both experimental and control clinics received training in counseling and provision of barrier methods, including the male condom, female condom, and foaming tablets. All clinics were considered to be high-quality facilities, identified from among MOHP and CSI clinics in three governorates of Upper and Lower Egypt. We used a variety of data collection techniques, discussed in detail below, to measure the acceptability and effectiveness of the intervention from the perspective of family planning clients and providers.

WOMEN'S SEXUAL HEALTH CONCERNS

Our first step was to understand women's sexual health concerns and to learn whether there was, in fact, a perceived need for sexuality counseling in this setting and how such counseling could be offered to appropriately meet women's needs. Focus-group discussions with Egyptian women who had used family planning services revealed that they experience a wide variety of sexual problems, many of which are related to family planning methods. These include problems with IUD threads bothering the husband during intercourse, extended periods of bleeding that affect the frequency of sex, and reduced sensation associated with male condom use, especially for the husband. According to participants, these problems can lead to considerable tension between husbands and wives, often forcing the woman to switch contraceptive methods or to stop using contraception altogether.

In addition, many women reported sexual problems not related to contraception, including a loss or lack of sexual desire, particularly at the end of a long day when they are too tired to have sex. Women noted that husbands often get offended and angry with their wives when they are unwilling to have sex. As one 22-year-old woman from Menia City said: "I once told him [her husband] I was tired . . . it's not that I don't want him. He got angry and he hit me. 'What do you mean by tired?' he asked. He just couldn't understand."

Perhaps not surprisingly, the taboos surrounding discussion of sexuality often hamper the resolution of such problems and further constrict the few sources of adequate sexual health information to which women in Egypt have access. One 40-year-old woman from a rural village in Upper Egypt summed up her feelings on the matter in this way: "No one can talk about those things [sexual problems]. Maybe it will go away . . . it's just too personal . . . it's not right to talk about it." Furthermore, women are often reluctant to initiate discussions with health care providers because they are embarrassed or afraid to act inappropriately. One woman, a 30-year-old participant from Gharbeya in Lower Egypt, said, "I had a problem for four years but was too embarrassed to mention it to the doctor."

Confidentiality is another significant concern for many women, especially in rural areas; they worry that their problems will become known to their relatives and friends, or feel uncomfortable talking to a provider who might also be a relative or neighbor. As one 35-year-old family planning client from Gharbeya noted, "People don't know me here [in this clinic]. I can say whatever I want. But with a doctor in my village, it would be embarrassing. We see each other all the time."

Women clearly had sexual health concerns that they were willing to share with us in the focus-group setting, where considerable care had been taken to make the atmosphere open and accepting. They were uncomfortable raising these issues in other settings, where confidentiality and acceptance of their feelings were not assured. They did, however, indicate that they would welcome the opportunity to discuss these issues with health care providers, and that some encouragement or prompting from doctors could help to minimize their embarrassment. For example, a 35-year-old woman from Gharbeya said, "We wish family planning doctors would talk to us about those things. . . . If the doctor asks us those questions we would tell her about our problems, but otherwise I would be embarrassed to tell her."

We also spoke with providers about whether there is a need for sexuality counseling, whether and how it is currently offered, and the obstacles to its provision.[3] They told us that women report a variety of sexual problems during counseling, including lack of sexual desire, pain during intercourse, and inability to reach orgasm. However, providers are often unable to engage clients in discussion about these issues, partly because of inadequate medical school training in matters related to sexuality, and partly because of social restrictions around open discussion of such topics. It is noteworthy that very little of the medical or nursing school curriculum in Egypt focuses on sexuality, and there are few opportunities to acquire this knowledge on the job. In addition, many providers lack the communication skills needed to initiate discussions with clients or to respond appropriately if a client raises a sexual concern. While client counseling has received a great deal of attention in the Egyptian family planning program during the past ten years, and improvement has been considerable, counseling protocols do not cover matters of sexuality, including how a contraceptive method might influence relations between a woman and her husband.

HELPING PROVIDERS ADDRESS SEXUALITY

We hypothesized that training family planning service providers in sexuality and counseling skills might improve their ability to serve and win the trust of their clients. Because of the sensitive nature of the subject, we took extreme care in preparing the training course. We convened a group of local experts in the fields of reproductive health, counseling, gender issues, capacity building, and program management to design the content and format of the course. They developed a three-day training program using modified versions of International Planned Parenthood Federation manuals for sexuality training (Gordon and Gordon 1992). The program was conducted at the Regional Center for Training, the leading training institution for family planning service providers in Egypt.

Trainers were carefully selected to ensure the credibility of the project and maintain MOHP input and involvement. One trainer was well known and respected by the MOHP, another was affiliated directly with the MOHP, and the third was a respected obstetrician/gynecologist from Al-Azhar University.[4] We also involved the MOHP by inviting senior MOHP staff to the opening session and family planning directors from each of the study governorates to attend the full training. Doing this ensured that they heard and saw for themselves what was being discussed and that the project was deemed appropriate and relevant. Further, the participation of the governorate family planning directors in the training and the attendance of senior staff at the opening session sent a clear message to participating providers that both their superiors and the MOHP approved of the program.

While the training was designed primarily to improve providers' skills and their capacity to discuss sexuality, all participating providers (ten physicians and 15 nurses) received an update on contraceptive methods to ensure a minimum level of technical knowledge. This update took place over two days and emphasized barrier methods, including the male condom, the diaphragm, foaming tablets, and the cervical cap. In addition, the female condom was introduced to providers for the first time.[5]

Providers in the intervention clinics received an additional three-day training course on matters related to sexuality counseling. A total of 17 providers (14 females and three males) participated in this workshop. Trainees included eight physicians and nine nurses. We trained men, women, and providers of different types jointly, with the intention of fostering teamwork and greater openness on sensitive subjects.

The training covered the following topics:

Definitions of sexuality and sexuality issues as they relate to family planning methods, and clarification of values related to male and female sexuality. We sought to bring all participants to a common understanding of sexuality and explain why it is important in the context of family planning service delivery and contraceptive use. We emphasized the personal biases and judgments that people bring to the topic of sexuality and the need to understand and overcome these when working with clients. In one exercise, we gave the participants cards with incomplete sentences and asked them to complete the sentence as they saw appropriate. For example, "To me sexuality is————," "When I talk with clients about sexual matters I feel————," and "The thing that scares me most when I talk with clients about sexual matters is————." This was followed by a discussion of participants' responses and of the factors that influence attitudes about sexuality. The second part of the session included a brainstorming exercise on the effect of different family planning methods on sexual relations and how a service provider's knowledge of relations between a husband and wife can influence the choice of a family planning method. Some of the responses were: "Most men would not accept the male condom because it interferes with sexual pleasure" and "Learning about husband–wife relations is important, but how can a provider do this?"

The human sexual response and sexual problems commonly encountered by family planning service providers. The session on human sexual response was largely technical and didactic. The trainer explained different phases of human sexual response as well as factors affecting it. Participants became more involved in the latter part of the session, when we discussed actual sexual problems they had encountered in their work and offered possible solutions, with input from the facilitators. For instance, we discussed the effects of female circumcision on sexual response and strategies for helping circumcised women enjoy more pleasurable sexual relations with their husbands.

Gender issues as they relate to sexuality and family planning. Because the context of most women's sexual experiences is profoundly affected by gender power differentials, considerable time was devoted to helping providers understand gender issues. The training emphasized that sexual pleasure is as important to women as it is to men. One exercise included discussing basic characteristics of being a man and of being a woman. On a flip chart, the facilitators wrote each characteristic mentioned by participants and the group discussed why they believed this characteristic was specific to men or women. In another exercise, a series of statements was read to participants, and they were asked to agree or disagree with each. For example:

- A woman should not say no to her husband if he wants to have sex with her and she does not want to.
- Asking clients about their sexual history is an intrusion into their personal lives.
- Parents should speak with their children about sexual matters.

For each statement the trainer asked participants why they agreed or disagreed and then facilitated group discussion.

In a third exercise, participants were read a list of daily household activities and asked to indicate those the husband should do and those the wife should do. Examples included sewing, cooking, helping children with their studies, making decisions about children's education, and managing the budget. Again, facilitators helped participants examine their responses and question the roles assigned to men and women.

Husband–wife communication and negotiation skills, and strategies for enhancing spousal communication. To teach providers how to help clients overcome some of the barriers to talking about sex and using contraception, facilitators began the session with a discussion of the role of husbands in family planning and other decisions related to the health of their spouses. This was followed by a review of some of the negotiation strategies that providers could suggest that clients use with their husbands concerning family planning use and when and how sex is initiated. For example, providers recommended the "win–win" approach, that is, presenting a client's husband with the benefits he will gain from her family planning use or from his condom use. In that case they will both be "winners." Another strategy recommended was appealing to the husband's emotions, for example, expressing concern about how badly other contraceptive methods are affecting the wife's health and how grateful she would be if he helped by using a condom. The session also included two role-play exercises. In the first, participants were asked to play the role of a provider who is trying to convince a couple to use a condom because the woman has health problems that contraindicate her use of any other family planning method. The husband in this exercise is opposed to using a condom because he believes it will interfere with his sexual enjoyment. The provider uses various negotiation skills to convince the husband to use a condom and describes to the couple techniques they can use to decrease its negative impact on their sexual enjoyment. The second role-play involved a client who says that her husband is opposed to her use of family planning. The counselor discusses some of the strategies that the client can use to convince her husband, such as talking to him about the benefits that *he* will gain from her use of family planning, putting pressure on him through some other respected family member, or asking him to go to the clinic with her.

Technical and social issues related to the management of reproductive tract infections. In this more didactic session, the trainer presented refresher information on reproductive tract infections, including causes, prevention messages, diagnosis, and treatment. We also highlighted the role that different family planning methods play in protecting individuals from infection or exacerbating existing infections. Finally, we carried out brainstorming exercises to highlight some of the reasons a woman might not be able to protect herself from infection, might not seek care, or might not be able to ensure that her husband also takes a full course of treatment.

Incorporating sexuality issues into family planning counseling, including becoming comfortable with discussions of sexual issues, protocols for including sexuality issues, and taking a sexual history. With this session, we sought to help providers learn skills that would enable them to put their new knowledge about sexuality into practice. The first part of the session aimed to help participants get comfortable using sexual terms during family planning counseling. This was done through exercises that had participants frequently using both scientific and lay terms for male and female sexual organs. Participants labeled anatomical diagrams, made presentations, and described sexual acts such as vaginal sex, oral sex, and anal sex using lay terms. In the second half of the session participants were divided into two working groups. Each group was asked to develop a list of questions they believed should be included in history-taking during a family planning consultation. The two lists were then discussed by the full group of participants. This exercise was followed by a short lecture on basic steps in sexuality counseling.[6]

Participants were instructed on management of three problems: painful intercourse, premature ejaculation, and difficulty reaching orgasm. For difficulty reaching orgasm, participants were taught to give the following advice to female clients: (1) ask the woman to conduct a self-examination and encourage her to touch her body and discover the parts that give her pleasure; (2) encourage the woman to stimulate herself sexually; (3) when the woman feels comfortable doing these things she can teach her husband how to stimulate her in ways that she likes. For more complex cases—such as impotence with an organic cause or painful intercourse that does not respond to lubricants—participants were asked to refer the case to the nearest university or teaching hospital, where there is more likely to be an on-staff gynecologic specialist or, more rarely, a specialist in sexology.

The practice of female circumcision and women's sexual experience. Because female circumcision is almost universal in Egypt, we wanted providers to understand the effect circumcision has on sexuality and how they can help circumcised women who may have sexual concerns or problems. Consequently, we wove the topic into most of the sessions described above, either as an illustrative example or within exercises designed to increase providers' awareness of problems associated with the practice. We discussed its negative effects on sexual relations, as well as strategies circumcised women can use to improve sexual relations with their husbands. Participants were also given two pamphlets on the topic to take home as part of the course reading material.[7]

Finally, providers spent two hours at a family planning clinic, where they provided family planning counseling, including counseling on sexuality issues, to clients. Participants worked in teams, each having two providers (one offering the counseling, the other observing). Trainers rotated with the teams and took notes about their performance.[8] After this practical session, there was a period during which participants reported on their experience and trainers provided feedback.

Providers' Reactions to Training

At the beginning of the course, some providers, especially younger women, were visibly uncomfortable and reluctant to participate, clearly a response to the strong social norms against discussing issues of sexuality. One participant said that it was inappropriate for unmarried girls like herself to participate in such training. However, by the second or third session, participants became more relaxed—including the woman who said it was inappropriate for her to be there—and agreed that this type of training was greatly needed.

Overall, providers responded positively to the training. The majority (73 percent) indicated that most of the information they received was new to them, and many said they would like more information on the management of sexual problems (73 percent) and on human sexual response (33 percent). Trainers noted high levels of interaction with participants, although the session devoted to talking about sex clearly disturbed some providers. The mention of oral and anal sex was particularly repulsive to some. Discussions of female genital cutting revealed some ambivalence on the part of providers with regard to the practice. While most were convinced of its negative effects, some still believed that it should continue in the name of tradition. Two providers reported that they sometimes gave in to clients' requests to perform the operation on their daughters by cutting a very small piece of the clitoris. According to those providers, if they did not do so, the girls would otherwise be taken to a *daya* (traditional birth attendant) or another practitioner who would do her more harm.

The participants also made suggestions for improving the training course. More than 75 percent suggested that it should incorporate more hands-on, clinic-based training in handling clients' sexual problems. Twenty-two percent also suggested that the training be lengthened and that more problem-solving exercises be added. Trainers agreed with this assessment, especially with regard to the need for practical training.

Back in the Field: Ongoing In-service Support

In the six-week period following the training, we made several follow-up visits to the trained providers. During those visits, we inquired about sexuality-related problems they had discussed with their clients since the training period. We listened to how they had handled particular situations and gave them feedback and suggestions for improvement. For example, during one of the clinic visits we observed that a doctor did not explain to the client how the bleeding associated with the IUD might affect her sexual relations with her husband. In another clinic, the provider indicated that in spite of counseling, very few women chose the male condom because the majority thought that their husbands would refuse it. This provider was encouraged to suggest that these clients bring their husbands in, especially when clients could not use any other family planning method or if they were at risk of contracting sexually transmitted infections from their husbands.

TOOLS TO MEASURE CHANGE

We used several instruments to evaluate the effects of the training, including exit interviews with clients, a questionnaire administered to providers six weeks after training, visits of mystery clients to trained providers,[9] focus-group discussions, observations by project staff during provider training, and evaluation forms completed by providers after the training sessions (Abdel-Tawab et al. 2000). These instruments were used to assess the acceptability of sexuality counseling to clients, the acceptability of sexuality training to providers, providers' attitudes about offering sexuality counseling to clients, providers' counseling practices, and providers' and clients' acceptance of barrier methods.

Acceptability of sexuality counseling to clients. Clients were asked what sexuality-related problems they encounter and how they manage them, their views about presenting their problems to providers, and the characteristics of a service provider they feel is best suited to managing their problems. Clients' satisfaction with the service they received was also measured, including whether those who received sexuality counseling felt embarrassed by it. Finally, clients were asked what information the provider had given them and their level of satisfaction with the information provided, and to rate the provider on whether she or he encouraged the client to ask questions, listened to her, and treated her well.

Acceptability of sexuality training to providers. Providers were observed during the training to assess their reactions and were asked to evaluate the quality of each training session and the overall usefulness of the course. In addition, they were asked to make suggestions for future training courses. (Some of the results of this assessment were described above.)

Providers' attitudes about offering sexuality counseling to clients. Six weeks after training, we compared the responses of untrained and trained providers regarding their feelings about sexuality counseling. For example, providers in both categories were asked whether they agreed with such statements as, "I feel embarrassed to talk with clients about sexual issues," "Talking about sexual issues must be done only with those cases suffering from a clear problem," and "Most sexual problems require a specialist for their management."

Providers' counseling practices. Client exit interviews and mystery clients provided the opportunity to "get inside" the examination room, since other observations of provider–client interactions were not conducted. Comparisons were made between the provider–client exchanges of trained and untrained providers. Specifically, we examined whether any discussion took place on sexuality issues and barrier methods (including whether the provider discussed sexuality issues pertinent to using the method).

Mystery clients evaluated only the trained providers' counseling skills, especially their reactions and responses to questions about sexuality and barrier methods. They reported on the information provided regarding the problem or question presented, and evaluated the providers' objectivity and level of comfort in discussing sexuality issues.

Providers' and clients' acceptance of barrier methods. A wide range of statements was posed to providers to assess their attitudes toward the reliability, ease of use, acceptability, and other characteristics of barrier methods. For each type of barrier method, providers were asked whether they agreed with statements such as, "The [barrier method] is easy to use," "Talking about [barrier method] with the client is very embarrassing," "It is difficult to convince clients to use [barrier method]," and "Most husbands refuse [barrier method]." Clients were asked whether they agreed with a variety of statements about each type of barrier method, including "I'm afraid I would get pregnant while using [barrier method]," "[Barrier method] bothers the man during intercourse," "[Barrier method] interrupts intercourse," and so on. They were also asked whether they were leaving the clinic with a barrier method, whether they might use a barrier method in the future, and whether they approve of barrier methods but do not plan to use them.

THE EFFECTS OF THE SEXUALITY TRAINING

The intervention was a qualified success. Discussion of sexuality-related issues was acceptable to and desired by clients. Trained providers appeared to be more willing than untrained providers to raise sexuality issues with clients and to encourage clients to ask questions. Clients who saw trained providers were more likely to receive counseling on the possible effects their family planning method might have on sexual relations, and to be pleased with the amount of information provided. They were also more likely to receive a barrier method. Finally, women who were counseled by trained providers had more positive attitudes toward barrier methods than those who attended control clinics. These results are described in more detail below.

Effects on Providers' Attitudes and Counseling Practices

Trained providers were significantly more likely than untrained providers to discuss how a family planning method might affect a woman's sexual relations with her husband (41 percent of trained providers vs. 22 percent of untrained providers) and to discuss sexuality issues unrelated to a contraceptive method (44 percent vs. 18 percent). While less than half of trained providers discussed these sexuality issues with their clients, this improvement over the performance of untrained providers is substantial when considered in the context of a society characterized by rigid restrictions around discussing such issues.

Many trained providers responded appropriately to clients' concerns about their loss or lack of sexual desire. One client was told by a trained provider that she might not be experiencing sexual desire because of her circumcision. The nurse proceeded to tell the client about erogenous parts of the body other than the clitoris that her husband could touch during foreplay to arouse her. Another woman was told that her lack of desire might be due to insufficient foreplay and that she and her husband should consider engaging in more foreplay before intercourse. Yet another client was advised to switch from an injectable to the IUD because the injectable, like other hormonal methods, may dampen some women's interest in sex.

Interestingly, although trained providers appeared to change some of their sexuality counseling behaviors, the training had only a marginal effect on their attitudes toward sexuality counseling. While trained providers were significantly more likely than untrained providers to feel that sexuality issues should be raised with clients even if an obvious problem was not present (80 percent vs. 20 percent), they were as likely to feel embarrassed about such counseling as untrained providers and significantly *more* likely to feel that asking clients about their sexual history would be embarrassing to the client (60 percent vs. 10 percent). It is evident that three days of training cannot counter the powerful social norms surrounding this topic, even when the training is reinforced with several weeks of follow-up support. While providers' behaviors did change to a limited extent, their attitudes toward sexuality counseling remained entrenched. Nevertheless, all providers who received training felt that their style of counseling had changed as a result of the training, and, notwithstanding their concerns about their own or their clients' embarrassment, more than half (53 percent) said they were more likely to discuss sexual subjects with clients.

Unfortunately, even trained providers still appeared to lack key technical information. A number of clients were told that family planning methods have no effect on a woman's level of sexual desire and that sexual desire "comes from within." Some providers were insensitive to women's social context. One woman, who said that she was embarrassed to have sex with her husband because her in-laws lived in the same house, was still advised to "get herself in the mood" by dressing nicely. Another was told that her loss of desire was due to a vaginal infection, but the physician did not prescribe any medication to treat her condition or provide her with any additional information. And still another was advised to switch from injectables to the IUD, not because injectables could be causing her loss of desire, but because they could delay her return to fertility in case she decided to become pregnant; the provider assumed that she would soon make such a decision, based solely on the fact that she was in her early 20s and had two children. Finally, although some providers made the link between female circumcision and difficulty in reaching orgasm, and even advised women on how they might overcome this, none seized the opportunity to advise clients against circumcising their daughters.

Effects on Barrier Method Use

The training appeared to improve providers' attitudes toward barrier methods. Attitude scores for each barrier method were higher among trained than among untrained providers (this difference in attitude scores was statistically significant only for the female condom). Yet, these improvements in attitudes did not appear to translate into substantial changes in providers' counseling practices. Trained providers were somewhat more likely than untrained providers to mention the male condom (100 percent vs. 89 percent), but there was virtually no difference in their tendency to mention the female condom (85 percent vs. 87 percent). These differences were not statistically significant. On the other hand, trained providers were significantly more likely to mention foaming tablets to clients than were untrained providers (77 percent vs. 62 percent). In addition, untrained providers gave significantly more complete information on foaming tablets[10] and the female condom than did trained providers; providers did not differ in the amount of information they provided on the male condom. These similarities may be due to the fact that all providers received training in barrier methods, while only those in the intervention group received additional training that focused on sexuality. Perhaps providers in the intervention group were more focused on the sexuality counseling, which was the more significant new component of their counseling protocol, whereas providers in the control group focused on barrier methods, especially the female condom, which were the "new element" in theirs.

Clients who visited trained providers were significantly more likely to leave the clinic with a barrier method than those who saw untrained providers (9 percent vs. 2 percent). It should also be noted that only 33 percent of clients who received a barrier method chose the method themselves; in 3 percent of cases the client and provider selected the method jointly; and in 64 percent of cases the provider chose the method, often because other methods were contraindicated. Apparently, barrier methods were often prescribed as a transitional method—51 percent of users expected to use the method for one month or less or temporarily (until cured of a reproductive tract infection or until their next menses), indicating that providers and/or clients do not have confidence in barrier methods as a long-term method of contraception. Finally, among clients who said they would not consider using a barrier method in the future, those who were counseled by trained providers still had significantly better attitudes toward each of the three methods (male condom, female condom, and foaming tablets) than clients who attended control clinics.

Clients' Reactions to Sexuality Counseling

The vast majority of clients of both trained and untrained providers felt that the providers listened to them and treated them well. However, trained providers were significantly more likely to encourage their clients to ask questions than were untrained providers (95 percent vs. 84 percent). Clients who met with trained providers were also significantly more likely to say that they received all the information they were expecting. Most mystery clients were reportedly pleased with the competence with which the providers had dealt with their sexual concerns.[11] One mystery client said she experienced a burning sensation and dizziness after intercourse. The client said that the doctor provided her with all the information she needed about her condition, explaining that she had a vaginal infection, and prescribed treatment. The woman trusted the doctor's knowledge and was satisfied with the care she received.

Less than one-third of the clients (29 percent) felt embarrassed by sexuality discussions they had with providers. Interestingly, clients who saw trained providers were significantly more likely to have been embarrassed than those who met with untrained providers (33 percent vs. 15 percent), perhaps because the trained providers were more open or explicit during the discussion. Nonetheless, since clients who saw trained providers were more likely to have received the information they wanted, this may indicate that they were more satisfied with their exchange with the provider even if embarrassed by it. Moreover, once the silence surrounding these sensitive issues had been broken, many women appeared willing to discuss them more openly in the future. As one mystery client said, "This experience gave me the courage to ask about my sexual problems. If any question comes to my mind, I will go and ask my doctor."

Finally, clients were often satisfied with discussions of sexuality with providers even though the latter had supplied them with very little or even incorrect information. Thus, in any efforts to scale up and evaluate this intervention, it is important to use measures other than client satisfaction, such as direct or indirect observation of the family planning consultation, to assess providers' performance.

CONCLUSIONS

This project showed that sexuality-related questions and concerns are common among family planning clients in Egypt and that discussion of sexual issues is not only acceptable to but desired by clients. The experiment indicates that such interventions are feasible with public-sector family planning providers and that they can succeed in changing providers' attitudes regarding sexuality and its links to contraception. Effects went beyond attitudinal change: The sexuality training was successful in changing some of the providers' counseling behaviors. Trained providers were more likely to discuss sexuality issues with their clients and to have more positive attitudes regarding barrier methods. The project also suggests a small, positive association between training providers in sexuality counseling and clients' use of barrier methods.

The training, perhaps not surprisingly given its three-day duration, was less effective than had been hoped in improving providers' technical skills and countering some of the powerful social norms surrounding this topic. It did not seem to equip the providers with enough information to handle many problems appropriately, especially women's concerns about loss of sexual desire. Trained providers themselves recommended that the training be longer; in addition, they said that they would like more emphasis on role-plays, case studies, and other practical experience, as well as more post-training technical assistance to help them respond to clients' "real-life" concerns and questions. In addition to more intensive, participatory training and ongoing follow-up, providers need to know that their supervisors support this type of work. They also need to be fully convinced that their clients need sexuality counseling and will not object if the provider initiates a discussion of sexual matters, as long as it is done in a sensitive manner.

The results of the study were well received by the Ministry of Health and Population and the Clinical Services Improvement Project. The Regional Center for Training has already included the sexuality module in its core family planning training curriculum. The MOHP is currently revising its training curricula and counseling protocols to include a component on sexuality counseling. A committee consisting of representatives from senior levels of the MOHP and the Population Council, as well as other experts in the field, will be convened to develop culturally sensitive counseling protocols that take into account issues of sexuality, gender, and communication between spouses[12] as well as some of the constraints facing family planning service providers in Egypt.

Some MOHP senior staff have expressed concerns about the effects that integration of sexuality issues could have on family planning services themselves. They worry that staff may become overburdened, that sexuality matters may detract from contraceptive service provision, and that clients will not accept being asked routine questions about sexual relations. The results of this study have helped to allay some of these concerns, but it will be important to consider and address the unease of skeptics as this work is replicated on a larger scale.

Despite the limitations of devoting only three days of training (supplemented by follow-up in-service support) to such a complex and sensitive topic as sexuality, the intervention demonstrated that sexuality training and counseling is feasible and acceptable even in a conservative setting. It also succeeded in positioning the topic and pilot program in a manner that laid the groundwork for its broad expansion throughout the government health system.

Acknowledgments

The authors acknowledge the substantial contribution of Susan Lee in the preparation of early drafts of this chapter. The study was conducted as an in-house activity by the staff of the Frontiers in Reproductive Health Program in Cairo with funds from USAID/Washington. We also thank the Ministry of Health and Population, the Clinical Services Improvement Project, the USAID Population Office, and the Regional Center for Training. Finally, we thank the trainers and staff of the study clinics, as well as the clients who participated in the project.

Notes

1 According to the 1995 Demographic and Health Survey, 97 percent of married Egyptian women ages 15–49 are circumcised (El-Zanaty et al. 1996). In Egypt, this procedure typically involves removal of the clitoris and sometimes part or all of the labia minora. While these parts of the female genitalia play an important role in sexual arousal and orgasm, most, if not all, circumcised women can have satisfactory sexual and emotional relationships regardless of the degree of their circumcision (Toubia 1999).

2 Male condoms (used by about 3 percent of currently married women using a contraceptive method) are more widely available than other barrier methods, but they are often associated with extramarital affairs rather than with the prevention of pregnancy within marriage. Other methods, like foaming tablets and cervical caps, are rarely available and only rarely used—less than 1 percent of contraceptive users use the diaphragm, foam, or jelly (El-Zanaty et al. 1996). The female condom was not available in Egypt before this project.

3   We spoke with providers about these topics during the training course described later in the chapter.

4   Al-Azhar University is a prestigious Islamic university in Egypt, with departments of Islamic studies and secular studies such as medicine, agriculture, and engineering.

5   Unfortunately, because supplies of the female condom were limited, clinics were not able to offer it to clients during the intervention. Instead, samples given to each clinic were shown to clients, who were told that the method would be available soon. It became available after the study was completed.

6   The project used a simple sexuality counseling model known as PLISSIT, which stands for Permission (i.e., help the client realize that his or her feelings are acceptable to the counselor) Limited Information (i.e., give the client relevant information that he or she can understand) Specific Suggestions (i.e., suggestions that help the client overcome the problem) Intensive Therapy (i.e., for more complex cases) (Gordon and Gordon 1992).

7   The pamphlets, "Medical facts about FGM" and "FGM from the point of view of Islam," were produced by the Egyptian Society for the Prevention of Harmful Traditional Practices Against Woman and Child.

8   The trainer obtained client consent in the following way: "These are providers from another clinic and they are here for a training course on family planning counseling. They have learned a new counseling technique. If you agree to be seen by them, one of them will counsel you while the other observes. I will be present during the consultation, in case any information needs to be added or you want to ask me a question. If you do not want to be seen by these visitors please feel free to say so. You will still receive services from one of this clinic's staff members."

9   Rather than conducting our own direct observation of service providers, we recruited "mystery clients" to undertake this task. These clients were selected from among family planning clients who, during focus-group discussions, had expressed a sexuality-related problem or concern. They were recruited only from control clinics, and participated only if they had never been to an intervention clinic. We helped each client phrase her questions for the provider but did not accompany her to the clinic. Mystery clients were asked not to mention any affiliation with the study and to observe and report back on everything the provider did or said. We interviewed these clients immediately after their consultations, either at a nearby coffee shop or at another clinic.

10   This contradicted the finding that untrained providers were less likely to mention foaming tablets to clients than trained providers; however, it may be that untrained providers were less likely to mention this method to clients but provided more complete information when they did mention it.

11   Because mystery clients visited only trained providers, qualitative evaluation of counseling by untrained providers is not available.

12   Because of the sensitivity of matters related to sexuality and social restrictions on sexual relations outside marriage, this type of counseling will be restricted to married couples.

References

Abdel-Tawab, Nahla, Laila Nawar, Hala Youssef, and Dale Huntington. 2000. "Integrating issues of sexuality into Egyptian family planning counseling," final report. Cairo: Population Council, Frontiers in Reproductive Health Project.

Dixon-Mueller, Ruth. 1993. "The sexuality connection in reproductive health," *Studies in Family Planning* 24(5): 269–282.

El-Zanaty, Fatma, Enas M. Hussein, Gihan A. Shawky, Ann A. Way, and Sunita Kishor. 1996. *Egypt Demographic and Health Survey 1995*. Calverton, MD: National Population Council (Egypt) and Macro International, Inc.

Gordon, Gill and Peter Gordon. 1992. *Counseling and Sexuality: A Training Resource*. London: International Planned Parenthood Federation.

Haffner, Debra W. and William R. Stayton. 1998. "Sexuality and reproductive health," in Robert A. Hatcher, James Trussell, Felicia Stewart, Willard Cates, Jr., Gary K. Stewart, Felicia Guest, and Deborah Kowal (eds.), *Contraceptive Technology*, 17th ed. New York: Ardent Media, pp. 13–41.

Helmy, Magdy. 1999. "Female genital mutilation in Egypt," report submitted to UNICEF. Cairo: UNICEF.

Khattab, Hind. 1992. *The Silent Endurance: Social Conditions of Women's Reproductive Health in Rural Egypt*. Cairo: UNICEF

Moore, Kirsten and Judith F. Helzner. 1996. *What's Sex Got to Do With It? Challenges for Incorporating Sexuality into Family Planning Programs*. New York: Population Council and International Planned Parenthood Federation/Western Hemisphere Region.

Stewart, Felicia. 1998. "Vaginal barriers," in Robert A. Hatcher, James Trussell, Felicia Stewart, Willard Cates, Jr., Gary K. Stewart, Felicia Guest, and Deborah Kowal (eds.), *Contraceptive Technology*, 17th ed. New York: Ardent Media, pp. 371–404.

Toubia, Nahid. 1999. *Caring for Women with Circumcision: A Technical Manual for Health Care Providers*. New York: Rainbo.

Zeidenstein, Sondra and Kirsten Moore (eds.). 1996. *Learning About Sexuality: A Practical Beginning*. New York: Population Council.

Contact information

Nahla Abdel-Tawab
Consultant
5 Sabry Abou Alam Street
Apartment 10
Bab El-Louk
Cairo, Egypt
e-mail: nabdeltawab@yahoo.com

Laila Nawar
Regional Advisor
Frontiers in Reproductive Health
Population Council
6A Giza Street
P.O. Box 115
Dokki 12211
Cairo, Egypt
e-mail: lnawar@pccairo.org

10

Recovery from Abortion and Miscarriage in Egypt: Does Counseling Husbands Help?

Nahla Abdel-Tawab, Dale Huntington, Ezzeldin Osman,
Hala Youssef, and Laila Nawar

Public hospitals in Egypt admit a steady stream of women suffering from the consequences of both spontaneous and unsafely induced abortion. While country-level statistics on the incidence of abortion are lacking, a nationally representative study demonstrated that one out of every five admissions to obstetrics/gynecology wards is a postabortion patient, including women who have had induced abortions or spontaneous miscarriages (Huntington et al. 1998). (The term postabortion will be used in this chapter to refer to the time following induced or spontaneous abortions.)

Egyptian abortion laws are restrictive compared to those of other countries. The Egyptian Penal Law of 1937, still in effect, explicitly prohibits acts that cause abortion and imposes stiff penalties on medical professionals who induce abortion (Azer 1979). Other articles of the law, however, permit women to obtain necessary medical services for life-threatening conditions. These articles are generally interpreted to permit abortion in the presence of serious maternal health risks.

The legal dimensions of induced abortion in Egypt are strongly moderated by religious considerations. Approaches to Islamic jurisprudence vary widely, and positions on abortion are divergent, ranging from complete prohibition by one school of the Sunni tradition to complete permissibility by a Shi'i school (Brown 1997). Islamic theologians in Egypt generally hold that the termination of a pregnancy is acceptable in order to save a woman's life. Nonetheless, regardless of whether a pregnancy aborts spontaneously or is terminated to protect the pregnant woman's health, abortion is an extremely delicate and sensitive topic in Egypt.

Added to the sensitive nature of abortion in Egypt are issues surrounding the status of women. Many marital relationships are based firmly in patriarchal tradition, although the degree to which this is true varies across the country. Men are expected to be primary breadwinners while women are expected to take primary responsibility for domestic matters. Decisionmaking is considered a male prerogative by the majority of men and women in Egypt—indeed women rarely have the final say in any decisions except those related to domestic activities (El-Zanaty et al. 1996). About 49 percent of women have no influence on household budget decisions (El-Zanaty et al. 1996). Social norms also enforce a strict segregation of gender roles; men are discouraged from performing household chores, while women are discouraged from working outside the home. Women have more say than men in reproductive health matters (Nawar, Lloyd, and Ibrahim 1995). About two-thirds (65 percent) make decisions on contraceptive use in consultation with their husbands, and another 13 percent have the final say (El-Zanaty et al. 1996).

Not surprisingly, women's roles as wives and mothers are highly valued in Egyptian society. Although more roles are available to women in Egypt today than in the past, the majority of men and women still consider the roles of wife and mother to be the embodiment of ideal womanhood. Consequently, a woman's capacity to conceive and bear children is a critical component of her identity and, by extension, of her status with her husband, within his family, and within society at large. An abortion, regardless of whether it is spontaneous or induced, is often perceived as a woman's failure and raises doubts about her ability to fulfill her ascribed role.

Given the centrality of childbearing to a woman's status, it is perhaps not surprising that an abortion can cause a woman significant stress that could hamper her recovery. The project described in this chapter attempted to address some of the difficulties faced by Egyptian postabortion patients during their recovery by providing their husbands with appropriate counseling. The premise was that husbands who had received information about their wives' needs during recovery would provide more support to their wives and thus enhance their recovery. It was also believed that spousal counseling would help those women who did not want to become pregnant following recovery to use contraception.

THE PROJECT SETTING

Menia Governorate, where the project described in this chapter was implemented, is a predominantly rural province of southern Egypt. The overall level of education is low. Boys are frequently pulled out of school to help with family agricultural activities. Girls' education is not a priority for many families; one-third of 10-year-old girls have never attended school (compared to 13 percent nationally) (El Tawila et al. 1999). Poverty is common in this part of the country, and families, often in extended households, are typically involved in agriculture. The majority of couples live with the husband's parents and siblings. In such households, the mother-in-law is an authority figure and assigns household chores and responsibilities to her daughters-in-law.

Traditional values hold sway: Marriage and childbearing are expected to begin early for women, who are restricted in their movement outside the home. Only 58 percent of women in this setting are permitted to go alone to their local health center/doctor (El-Zanaty et al. 1996). Usually, a woman is escorted to routine medical visits by her mother, mother-in-law, or husband; in emergencies, or when a woman needs to be admitted to a hospital, she is generally accompanied by her husband.

The project was conducted in six hospitals (five public hospitals and one university hospital). Women receiving postabortion care in these hospitals are typically not employed outside the home (95 percent) and only 19 percent have completed primary school or a higher level of education. Although husbands are likely to have more education than their wives, the majority (63 percent) have little or no schooling. Most of the women come from rural areas (79 percent) and low-income households, and almost half of their husbands (40 percent) are farmers (Egyptian Fertility Care Society 1995).

WOMEN'S EXPERIENCE OF THE POSTABORTION PERIOD

The majority of postabortion patients in Egypt (86 percent) present to the hospital with mild to moderate bleeding. The remainder (14 percent) present with severe hemorrhaging. About 1 percent show signs of trauma, such as vaginal or cervical tears, and 5 percent have one or more signs of infection (Huntington et al. 1998). On average, because of the low incidence of serious complications, women remain in the hospital for about half a day.

Women who experience a miscarriage or abortion in Egypt may receive inadequate care after they are discharged from the hospital. The physical demands placed on an Egyptian woman during a typical day are considerable. Women recovering from an abortion are not always able to obtain the rest that they need; most resume their domestic responsibilities prematurely. While early resumption of household activities is not normally contraindicated for women recovering from abortion,[1] many women in this setting already have compromised health—because of preexisting conditions such as anemia and malnutrition—which makes their recovery more difficult.

As a postabortion patient in an earlier study stated, "To get back to her normal condition, a woman needs a proper diet and a place to relax and rest. But how can I get that? Where I come from [a rural area], women have to work hard, and we also have to provide all that we can for our children" (Huntington, Nawar, and Hady 1995).

While women in extended family settings can sometimes rely on other adult women to take up at least part of their workload during their recovery, women in nuclear family households—42 percent of households in Egypt and 34 percent in southern Egypt (El-Zanaty et al. 1996)—often do not have such assistance. As one woman commented: "I know that the most important thing is resting . . . so that I can get back my original health. The only problem in doing this is that there is no one to help me during that time."

In addition, women's husbands and families may simply not understand postabortion patients' physical or emotional needs. Women themselves do not receive much information on their condition. With hospital environments typically hostile to the presence of husbands, and providers not in the habit of giving information to the presenting client, much less those accompanying her, husbands' lack of understanding of their wives' condition is to be expected. Moreover, research has shown that because an abortion does not result in the delivery of a baby, a woman who has an abortion rarely receives the same attention and care that she would following a live birth, when she is served protein-rich meals, pampered by her husband and in-laws, and excused from housework for up to 40 days. Because they did not deliver a living baby, many women feel that they cannot ask their families for necessary support during their recovery period (Huntington 1997).

Psychological stress poses another threat to a woman's ability to recover from a miscarriage. Because so much of an Egyptian woman's sense of her "proper" role is connected with bearing and raising children, the possibility that she might be unable to fulfill this role can cause her considerable anxiety. Many women worry that a miscarriage signals a serious health problem and are afraid they might miscarry again. One woman said: "Losing a pregnancy affects a woman's future ability to have a child. If the body did not accept a child once, it will never accept it again."

One of the most stressful issues for women following a spontaneous abortion appears to be their inability to perceive a "logical" reason for the miscarriage. As one woman stated: "I just want to know how. This is my only problem. Some people say that I will keep aborting every time I get pregnant and I do not want that to happen to me." Another commented: "I really need to know what happened so that I can avoid it in the future."

Women who have induced an abortion are less likely than women who have experienced spontaneous abortion to dwell on issues around the "ensoulment of the fetus." They tend to view their loss as the loss of a potential child, rather than a living baby, and to be concerned first and foremost with recovering fully for the sake of the children they already have. One woman remarked: "I know that inducing an abortion is sinful. But I had to sacrifice myself for the sake of my children and my husband. What else could I have done?"

Regardless of whether a woman experiences a spontaneous or an induced abortion, many postabortion patients also have to contend with questions, judgments, and doubts from their husbands and in-laws regarding their ability to conceive again or to carry a pregnancy to term. They also worry that their family members will dwell on issues concerning the "ensoulment of the fetus." The following comments from women in our study are typical:

The first time [I lost a pregnancy], they [the in-laws] told me it would have been much better if the buffalo had died [than to] have the abortion. Now they will annoy me all the more, and I have to be ready for this.

I will still have to face some other problems, like what people will say about me when they know I have lost the pregnancy.

Many women go through a lot of psychological pain, especially if the husband is not appreciative of the situation and does not act like he understands what the woman has gone through. . . . Many husbands think that the woman has induced the abortion.

Some women are concerned that other family members will find out they have lost a pregnancy, and those who induce abortion often claim that it was spontaneous. Given this concern, women's low status, and restrictive abortion laws, any intervention or research surrounding postabortion care in this context must pay strict attention to ensuring women's safety and privacy.

RESPONSE OF THE EGYPTIAN HEALTH CARE SYSTEM TO PREGNANCY LOSS

Medical care in Egypt tends to focus almost exclusively on the physiological aspects of health while ignoring its psychosocial dimensions. Little value is placed on interpersonal interactions, and medical staff rarely receive training in counseling techniques either in medical school or during in-service training. While family planning client counseling has received considerable attention in recent years, this emphasis has not been extended to women receiving other types of reproductive health services. Physicians have heavy workloads and little time and motivation to interact with their patients. Although nurses have more time and are more approachable, their low social status limits their credibility as sources of information.

The provision of postabortion care to women is complicated by the socio-religious and legal climate surrounding abortion in Egypt. Despite the steady stream of postabortion patients in public hospitals, physicians lack knowledge of common postabortion complications and consequences (Egyptian Fertility Care Society 1995). Combined with physicians' lack of counseling skills and time, it is perhaps not surprising that women receive little information about their condition. Even family planning services are typically not offered to postabortion patients who want to delay or cease childbearing. Furthermore, the concerns and questions of women who lose wanted pregnancies are not addressed, and they are rarely referred to other providers for treatment of repeat pregnancy loss, toxoplasmosis, or other medical conditions, even when such treatment is clearly appropriate.

Even less has been done to involve men in matters related to their wives' health care, despite the documented role of husbands in contraceptive use and method selection (Abdel-Aziz, El-Zanaty, and Cross 1992; Ali 1996). Women are rarely provided with information; their husbands receive none.

The hospital environment itself poses a challenge to the involvement of husbands in their wives' health care. Interested husbands have to contend with a number of obstacles, including a lack of waiting areas for men and staff who are unfriendly or even hostile to their presence. Many hospitals bar men from the obstetrics/gynecology ward. One husband interviewed during this project described his experience as follows: "I spent two nights in the hallway; it was so inconvenient. Every few hours the janitors would come and ask me to go away because they needed to scrub the floors." These barriers make it difficult for men to get involved even if they want to, and may discourage many from even visiting their wives at the hospital.

DEVELOPING A PLAN TO PROVIDE POSTABORTION CARE

Staff from the Egyptian Fertility Care Society (EFCS) and the Population Council's Asia and Near East Operations Research Project had begun collaborating on a project to improve the quality of postabortion care in Egyptian public hospitals. Major components of this project included the introduction of manual vacuum aspiration and enhanced counseling for women receiving postabortion care.

Women presenting with bleeding related to pregnancy loss at Egyptian hospitals include a mix of spontaneous and induced abortion cases.[2] An earlier study (Huntington et al. 1998) showed the distribution of postabortion patients admitted to public hospitals to be as follows: 5 percent certainly induced, 2 percent probably induced, 58 percent possibly induced, and 35 percent spontaneous.[3] Researchers therefore estimated that a substantial proportion of the women in this project were likely to have induced the abortion.[4] Among those women who had spontaneously miscarried, in some cases the pregnancy was wanted while in others it was unplanned or unwanted. The pool of women seeking postabortion care is, therefore, diverse, but all have urgent psychological and physiological needs. All are bleeding. Those who have induced the abortion may be fearful of the consequences of being discovered and eager to ensure that their unwanted pregnancy has been terminated. Those who have miscar-ried—especially those who desired the pregnancy—are experiencing the grief of preg-nancy loss.

Interviews with postabortion patients during this project revealed that the most salient issue confronting them was physical survival. As one woman said, "After an abor-tion, a woman has many worries about her future health, such as: Will she survive the experience or will her body get back to its normal condition?" The women understood the need for rest and recuperation and were troubled by the need to return immediately to their physically demanding routines. The interviews made it apparent that without special preparation and a supportive family environment, women were unlikely to re-ceive adequate physical and emotional support during the postabortion period.

In order to create a more supportive environment in which women could conva-lesce, the project staff began counseling husbands—but only in cases in which the women permitted such contact. We hypothesized that husbands who received coun-seling might be more attuned to their wives' needs during recovery and that their involvement in the recovery would improve their wives' outcomes. A husband who received counseling might offer emotional support; ensure that his wife had plenty of nutritious food available; help to obtain any required medication; and help to mini-mize her workload by assisting with household chores, arranging for other women in the family to perform some of these chores, or convincing his mother to reduce her demands on his wife during her recovery.

The project staff also hypothesized that counseling patients' husbands would re-duce the stress women felt over their return to fertility and the extent to which they were pressured to return to sexual activity before they were ready. Finally, the staff hypoth-esized that counseling husbands would help each couple to define and reach their par-ticular reproductive goals. Some would seek, after the recovery period, to prevent unwanted pregnancies by using contraception. Others would be eager for the woman to get preg-nant again. Women in the latter group may have suffered from repeat miscarriage and would need special help to achieve and sustain a wanted pregnancy.

The counseling intervention used an experimental design that involved all of the women who were admitted to the six hospitals with bleeding during or following preg-nancy loss. A total of 366 women were enrolled. After completing a baseline interview and an informed consent procedure (described below), the women were randomized into a control group and an intervention group. Women in the control group received improved care and counseling, but their husbands were not counseled. Women in the intervention group received improved counseling and care, and their husbands also re-ceived counseling. The counseling was provided to each partner separately.

Of the 366 women initially enrolled, 293 completed the study (136 in the intervention group and 157 in the control group). The remaining 73 women were excluded from the study because they were lost to follow-up, their husbands were absent during the entire follow-up period, or their husbands did not come to the hospital at the time of their discharge.

Maintaining women's confidentiality and rights was a major challenge throughout the intervention design and the study. Because of the sensitive nature of abortion in Egypt and the possibility that involved husbands might gain information about their wives' medical condition that could pose a risk to these women (e.g., a husband might learn that his wife had induced the abortion without his knowledge or that she had concealed the pregnancy from him), considerable attention was devoted to establishing strict ethical guidelines and procedures, as outlined below.

Follow-up interviews were conducted with women one month after hospital discharge. The interview included a questionnaire exploring the women's physical health, psychological well-being, contraceptive practices, and the extent of their husbands' emotional and tangible support during their recovery. Tangible support included help with household activities, buying or preparing food, and securing such support from other women in the family. Measures of emotional support were based on the husband's reaction to the lost pregnancy and his understanding of his wife's physical and emotional needs during recovery. In addition, in-depth interviews were conducted with 16 of the 136 husbands in the intervention group to learn their opinions of the counseling they had received.

PROJECT OPERATION

Training of Physicians and Nurses

Thirty senior physicians (five from each hospital) received one day of training on postabortion counseling procedures and content. Only physicians were trained because of their higher status and credibility: In formative research interviews, husbands expressed a preference for counseling from physicians, but expressed no preference regarding the sex of the provider. The majority of the physicians trained were male (64 percent).

The content of counseling procedures was developed jointly by investigators from EFCS and the Population Council following review of relevant literature and an assessment, conducted in two of the study hospitals, of the needs of women and their husbands following abortion. The training was done in conjunction with five days of training for the larger postabortion project and included training in manual vacuum aspiration, postabortion complications and warning signs, counseling in reproductive health care and contraceptive methods, and the psychological and religious dimensions of postabortion care. The session on counseling focused on creating a cadre of trained supervisors who would then train their colleagues and provide daily, onsite supervision and follow-up. Topics included the role of husbands in reproductive health, the role of physicians as counselors, protection of women's privacy, and constraints to counseling husbands.

This training was followed by three months of on-the-job practice during which the five supervisors in each hospital trained and supervised other physicians and nurses in procedures for counseling husbands. The training of nurses focused on patient enrollment procedures and obtaining informed consent.

A study coordinator, usually the senior obstetrician/gynecologist in each hospital, monitored the hospital's training activities. In addition, staff from EFCS and the Population Council made weekly visits to monitor the quality of the on-the-job training and adherence to informed consent and confidentiality procedures.

Protecting Patient Confidentiality

The following enrollment procedures were developed through extensive pretesting to ensure the protection of patient privacy while maximizing the number of husbands who would receive counseling:

Patient admission procedures. If the woman's husband brought her to the hospital, the nurse in charge asked him to return at discharge to pick up and assist his wife. A husband did not receive counseling at this point; he was counseled only after the woman gave her informed consent.

Obtaining women's informed consent. The nurse in charge sought the woman's permission for the doctor to speak to her husband about her medical condition. Consent was sought after the woman had received complete medical treatment, including counseling, and only after the attending physician had confirmed that the woman was in stable physical and emotional condition. Standard procedures for obtaining informed consent were adapted to suit the Egyptian context. Because most female patients at Egyptian public hospitals are illiterate and obtaining written consent is thus not feasible, the nurse read each woman a standardized consent statement (see Box 1). Moreover, since obtaining informed consent is not standard practice in Egypt, patients may feel intimidated by the form and the informed consent procedure. As a result, the nurses were trained to request consent in a more informal, conversational manner. Thus, in most cases, the consent statement was not read verbatim, but the information it contained was transmitted accurately. In order to minimize the possibility of coercion, all of the nurses in charge of enrolling women were paid a flat monthly fee for their involvement in the study, regardless of how many women they enrolled. About 4 percent of the women approached did not consent to participate.

Box 1. Informed consent statement

Hello, my name is ———, and I am collecting information from postabortion patients from several hospitals in Menia with the purpose of improving quality of care in those hospitals. I want to ask for your permission to participate in our study. I would like you to know that it is up to you to participate in the study: No one will charge you or pay you any money to participate; you will receive complete medical care if you do not participate. You can withdraw from the study at any time.

If you agree to participate, the doctor might meet with your husband and give him some instructions on the care that you need after discharge. It is important for you to know that even if you agree to participate, the doctor may still not meet with your husband; this will be determined by study procedures.

Do you agree or disagree to have the doctor talk to your husband?

(1) Agree (2) Disagree

Also, if you agree to participate, a female researcher will conduct a follow-up interview with you about one month from now to ask you questions about your health and your recovery. The interview could be done at your home or at the hospital if you want. The interview will be private and the arrangements for the follow-up interview will be confidential.

Do you agree or disagree to have a follow-up interview?

(1) Agree (2) Disagree

If you have any questions, you may ask me or any of the physicians in the hospital's obstetrics/ gynecology department at any time.

During pilot testing of the study instruments and procedures, the study team noticed that some nurses misunderstood the idea of obtaining the women's informed consent and instead asked the consent of the husband to speak to his wife. As mentioned above, informed consent procedures are not routinely used in Egypt except in large private hospitals. Also, the norm in patriarchal societies like Egypt is that permission is sought from the husband. Seeking permission from a woman to speak to her husband was inconceivable to some of the nurses. With more training they came to understand the logic behind the procedures.

Contacting the husband. The project team found that family members often go back and forth between home and the hospital while the woman is hospitalized, even when her stay lasts only a few hours. Thus, it was relatively easy to contact those husbands who had not accompanied their wives upon admission. Attending relatives or companions of a consenting woman were asked to send for the husband to pick her up at discharge. Husbands were generally expected to come anyway, in order to take the woman home and pay tips to hospital staff.

Procedures at discharge. The attending physician commonly signs the discharge forms and gives the woman any remaining instructions for postabortion care. If the woman had agreed to have her husband counseled, was in the intervention group, and her husband was present at discharge, the nurse would ensure that he met with the physician.

Counseling Women

Following treatment, the attending physician counseled the woman. Counseling emphasized the woman's physical and nutritional needs during the recovery period, the warning signs of complications, and instructions about what to do if any problems arose. Women also received counseling about family planning methods. Use of family planning was recommended even for women with repeat miscarriage in order to allow time for the cause of the abortion to be determined and treated. These women were reassured and told not to blame themselves, counseled on possible causes, and, when appropriate, referred to private labs for toxoplasmosis and Rh incompatibility testing, tests not available in public hospitals. Women in the intervention group were also told that their husbands would be counseled and given similar information so that they would better understand their wives' recovery needs.

Counseling Husbands

As noted above, the attending physician counseled the husbands separately when their wives were ready to be discharged from the hospital and after the wives' informed consent had been obtained. Physicians had been encouraged to have a lengthy exchange with each husband and to tailor the content of the discussion to the needs of each couple. The core messages focused on the following topics: (1) the woman's need for rest and adequate nutrition, emphasizing inexpensive, nutritious food; (2) postabortion warning signs indicating need for follow-up care; (3) the woman's return to fertility within two weeks; (4) the need for contraception to avoid unwanted or mistimed pregnancies; and (5) the cause of miscarriage, if appropriate, and sources for referral care if necessary.

Follow-up Interviews

Follow-up interviews with women were conducted one month after discharge from the hospital in order to assess the extent of husbands' involvement in their wives' recovery, the physical and emotional status of the women themselves, and the use of contraception. Unless a woman had indicated a preference for the interview to take place at the hospital, follow-up interviews were conducted in the woman's home.

DOES COUNSELING OF HUSBANDS WORK?

This project demonstrated the feasibility and effectiveness of a postabortion care counseling intervention aimed at husbands. The counseling, well received by both husbands and wives, had a measurable and positive effect on husbands' behavior and their wives' recovery.[5] These outcomes are described in more detail below.

Husbands' and Women's Reactions

Husbands unanimously expressed a desire to be with their wives at the hospital. It was also clear in follow-up interviews that the men greatly appreciated the attention and information that the doctor provided to them. In particular, they felt it was very important for a husband to receive information about his wife's condition and how to provide proper care because he is the primary decisionmaker and is responsible for his wife. For example, one man said: "Some husbands will not believe their wife if she says that the doctor asked her to stay in bed . . . it is therefore better if the doctor speaks to him in person so he would be responsible if anything happens to her afterward."

While most husbands thought it was important that both they and their wives receive counseling, some thought that counseling the husband was most important because men "would understand the doctor's instructions better" than their wives would. Indeed the project team found that the doctors often preferred communicating with husbands, perceiving them to be more educated and better able to understand the information conveyed. Whether or not this preference led doctors to spend more time counseling husbands than counseling the women themselves is not known. This issue merits attention in future projects of this type.

Some husbands indicated that the doctor had given them information they knew already, particularly about the need for adequate nutrition and rest. For example, one husband said, "It goes without saying that someone who has undergone surgery needs good nutrition." However, the reinforcement of this knowledge was appreciated by some: "Although I had already known that after an abortion or a delivery a woman would need to eat well, I made an extra effort after the doctor's advice to me. Instead of having her come directly to our house I let her go to her mother's. I also delayed sex as the doctor advised me."

In general, the husbands felt that the counseling was acceptable and helpful, and that all husbands of postabortion patients should receive it. Although the venue in which counseling was provided was not ideal—typically five minutes in the hallway while the doctor was on his or her way to see another patient, according to husbands' reports—husbands appreciated the fact that the doctor took the time to talk to them. They also suggested a number of improvements to the content of the messages, including elaborating on the information provided about the resumption of sexual activity and use of family planning.

Wives were also pleased to have their husbands learn about their condition and their need for care directly from the doctor, which they felt increased the likelihood that their husbands would take the information seriously. In particular, they wanted doctors to talk to their husbands about family planning, to reassure them about women's fertility following an abortion, and to encourage their husbands to take good care of them.

Effects on Husbands' Support, Women's Recovery, and Use of Contraception

As described above, follow-up interviews with participating women were conducted one month after their discharge from the hospital to assess their emotional and physical recovery and the extent to which their husbands supported them during the recovery period.

After controlling for other patient and husband characteristics, such as the woman's medical condition, household composition, husband's education, and number of living children, husbands who were counseled were 50 percent more likely to provide a high level of tangible support to their wives, 30 percent more likely to provide their wives with a high level of emotional support, and 60 percent more likely to provide a high level of support for the use of family planning than husbands who were not counseled, although only the association with family planning support is statistically significant. The effects of a range of sociodemographic and other characteristics on the likelihood of husbands' support were also assessed. Selected results are presented in Table 1.

Husbands in nuclear households were 2.6 times as likely to offer a high level of tangible support to their wives than husbands in extended households, implying that husbands may be more willing to help if no other women are available to provide support. Husbands were almost three times as likely to provide a high level of emotional support to their wives if the last pregnancy was planned than if it was not. Husbands with secondary education or above were 2.5 times as likely to provide a high level of family planning support than husbands who had completed less than a secondary education. Through the above analysis, the project staff were able to identify subgroups of husbands who are significantly less likely to support their wives during their recovery. For example, a woman with fewer living children was less likely to receive emotional and family planning support from her husband; a woman whose pregnancy was not planned was also less likely to receive emotional support; and a woman whose husband had less education was considerably less likely to receive support in using contraception.

The effects of husbands' support on women's recovery and use of contraception was also assessed (see Table 2). Husbands' emotional support proved to be a particularly important predictor of women's recovery from abortion complications, affecting both her physical and emotional recuperation. When other variables—including the severity of postabortion complications—were controlled for, women who received high levels of emotional support from their husbands were 70 percent more likely to report good physical recovery; that is, they were less likely to report having had such symptoms as fever, bleeding, offensive discharge, shortness of breath, abdominal or pelvic pain, and weakness. Furthermore, women who received high levels of emo-

Table 1. Adjusted odds ratios for high tangible, emotional, and family planning support (n = 293)

	Adjusted odds ratio
Variables associated with high tangible support	
Husband received counseling	1.5
Household composition (nuclear)	2.6*
Complications during recovery (yes)	1.8*
Husband's education (secondary or above)	1.7
Group A hospital[a] and husband counseled	0.5*[b]
Variables associated with high emotional support	
Husband counseled (yes)	1.3
Husband and wife blood relatives (yes)	1.9*
Most recent pregnancy planned (yes)	2.8*
Number of living children (≥3)	2.0*
Variables associated with high family planning support	
Husband counseled (yes)	1.6*
Desire for more children (no)	5.0*
Husband's education (secondary or above)	2.5*
Number of living children (≥3)	2.5*
Group A hospital[a]	1.7*

* Statistically significant at $p = 0.1$.

[a] In smaller Group A hospitals, a higher proportion of physicians received direct training from project staff as opposed to on-the-job training from colleagues.

[b] A surprising finding was that husbands who received counseling in Group A hospitals were less likely to provide tangible support to their wives during the postabortion recovery period. It is possible that providers in Group A hospitals focused on counseling regarding emotional and family planning support, believing that women were likely to receive the tangible support they needed from other women in the household. Alternatively some characteristic of the individuals/couples concerned (e.g., husband's occupation or duration of marriage) may not have been adequately controlled for and may have confounded the relationship between counseling and tangible support.

tional support from their husbands were twice as likely to report good emotional recovery as women who did not receive such support.

The strongest predictor of use of or intention to use a contraceptive method was a husband's support for his wife's contraceptive use. Women whose husbands provided a high level of support for their use of family planning were almost six times as likely to use or intend to use contraceptives, a finding that supports the conclusions of previous research (Joesoef, Baughman, and Utomo 1988; Terefe and Larson 1993). Unfortunately, couples in these hospitals cannot obtain a family planning method without some effort. Because contraceptives are not provided by the obstetrics/gynecology ward, couples must go to the family planning clinic, which, while located in the same hospital, requires a walk and a wait. While the study did not assess whether or not any individuals chose to go to the clinic immediately after discharge, this is believed to be unlikely.

Table 2. Adjusted odds ratios for women's recovery and contraceptive use (n = 293)

	Adjusted odds ratio
Variables associated with good physical recovery	
Husband's emotional support (high)	1.7*
Husband's tangible support (high)	1.1
Variables associated with good emotional recovery	
Husband's emotional support (high)	2.0*
Variables associated with use of or intention to use family planning	
Husband's family planning support (high)	5.9*

* Statistically significant at p = 0.1.

It should be noted that some of the postabortion patients did not want to avoid pregnancy. They may have been trying to get pregnant, some following previous miscarriages. Indeed, about half of the women in both study groups reported one or more previous miscarriages. These women were counseled and referred as described above. The project team was not able to assess whether or not referred women sought or received treatment.

The study also found that counseling of husbands was associated with more positive family planning outcomes at some hospitals than at others. Counseling a woman's husband per se did not have any effect on women's use of or intention to use contraception. However, women who had been admitted to and whose husbands had been counseled at Group A hospitals (smaller hospitals in which a higher proportion of physicians received direct training from project staff as opposed to on-the-job training from their colleagues) were almost four times as likely to use or intend to use family planning as women who had been admitted to and whose husbands had been counseled at Group B hospitals (larger hospitals where a higher proportion of physicians received on-the-job as opposed to direct training), although family planning services were equally accessible in both types of hospitals. This finding suggests differences in the quality of counseling provided by physicians trained by these two methods. Providers in Group A hospitals seemed to be more enthusiastic about offering the counseling, which was probably reflected in more time spent with husbands and the provision of more complete information.

Sustaining the Project's Effects

These findings were well received by officials of the Ministry of Health and Population (MOHP), nongovernmental organizations, and university hospitals, who acknowledged the need for the hospital environment to be more supportive of husbands.

Senior MOHP officials have indicated that the ministry is conducting training to increase provider awareness of the importance of involving men in matters related to their spouses' reproductive health, and is revising standards of practice and the training curriculum to take into account the role of husbands in family planning. Efforts have been made to ensure that MOHP officials view the counseling of husbands as a supplement to—rather than a substitute for—direct counseling of women receiving postabortion care. In a meeting held with staff from the six study hospitals six months after the completion of data collection, several staff members indicated that counseling of husbands is now done routinely in their hospitals. However, it was clear from their statements that counseling of husbands is left to the initiative of the provider and that husbands are not systematically contacted to participate in postabortion counseling. The development and use of specific counseling protocols would greatly increase counseling by providers.

CONCLUSIONS

Counseling husbands works. Counseling husbands is feasible and effective in increasing the support Egyptian women receive during postabortion recovery. It is likely that a similar intervention would work in other settings, although the content of counseling messages would need to be tailored to the specific needs of women in those settings.

Counseling of husbands should become an integral component of postabortion services in settings where women desire it. In this experiment, women reacted positively to having their husbands counseled, and the counseling appears to have benefited women's health. Providers should establish two-way communication with husbands in order to identify those who are less likely to provide support to their wives. A special effort should be made during counseling sessions to identify such husbands and provide them with more intensive counseling.

The hospital environment may need to change. Expanded husband counseling programs may require changes in hospital policies and staff attitudes regarding the presence of men as well as changes to the physical setup of obstetrics/gynecology wards in many hospitals. Making the hospital environment more welcoming to husbands would encourage men's involvement in their wives' health care.

Attention to the quality of counseling is warranted. In this project, counseling had a greater impact on husbands' behavior if it was provided by senior hospital staff who had received training directly from project staff rather than on-the-job training. More direct training of hospital staff and the monitoring of individual counseling sessions might make results more consistent across hospitals. The project findings also suggest that the training-of-trainers approach may not be as effective as direct training of all providers, although the former is less expensive and, therefore, more easily replicable. More intensive monitoring to ensure that trained trainers are doing their jobs effectively may help reduce differential effects.

Family planning services should be more fully integrated into postabortion care to help couples achieve their reproductive goals. Offering family planning services to postabortion patients in the obstetrics/gynecology ward would save them from having to make a separate visit to the family planning clinic to obtain a method and would thus help couples translate their intentions to use contraception into action.

Referral services should be made available to women with repeat miscarriages in order to diagnose and treat the cause of miscarriage. Doctors who provide care following a miscarriage should manage the immediate complications and also provide the woman with appropriate counseling and advise her to see a specialist or to undergo appropriate tests. Some links may also need to be established between public and university hospitals so that some of the more expensive tests, such as that for toxoplasmosis, can be made available to poor women at lower cost.

Counseling husbands should never be seen as a substitute for counseling female patients, a danger that exists in settings with entrenched patriarchal social structures. Some of the attitudes of husbands and providers indicated that this could be a cause for concern in Egypt. Counseling of husbands should be perceived and implemented as an additional service for those women who choose to involve their husbands. In all instances, precautions to protect women's privacy and confidentiality should be mandatory.

Acknowledgments

We acknowledge the substantial contribution of Susan Lee in the preparation of early drafts of this chapter. Input provided by Beverly Winikoff and Anrudh Jain assisted us in clarifying many of the ethical issues surrounding interaction with postabortion patients. The willingness of the Egyptian physicians to critically review the ethical dimensions of postabortion care contributed to the development of the ethical procedures described here. This study was supported by the Population Council's Asia and Near East Operations Research and Technical Assistance Project with funds from the United States Agency for International Development, Office of Population, under contract number DPE-C-00-90-0002-10.

Notes

1   Recommendations regarding rest and the resumption of household activities for postabortion patients vary based on the length of gestation at the time of the abortion and the seriousness of any complications. As noted, the majority of postabortion patients in Egypt present with fairly minor complications (Huntington et al. 1998).

2   Because abortion is illegal in Egypt, no attempt was made to distinguish between spontaneous and induced abortion during the conduct of the project.

3   A protocol recommended by the World Health Organization Task Force on Safety and Efficacy of Fertility Regulating Methods was used to distinguish among the four groups of patients. A patient's abortion was classified as (a) certainly induced if she herself reported inducing the abortion or when

there was evidence of trauma; (b) probably induced if there was evidence of sepsis or peritonitis, and the woman indicated that the pregnancy was unplanned; (c) possibly induced if only one of the two conditions in category (b) was present; and (d) spontaneous if none of the previous conditions was present or the woman stated that the pregnancy was planned or desired (WHO 1987).

4   The low incidence of trauma and infection among postabortion patients in Egypt (Huntington et al. 1998) suggests that women who induce abortion are more likely to use menstrual regulation techniques than sharp instruments.

5   Twelve percent of the husbands of women in the intervention group did not show up when their wives were discharged from the hospital and, therefore, did not receive counseling; the wives of these men did not receive follow-up interviews and were not included in the analysis. The reasons men did not show up at discharge were not determined. Women in the control group, however, were not excluded from follow-up interviews and analysis if their husbands did not show up at discharge. When asked why their husbands were absent, women in the control group reported that their husbands were traveling or were absent for other compelling reasons. To the extent that men who did return were more motivated to help their wives than men who did not, including all control group women in the analysis, but only intervention group women whose husbands returned at discharge, would tend to exaggerate findings regarding the intervention's effects.

References

Abdel-Aziz, H., F. El-Zanaty, and A. Cross. 1992. *Egypt Male Survey 1991*. Calverton, MD: Macro International, Inc.

Ali, Kamran Asdar. 1996. "Notes on rethinking masculinities: An Egyptian case," in Sondra Zeidenstein and Kirsten Moore (eds.), *Learning About Sexuality: A Practical Beginning*. New York: Population Council, pp. 98–109.

Azer, A. 1979. "Law as an instrument for social change: An illustration from population policy," *Cairo Papers in Social Science* 2(4): 60–96.

Brown, Donna Lee. 1997. "Abortion, Islam, and the 1994 Cairo Population Conference," *International Journal of Middle East Studies* 29(2): 161–184.

Egyptian Fertility Care Society. 1995. "Improving the counseling and medical care of postabortion patients in Egypt: Final report." Cairo: Egyptian Fertility Care Society and Population Council, Asia and Near East Operations Research and Technical Assistance Project.

El Tawila, Sahar, Barbara Ibrahim, Omaima El-Gibaly, Fikrat El Sahn, Sunny Sallam, Susan M. Lee, Barbara Mensch, Hind Wassef, Sarah Bukhari, and Osman Galal. 1999. *Transitions to Adulthood: A National Survey of Egyptian Adolescents*. Cairo: Population Council.

El-Zanaty, Fatma, Enas M. Hussein, Gihan A. Shawky, Ann A. Way, and Sunita Kishor. 1996. *Egypt Demographic and Health Survey 1995*. Calverton, MD: National Population Council (Egypt) and Macro International Inc.

Huntington, Dale. 1997. "Abortion in Egypt," paper presented at the seminar "Cultural Perspectives on Reproductive Health," at the International Union for the Scientific Study of Population, Rustenburg, South Africa, 16–19 June.

Huntington, Dale, Laila Nawar, and D. Abdel Hady. 1995. "An exploratory study of the psycho-social stress associated with abortions in Egypt." Cairo: Population Council.

Huntington, Dale, Laila Nawar, Ezzeldin Osman Hassan, Hala Youssef, and Nahla Abdel-Tawab. 1998. "Postabortion caseload study in Egyptian hospitals," *International Family Planning Perspectives* 24(1): 25–31.

Joesoef, Mohamad R., Andrew L. Baughman, and Budi Utomo. 1988. "Husband's approval of contraceptive use in metropolitan Indonesia: Program implications," *Studies in Family Planning* 19(3): 162–168.

Nawar, Laila, Cynthia Lloyd, and Barbara Ibrahim. 1995. "Women's autonomy and gender roles in Egyptian families," in Carla Makhlouf Obermeyer (ed.), *Family, Gender, and Population in the Middle East.* Cairo: American University in Cairo Press, pp. 147–178.

Terefe, A. and C.P. Larson. 1993. "Modern contraception use in Ethiopia: Does involving husbands make a difference?" *American Journal of Public Health* 83(11): 1567–1571.

World Health Organization. 1987. "Protocol for hospital-based descriptive studies of mortality, morbidity related to induced abortion," WHO project no. 86912. Geneva: WHO.

Contact information

Nahla Abdel-Tawab
Consultant
5 Sabry Abou Alam Street
Apartment 10
Bab El-Louk
Cairo, Egypt
e-mail: nabdeltawab@yahoo.com

Laila Nawar
Regional Advisor
Frontiers in Reproductive Health
Population Council
6A Giza Street
P.O. Box 115
Dokki 12211
Cairo, Egypt
e-mail: lnawar@pccairo.org

Dale Huntington
Associate Director, South and
    East Asia Region
Frontiers in Reproductive Health
Population Council
Zone 5A, Ground Floor
India Habitat Centre, Lodi Road
New Delhi 110 003, India
e-mail: dhuntington@pcindia.org

11

Promoting Postpartum Health in Turkey: The Role of the Father

Janet Molzan Turan, Hacer Nalbant, Ayşen Bulut,
W. Henry Mosley, and Gülbin Gökçay

The international community is coming to realize that reproductive health cannot be achieved by focusing exclusively on women. The Programme of Action from the 1994 International Conference on Population and Development commits nations to "encourage men's responsibility for sexual and reproductive behavior, and increase male participation in family planning" (ICPD Programme of Action 1994). Since the mid-1990s, the international health community has begun to focus more attention on male involvement in reproductive health (Drennan 1998). Few strategies that address the circumstances of men or couples have been tested, however (Becker 1996).

Programs that include expectant fathers in antenatal education and care are still rare, especially in developing countries. In Sweden, fathers have been included in antenatal classes since the 1970s, and separate groups for expectant fathers have recently been introduced (Swedin 1996). In a program in the United States, expectant fathers learn about parenting from experienced fathers at "bootie camp" (McGee 1998). A study of the effects of including unwed prospective adolescent fathers in antenatal classes in the United States found that fathers' knowledge of pregnancy, antenatal care, infant development, and child care increased significantly among those who participated (Westney, Jackson, and Munford 1988). In turn, fathers who were better informed tended to be more supportive of the mother and infant. Similar programs in developing countries are uncommon. One clinic in southern India tested the effects of educating expectant fathers about how they could support their wives during pregnancy, childbirth, and the postpartum period (Bhalerao et al. 1984). Researchers there found that the group in which expectant fathers were educated made significantly more antenatal visits and experienced lower perinatal mortality than the group in which expectant fathers were not educated.

THE SETTING

This chapter describes efforts made after the Cairo conference to involve fathers in promoting postpartum health in Istanbul, Turkey. Although indicators of reproductive health status have steadily improved in Turkey over the past 50 years, some problems persist. In the Turkish Demographic and Health Survey (TDHS) conducted in 1998, the infant mortality rate was estimated at 43 per 1,000 live births, a relatively high rate considering Turkey's level of development (Hacettepe University and Macro International 1999). Although Turkey's total fertility rate is relatively low (2.6 children per woman), a substantial amount of unwanted pregnancy exists, a situation that results in high rates of unwanted births and induced abortions (14.5 induced abortions for every 100 live births).[1] According to the 1998 TDHS, 68 percent of women who gave birth in the five years preceding the survey had at least one antenatal care visit with a trained health care worker, and 72 percent of births occurred in a health facility. In addition, the survey discerned a trend toward unnecessary reliance on cesarean section, especially in the western region of the country (22 percent of births).

Reproductive health services can be obtained from a variety of public and private sources in Turkey. The Ministry of Health has a large network of hospitals, maternal and child health/family planning centers, and local health centers that deliver services at low or no cost. In urban areas there are many private hospitals, clinics, and doctors. However, a situation analysis of selected reproductive health care services in Turkey conducted in 1994 found that although facilities, equipment, and supplies were adequate, other aspects of service quality were deficient (Ministry of Health, Population Council, and AVSC International 1995). In addition, men are rarely specifically included in these maternal and child health services.

With a population of around 10 million, Istanbul is the largest and most cosmopolitan city in Turkey. The city is growing rapidly, largely because of migration from other parts of the country. The city government has been unable to keep pace with this rapid urban growth, and, as a result, public services are inadequate in many areas. This is especially true in squatter settlements inhabited by recent immigrants to the city. Given the high rate of inflation and other economic problems, raising children is expensive and desired family size is now quite low.

The project described in this chapter was carried out by the Istanbul Medical School Woman and Child Health Research and Training Unit (hereafter the Woman and Child Health Unit). The unit provides education and services and conducts research in the area of reproductive health. Integrated clinical services, information, and counseling are offered in the areas of antenatal care, well-baby care, family planning, pregnancy termination, women's health, and infertility. One of the unit's special concerns in recent years has been family health during the postpartum period, defined here as the first six months after a woman gives birth. As a result, an intervention was designed to include expectant fathers in an antenatal information and counseling program to promote postpartum health. It was carried out by a multidisciplinary team that included physicians (specialists in pediatrics, public health, and obstetrics/gynecology), nurses, and social scientists (from the disciplines of sociology, public health, and education).

Participants in the project were clients of the Istanbul Medical School Hospital at Çapa. This large government university teaching hospital serves clients from a variety of socioeconomic groups. Fees are low, relative to those charged by private providers. Government employees and patients referred through the social security system are charged reduced fees. Thus, a sizable percentage of the hospital's clients are low-level, low-income government employees.

WHAT WAS KNOWN

An earlier diagnostic study of postpartum health needs in Istanbul, which included interviews with 183 women at 1–2 and 5–6 months after giving birth, provided us with preliminary information on postpartum behavior. In the formative stage of this project, we used qualitative methods to improve our understanding of the roles of various family members in postpartum decisionmaking and behavior. Methods used included focus groups (four with new parents and five with expectant parents), in-depth interviews of ten new mothers and ten new fathers, and brief telephone interviews with 17 expectant fathers and 21 expectant mothers.

What Postpartum Health Problems Exist?

The earlier diagnostic study had found that at 1–2 months postpartum, 26 percent of women had had postpartum checkups and 11 percent were exclusively breastfeeding. Despite the fact that most women stated an intention to use a modern contraceptive method soon after the birth, only 34 percent were doing so when interviewed at 5–6 months after the birth (Bulut and Turan 1995).

Do Husbands and Wives Communicate?

In the formative qualitative phase of the project, we found that young, newly married couples rarely talk to each other about reproductive health topics. Young women expressed expectations for communication, understanding, and emotional support from the fathers of their children, rather than for physical assistance with the tasks of motherhood. The father's financial support of the family appeared to be taken for granted and was rarely discussed. Women said that men work hard outside the home and thus should be excused from much involvement in housework and childcare. As one 22-year-old pregnant woman put it: "It's important for the father to be helpful at home. Not in terms of the work, but in terms of psychological support. At home friendship is important, sharing and taking an interest is important, talking is important."

How Involved Are Men?

Not surprisingly, men experienced fewer changes in their lives during the pregnancy than did women. In fact, some men experienced no changes in their normal routine. In other cases, men began to pay more attention to their wives and to help with heavy tasks around the home. Many expectant fathers take their wives to see the doctor during pregnancy. In general, the expectant father's participation in antenatal visits is limited to accompanying his wife to the clinic and dealing with the clinic bureaucracy. At antenatal clinics men are often seen smoking outside or relaxing in waiting rooms. The expectant father is rarely an active participant in the interaction with the health care provider. Even if men want to participate, they may be discouraged by health workers or by the largely "female atmosphere" of the clinic. Some men express the idea that antenatal visits are private and that men should not be present. As one 31-year-old factory manager said: "Usually she went with her mother. I went once or twice, but it's hard for me to get off from work. It was more appropriate for her to go with her mother. They might talk about private things."

Men are more involved in some aspects of postpartum health care. These include visits to health care facilities and preventing pregnancy after the birth. Many fathers accompany their wives and children on visits to health care facilities and are involved in decisionmaking regarding when, where, and how to seek health care. However, while men often bring their families to the clinic, deal with the bureaucracy, and pay for the visit, they are rarely invited into the counseling or examination room. Most couples said they made decisions about contraception jointly. Moreover, many couples use male methods, such as withdrawal or condoms, as their first postpartum family planning method. A 27-year-old new father described his situation: "Up until now we never protected ourselves. Before the birth we used our own willpower. After the birth we chose the IUD because it is more reliable. We heard that pills are habit-forming and cause infertility and that some condoms have holes in them. My wife and I decided together."

What Role Do Fathers Play in Infant Care?

The father's role in infant care is usually seen as supplementary. The mother usually makes daily decisions about infant feeding and care, with important input from relatives, doctors, neighbors, and others. Fathers may be informed and consulted at times, but they are often not present when decisions need to be made. The main responsibility of a man is seen as earning the income to provide his family with a good standard of living. One 30-year-old man summarized a father's responsibilities in the following manner: "The father should fill in when the mother can't do everything and provide economically for the child's future."

Is There Potential for Greater Involvement by Fathers?

Norms and expectations about fatherhood are changing in Istanbul. Young men are being told by their wives and the media that fathers should be more involved with their families. Young women are also demanding close, supportive, and communicative relationships with the fathers of their children. In addition, many young men do not want to replicate the distant relationships their own fathers had with their wives and children. As a result, many young fathers are willing to help out in areas traditionally defined as the mother's responsibility. Unfortunately, they have little information and few role models on which to base such behavior, and they face significant barriers in the extended family and in the health care system. Family health clinics largely cater to women and children, and special efforts to include men (such as male counselors, evening and weekend hours, or invitations to enter the doctor's office) are rarely made. As one 24-year-old man said: "At home we help out with some jobs, but beyond that we don't have any information about feeding or about how we can be helpful to our wives. It's like this: I don't know what she is feeling. Nobody taught me. I didn't get any information."

DESIGNING A PROGRAM TO INVOLVE YOUNG FATHERS

On the basis of these lessons, staff at the Woman and Child Health Unit designed a service intervention that would support use of preventive health services, exclusive breastfeeding, and family planning during the postpartum period. The strategy underlying the intervention was to meet couples' expressed need for information about postpartum health topics and women's desire for communication and understanding from their partners. In addition to providing factual information, emphasis was placed on describing the important role that fathers can play in supporting women during pregnancy, delivery, and the postpartum period. The main components of this information and support intervention were as follows:

- Four antenatal group education sessions covering pregnancy, childbirth, infant feeding and care, and postpartum women's health and family planning;
- A booklet containing answers to frequently asked questions about health during pregnancy, childbirth, and the postpartum period; and
- Access to a telephone counseling service during the postpartum period.

The project staff were not certain that providing services to couples rather than to women alone would automatically lead to better outcomes. For this reason, they developed an experimental design, which involved 333 women expecting a first birth who were attending the Woman and Child Health Unit for antenatal care. After completing a baseline interview and giving their informed consent, the women were randomized into three groups. In the first (hereafter referred to as the couples group) mothers and fathers were invited to participate in the information and counseling activities together. In the second group (the mothers-only group) mothers alone were invited to participate. Members of the third group (the control group) were not invited to participate in the intervention, but could take advantage of the regular services offered by the unit.[2]

Details on the development and operation of each of the information and counseling interventions are provided below.

Group Education and Information Sessions

Topics covered by the group sessions were determined on the basis of information needs identified during the initial assessment. We realized that participants would have limited time to spend at the clinic, so we decided to offer four sessions, each lasting approximately 1.5 hours. Topics covered in the group sessions are described in Box 1. An education specialist collaborated with physicians and nurses on the project team to develop standard education modules for each of the four sessions. In practice, however, the sessions tended to differ according to the needs, interests, and questions of the women and couples in attendance. Each session was offered on the same day of the week at the same time (10:30 a.m. for the couples group and noon for the mothers-only group). Group leaders were flexible, however, and often held sessions at other hours to suit the participants' schedules. Most sessions were conducted jointly by the education specialist and a nurse. Telephone calls, mailings, and doctor reminders were used to encourage participants to attend sessions.

Booklet of Questions and Answers for New Parents

The focus groups and interviews had helped the project team identify common problems and commonly asked questions. A booklet was designed to address questions on pregnancy, childbirth, infant feeding and care, and postpartum women's health and family planning. Experts in obstetrics/gynecology, pediatrics, family planning, and women's health wrote answers to the questions, which were edited and revised by a psychologist who had training in maternal and child health. The booklets were sent by mail to all participants in the mothers-only group and the couples group. While booklets sent to households of the mothers-only group were addressed to the woman only,

Box 1. Topics covered in group education and information sessions

Pregnancy
- Signs of pregnancy
- Women's reproductive anatomy
- Process of fertilization
- Baby's development in the womb
- Importance and content of antenatal care
- Taking care of the mother and baby during pregnancy
- Common symptoms and complaints during pregnancy (nausea, constipation, etc.)
- Situations in which women need to go to the doctor/hospital immediately

Main messages
- An expectant mother needs special care during pregnancy
- Regular medical checkups during pregnancy are important
- A balanced diet and adequate rest are necessary
- In some situations, it is necessary to go to the doctor/hospital immediately

Birth
- Planning for the birth (place, list of items to take to the hospital)
- Signs that labor is starting
- Stages of labor and delivery
- Breathing and pushing techniques
- Episiotomy
- Risks to the mother and/or baby
- Cesarean section and vacuum extraction
- Care of the baby and mother in the hospital after the birth
- Relaxation exercises

Main messages
- Birth is a normal, healthy process
- Support from the husband and other people makes birth easier
- Work with health care providers; trust their experience and knowledge
- Planning and preparing for the birth makes it easier and less frightening

Infant care and feeding
- Baby's needs (nutrition, sleep, hygiene, communication, love, etc.)
- Breastfeeding
- Prevention of common infant illnesses
- How to handle some common infant illnesses (fever, jaundice, diarrhea, etc.)
- Infant development during the first six months
- Basics of infant care (bathing, diapers, clothing, sleep, etc.)
- Things to be careful of in the home (potential accidents)

Main messages
- Breastfeeding is best
- Every mother can breastfeed successfully
- A baby can be fed exclusively with breastmilk for at least four months, and for up to six months if the baby continues to gain weight steadily
- Regular checkups help to monitor the baby's growth and prevent illnesses

Postpartum women's health and family planning
- Postpartum traditions
- Care of the mother after the birth
- Changes in a woman's body after birth and the return to fertility
- Reproductive anatomy and processes
- Methods for preventing unwanted pregnancy
- Common rumors about family planning methods

Main messages
- It takes a while for a woman's body to recover after a birth
- Postpartum women need support and care from people in their family and community
- Every mother should get a postpartum checkup by six weeks after the birth
- Getting pregnant again soon after a birth is bad for the health of both the mother and the baby
- There are several effective contraceptive methods that can be used soon after a birth; start planning now

---

Box 2. Excerpts from the booklet of questions and answers for new parents

Can we have sex during pregnancy? What about frequency and positions?

In general, there is no reason to limit your sex life during pregnancy. In terms of frequency and positions, couples can feel free to choose without limitations. However, in some special situations, such as miscarriage risk, premature labor risk, bleeding, premature breaking of water [rupture of the membranes], small uterine opening, previous miscarriage, or premature labor, it may be necessary to limit sexual activity.

Can I fast for religious reasons during pregnancy?

During pregnancy it is necessary to eat small amounts during frequent meals. This is necessary to meet the nutritional requirements of the mother and the baby. The expectant mother's body cannot withstand long periods without eating. In addition, the pregnant woman may experience nausea, vomiting, and heartburn. These complaints may increase if she doesn't eat for long periods of time. For these reasons, fasting is not good for maternal and child health. Although some mothers who fast during pregnancy have healthy pregnancies and give birth to healthy babies, fasting during pregnancy is not recommended.

What can my husband and I do when my labor pains start?

First, remain calm. There will be sufficient time between the start of your labor pains and the actual birth. For this reason, you don't need to go to the hospital immediately. Wait until the pains become more frequent and then gather your medical records and other items listed later in this booklet and go to the hospital where you received antenatal care. After they examine you, hospital personnel will give you the necessary information about your situation. Currently husbands are not allowed in the delivery room in public hospitals and most private hospitals. This practice may change in the near future, however. The husband's presence in the delivery room can provide important psychological support to the mother who is experiencing labor pains. Even if today's fathers are not allowed in the delivery room, they can provide important support to the mother when her labor pains start at home, at the hospital before going into the delivery room, and right after the birth. Such support can include monitoring the amount of time between contractions, giving the mother a soft lower-back massage, practicing breathing techniques with her, helping her take a shower, and giving her encouragement and support with verbal and nonverbal communication.

---

those mailed to households of the couples group were addressed to both the husband and wife. Sample questions and answers from the booklet are presented in Box 2. No booklets were sent to members of the control group.

Postpartum Telephone Counseling Service

Project staff established a postpartum telephone counseling service, with a dedicated telephone number, to function during clinic working hours (Monday–Friday, 8:30 a.m.–4:30 p.m.). The number was mailed and/or given to women in the mothers-only group and to both mothers and fathers in the couples group, but not to members of the control group. Educators were available to answer questions, and clinic doctors were available for consultation when an expert opinion was deemed necessary. The educators filled out a form for each phone call, recording information about the caller, the questions asked, and the advice/information given.

TO WHAT EXTENT DID MEN AND WOMEN USE THE INFORMATION AND COUNSELING SERVICES?

Of the 333 couples who participated in the project, 279 new mothers and 253 new fathers completed questionnaires four months after delivery. In addition to questions about postpartum health attitudes, beliefs, and behaviors, 187 couples in the mothers-only and couples groups combined answered questions about their use of the information and counseling services offered. The team reviewed the questionnaires and project records to assess the extent to which eligible women or couples had taken advantage of the new services. The vast majority (83 percent) reported that they had used at least one of the services (attending one or more education sessions, reading some or all of the booklet, or calling the telephone counseling service). A more detailed look at each group's participation in these interventions is provided below.

Group Education and Information Sessions

Despite special efforts, participation of expectant fathers was lower than expected. Of the 84 fathers responding to the follow-up interview who had been invited to attend the couples group, only 26 percent had attended one or more sessions. Furthermore, women's attendance at one or more sessions was significantly higher for the mothers-only group (54 percent) than for the couples group (40 percent), suggesting that insisting on husbands' involvement may create a barrier to some women's participation.

The men who attended the group sessions tended to be better educated, older, more likely to have a wife who works outside the home, and more likely to have some form of health insurance than were men who did not participate. Their wives had wider social support networks and were also significantly more likely to predict that their husbands would be interested in such sessions than were the wives of men who did not attend (84 percent vs. 62 percent).

Booklet of Questions and Answers for New Parents

The booklet reached a greater number of both women and men than did the group sessions. Overall, 74 percent of mothers and 63 percent of fathers in the mothers-only and couples groups combined reported having received the booklet. Of those who reported receiving it, 94 percent of mothers (n = 140) and 84 percent of fathers (n = 105) reported having read some or all of it.

The fathers in the couples group were significantly more likely to report having received and read the booklet than those whose wives were in the mothers-only group (see Table 1). Addressing the booklets to the fathers may have encouraged them to read them (or pressured them into reporting that they had done so). There was no

Table 1. Percentage of women and men who received and read booklet, by intervention group and sex

	Couples group		Mothers-only group	
	Women (n = 94)	Men (n = 84)	Women (n = 93)	Men (n = 84)
Received booklet	74 (79%)	62 (74%)	66 (71%)	44 (52%)
Read booklet	68 (72%)	52 (62%)	64 (69%)	36 (43%)

difference in background characteristics of fathers who said they had read the booklet and fathers who said that they had not. This may indicate that the booklet was equally accessible to all types of men enrolled in the project.

Postpartum Telephone Counseling Service

Thirty-two percent of participants (59 couples) in both groups reported that they had used the telephone counseling service at least once. No difference in telephone counseling service use was found between members of the couples group and the mothers-only group. In over 90 percent of cases, the new mother, rather than another member of the family, was the one who called the service. Only one new father (from the couples group) called the service. The most common types of questions asked over the phone were about infant care and health (50 percent), followed by questions on infant feeding (21 percent), women's health and family planning after the birth (14 percent), accessing health services (7 percent), childbirth (5 percent), and pregnancy (4 percent).

BARRIERS TO MALE PARTICIPATION

Through follow-up focus groups and interviews and a postintervention assessment, the project team identified some of the barriers to participation in the group education sessions. Chief among these was the research design, which required that individuals be assigned at random to the couples group, the mothers-only group, or the control group, and which prevented promotion of the sessions at the clinic. Another barrier was the regular mode of operation of the antenatal clinic. The clinic works on a first-come-first-served basis, which means that clients never know exactly when they will be called to see the doctor. Even though waits are generally long, this situation caused anxiety for those trying to attend an education session before seeing the doctor. Those who planned to attend a session after their visit with the doctor were often sent to another hospital building for medical tests and were not able to return in time. In addition, the sessions were a new type of service and some clients had a hard time believing that they would be provided without an extra fee. Men also experienced a number of institutional and social barriers to their participation: the general "female atmosphere" of the antenatal clinic, past experiences of being excluded from doctor visits, difficulties in getting time off from work, transportation difficulties, and lack of time.

Feedback from Fathers

In follow-up interviews, men who had used the information and counseling services were asked to comment on these services. In general, men who participated were pleased. The most common request was for even more detailed information on the health topics covered. Men often suggested that the program be advertised widely so that more people could benefit from it and that publications be reproduced in large numbers and distributed at work places. Some men felt that private sessions for couples would be more appropriate than group sessions. Those whose wives used the telephone counseling service were pleased. On the other hand, there were some complaints about access to the hotline, including busy signals and long waits.

EFFECTS OF THE INTERVENTION

Effects on Couple Communication and Decisionmaking

One goal of the intervention was to increase couple communication on issues related to pregnancy, childbirth, and postpartum health. The follow-up interviews indicate that it did stimulate conversation between partners. Seventy percent of wives who attended at least one group session said that they had talked to their husbands about the session afterward. In addition, 77 percent of husbands who attended at least one session talked to their wives afterward. Sixty-three percent of women and 79 percent of men who read the question-and-answer booklet said that they had talked to their spouse about it. The percentage of women who said they had talked to their husbands about the session was higher in the mothers-only group than in the couples group.

The project team also sought to encourage "joint decisionmaking" on postpartum health. In the follow-up questionnaires, mothers and fathers were asked who makes household decisions in four areas: infant feeding, infant health, postpartum women's health, and family planning. Contrary to our expectations, there were no differences in decisionmaking among the three groups. Members of the control group, who did not participate in the program at all, reported decisionmaking processes similar to those of the mothers-only and couples group members.[3] Fathers were significantly more likely to report involvement in decisionmaking than were mothers, particularly in the cases of postpartum women's health and family planning. For example, 24 percent of mothers reported joint decisionmaking about women's postpartum health, compared to 41 percent of fathers. Given the traditional role of Turkish men as family decisionmakers, it is not surprising that men report playing an active role in making these decisions.

Effects on Men's Sources of Health Information

After the birth, fathers were asked to report their most important sources of information on infant feeding, infant health, maternal health, and family planning. They were allowed to report up to five sources and were asked to give them in order of importance. As shown in Table 2, fathers reported many sources of information on postpartum health topics. Of interest is the fact that family members dominate as sources of infant feeding information (mentioned by virtually all fathers), although they are not as frequently mentioned as sources of other types of information. The area in which the highest percentage of fathers say they have no source of information is maternal health (14 percent). Friends are important sources of family planning information for fathers (59 percent), as are media channels (69 percent).

Fathers in both the couples and mothers-only groups were more likely to cite project sources (the Woman and Child Health Unit or the question-and-answer booklet) than were men in the control group, and fathers who participated in the couples group were more likely to cite these sources than were husbands of women in the mothers-only group. For example, 26 percent of men who participated in the couples group cited the unit as a source of information about infant feeding, compared to 21 percent of men whose wives participated in the mothers-only group, and only 12 percent of men in the control group. Thus, men who were purposefully included in the program were more likely to know how to obtain reliable information on postpartum health. Feedback from health workers at the Woman and Child Health Unit corroborated this finding. Staff noted that families who had previously participated in the intervention were "different" from those who had not (i.e., they were better informed and asked many questions during visits).

Effects on Postpartum Health Behaviors

Of the four postpartum health behaviors examined, only the use of modern contraceptives[4] was significantly higher in the intervention groups (62 percent for the couples group and 57 percent for the mothers-only group) as compared to the control group (45 percent). In addition, multivariate analysis revealed that use of modern methods in the couples group was significantly higher than use of modern methods in the other two groups. Thus, it appears that involvement of husbands is indeed a critical factor in

Table 2. Fathers' sources of information by postpartum health topic (percent of respondents mentioning the source; multiple responses allowed) (n = 253)

Source	Infant feeding	Infant health	Maternal health	Family planning
Community				
Family	99.6	67.9	45.1	23.9
Friends	22.9	23.3	6.7	58.6
Media[a]	53.0	41.5	14.2	68.5
Private doctor	16.2	25.7	11.9	4.8
Public doctor	10.3	20.9	19.4	3.2
Other	4.3	3.2	0	3.2
Intervention				
Woman and Child Health Unit[b]	19.8	27.7	17.8	16.3
Question-and-answer booklet	9.1	5.5	2.0	4.8
No source	1.2	3.6	13.8	6.0

[a] Includes newspapers, magazines, books, brochures, television, and radio.
[b] Includes Woman and Child Health Unit doctors, nurses, and educators.

supporting women's use of modern family planning methods after a birth. Infant feeding, infant checkups, and women's postpartum checkups were only slightly more common in the intervention groups as compared to the control group (differences were not statistically significant). The reasons for this are not clear, although the relatively small group sizes may have contributed to our inability to detect significant differences.

Some 99 percent of women said that they wanted to use a family planning method to postpone their next pregnancy. The results indicate that including expectant fathers in information and counseling activities may influence women's ability to select a family planning method after the birth.

Significant behavior change was not brought about in all the areas we had hoped. Possible reasons include small sample size, lower-than-expected attendance at the education sessions, and the need for a more intensive intervention to facilitate real behavior change. Nonetheless, the intervention may have helped fathers take the first steps toward becoming more involved in postpartum care. The project appears to have stimulated discussion between husbands and wives about reproductive health topics. For those involved in the couples group, the project increased men's awareness of reliable sources of information about postpartum health and women's success in negotiating use of modern contraceptive methods.

LESSONS LEARNED ABOUT MALE PARTICIPATION

The results of this project indicate that expectant fathers should be encouraged to participate in antenatal information and counseling programs, and that doing so may be effective in facilitating use of modern contraceptives. In the formative phase of this service experiment, we learned that young women want their husbands to be involved in information and counseling on maternal and child health. In implementing the intervention, however, we found it difficult to get men to participate. When designing reproductive health information and counseling programs for men and couples, the following lessons should be kept in mind:

- Barriers to men's attendance at education sessions included difficulties in getting time off from work, transportation difficulties, and lack of time.
- Institutional barriers for men included the general "female atmosphere" of the antenatal clinic and men's past experiences of being excluded from doctor visits.
- Men with low levels of education, young men, men whose wives do not work outside the home, men without health insurance, and men whose wives have limited social support networks may need special encouragement and recruitment efforts to participate in education sessions. It appears that women with more resources (e.g., those who work outside the home and have large social support networks) were better able to convince their husbands to attend the sessions.
- The question-and-answer booklet was the most effective channel for reaching the fathers targeted by this experiment. While only 26 percent of the fathers in the couples group attended a group education session, 62 percent found time to read the booklet. It appears that purposely addressing all invitations and encouragement regarding the project to both mothers and fathers in the couples group encouraged fathers to read the booklet.
- Even if men do not participate directly in project activities, they may learn indirectly from their wives. Around 70 percent of women who attended a session and 63 percent of women who read the booklet said that they discussed the information with their husbands afterward.
- Men's participation in education sessions should not be mandatory, as requiring the father to attend may be a barrier to participation for some women.

THE FUTURE

Antenatal information and counseling sessions have become a regular part of the services offered at the Woman and Child Health Unit. Sessions are open to and attended by expectant fathers as well as mothers-to-be. Promotional and educational materials are addressed to both men and women. The question-and-answer booklet for new mothers and fathers is distributed to the unit's clients.

A follow-up project testing a similar intervention for expectant parents in a community-based setting is underway in Istanbul. In designing it, the project team has taken into consideration the lessons learned in the service experiment described here. The project is being offered at a community center (not a health institution) in the hope that it will be easily accessible to both men and women. Members of the community are active in the planning and operation of the program, which includes information and counseling sessions for expectant mothers and fathers.

The project for expectant fathers was developed in partnership with the Mother Child Education Foundation, a Turkish foundation experienced in educating fathers. It is designed specifically by and for men, instead of simply incorporating men into a program designed by and for women. Based on the foundation's experience, a decision was made to offer a separate project for expectant fathers that would be taught exclusively by male educators, in addition to an existing program for women. Topics covered in the six-session program include fatherhood, communication techniques, pregnancy, childbirth, infant care and feeding, and family health after a birth. The program is held on Sunday afternoons to accommodate men's busy schedules. Preliminary results (Turan et al. 2001) indicate that this project more directly addresses the needs of expectant fathers and encourages them to support their families during the pregnancy, birth, and postpartum periods.

Acknowledgments

We thank EngenderHealth, the Population Council's Middle East Research Awards Program and the Robert H. Ebert Program on Critical Issues in Reproductive Health, and the Mellon Foundation for their financial support, without which this project would not have been possible. In addition, we acknowledge Joel Gittelsohn of Johns Hopkins University and Nükhet Sirman of Boğaziçi University for serving as advisors during the formative phase of the project. Füsun Kayatürk deserves thanks for her work as a focus-group moderator, in-depth interviewer, and editor of the question-and-answer booklet. We thank Olcay Neyzi for her advice and assistance throughout the project and, especially, for her review of the question-and-answer booklet. We also thank the other focus-group moderators and in-depth interviewers—Tuğrul Erbaydar, Sinan Yolsal, and Ali Riza Erdoğan. We acknowledge the excellent work of Ayşe Köybaşıoğlu Güngör and Gamze Dalgalı, who developed and led the group education sessions; and Yegane Gülerman, Gülten Tahtakiliç, Nezahat Bayır, Hulya Işler, Özlem Barsbay, Mehmet Barutçugil, Barçın Barlas, and Gökhan Teker, who worked as interviewers for the baseline and follow-up surveys. We thank the staff of the Istanbul Medical School Woman and Child Health Research and Training Unit for their support throughout the project. We acknowledge Bülent Turan's advice regarding the statistical analyses.

Notes

1 Since 1983 induced abortion has been legal in Turkey up to the tenth week of pregnancy. If a woman is married, her husband's consent is required.

2   Antenatal care was provided to women in all three groups by doctors in training who rotated every three months. A woman was likely to see a different doctor on each antenatal visit. Very little information and counseling were provided. Other services provided by the Woman and Child Health Unit included family planning counseling and services, well-baby checkups, postpartum well-woman checkups, breastfeeding counseling, and induced abortion.

3   Participants' decisionmaking processes and perspectives may have been too complex to be captured by simple questions on a structured questionnaire.

4   The term "modern contraceptives" is used in this case study to refer to methods that are offered through the medical system in Istanbul, including the IUD, pills, sterilization, and condoms.

References

Becker, Stan. 1996. "Couples and reproductive health: A review of couple studies," *Studies in Family Planning* 27(6): 291–306.

Bhalerao Vijaya R., Medha Galwankar, Shobha S. Kowli, Rajesh Kumar, and R.M. Chaturvedi. 1984. "Contribution of the education of the prospective fathers to the success of maternal health care programme," *Journal of Postgraduate Medicine* 30(1): 10–12.

Bulut, Ayşen and Janet Molzan Turan. 1995. "Postpartum family planning and health needs of women of low income in Istanbul," *Studies in Family Planning* 26(2): 88–100.

Drennan, Megan. 1998. "Reproductive health: New perspectives on men's participation," *Population Reports,* Series J, no. 46.

Hacettepe University, Institute of Population Studies, and Macro International. 1999. *Turkish Demographic and Health Survey 1998.* Ankara: Hacettepe University.

International Conference on Population and Development Programme of Action. 1994. United Nations document A/CONF.171/13. New York: United Nations.

McGee, Bill. 1998. "At ease, men! New dads prep for success at bootie camp," *Twins Magazine* (November/December): 26–27.

Ministry of Health (Turkey), Population Council, and AVSC International. 1995. *Turkey Situation Analysis Study of Selected Reproductive Health Care Services.* Ankara: Ministry of Health (Turkey).

Turan, Janet Molzan, Hacer Nalbant, Ayşen Bulut, and Yusuf Sahip. 2001. "Including expectant fathers in antenatal education programmes in Istanbul, Turkey," *Reproductive Health Matters* 9(18): 114–125.

Swedin, Göran. 1996. "Modern Swedish fatherhood: The challenges and the opportunities," *Reproductive Health Matters* 7: 25–33.

Westney, Ouida E., Cole O. Jackson, and Theodosia L. Munford. 1988. "The effects of prenatal education intervention on unwed prospective adolescent fathers," *Journal of Adolescent Health Care* 9: 214–218.

Contact information

Janet Molzan Turan
Family Health Department
Istanbul University Institute of Child Health
Cerrahi Monoblok Karşisi, Çapa 34390
Istanbul, Turkey
telephone: 90-212-533-1204
fax: 90-212-631-1710
e-mail: jmturan@attglobal.net

PART IV
ADDRESSING NEGLECTED
REPRODUCTIVE HEALTH CONCERNS

paragraph 7.5.a, Programme of Action

. . . To ensure that comprehensive and factual information and a full range of reproductive health-care services, including family planning, are accessible, affordable, acceptable and convenient to all users. . . .

How can programs that provide fragmented vertical services shift to the provision of an integrated reproductive health service package?

---

paragraph 8.25, Programme of Action

. . . In all cases, women should have access to quality services for the management of complications arising from abortion. Post-abortion counselling, education and family-planning services should be offered promptly. . . .

How can we provide appropriate postabortion care?

---

paragraph 7.35, Programme of Action

Violence against women, particularly domestic violence and rape, is widespread, and rising numbers of women are at risk from AIDS and other sexually transmitted diseases as a result of high-risk sexual behaviour on the part of their partners.

How can reproductive health workers acknowledge and address gender violence?

---

paragraph 7.30, Programme of Action

Reproductive health programmes should increase their efforts to prevent, detect and treat sexually transmitted diseases and other reproductive tract infections, especially at the primary health-care level.

How can we address the complexities of RTI management in low-resource settings?

12

A Hospital in Nigeria Reinvents Its Reproductive Health Care System

Oladapo Shittu, Dennis I. Ifenne, and Charlotte Hord

Conventionally configured family planning services have failed to gain acceptance among Nigeria's population, despite the desire of many to avoid unwanted pregnancy. Unmet need for contraception is estimated to be 21 percent, and contraceptive prevalence is about 6 percent (Nigeria Federal Office of Statistics and IRD/Macro International 1992). The extent of unwanted pregnancy is illustrated most dramatically by the fact that an estimated 610,000 Nigerian women resort to illegal induced abortion each year (Henshaw et al. 1998); many of these women suffer serious complications, and some do not survive. In addition, other reproductive health issues have been virtually ignored, despite a substantial burden of reproductive ill health. Sexually transmitted infections (STIs) are a serious concern, with some studies finding prevalence rates of 18 percent for gonorrhea (UNAIDS/WHO 1998) and 25 percent for trichomoniasis (Anosike et al. 1993) in non–sex worker populations.

In Zaria—a poor city of 600,000 in Kaduna State, northern Nigeria—reproductive health problems are perhaps more severe than in the country as a whole (Harrison 1985). Maternal mortality, obstetric fistulas, septic abortion, and cervical cancer are common. Women in this largely Muslim, culturally Hausa region are largely unemployed, illiterate, and impoverished. They have little power to make decisions about their fertility without the consent and financial backing of their husbands.

This state of affairs prompted a rethinking of family planning and reproductive health care strategies at the Ahmadu Bello University Teaching Hospital in Zaria. Ahmadu Bello Hospital serves the city and its environs as a primary, secondary, and tertiary care facility, accepting patients with advanced or complicated health problems from peripheral sites throughout Kaduna State. In 1995 the hospital launched an initiative to integrate its family planning and reproductive health services to promote a comprehensive, client-centered approach to reproductive health care. This initiative—inspired by the principles and recommendations of the 1994 International Conference on Population and Development (ICPD) in Cairo—aimed to improve women's reproductive health status and care, integrate family planning into the reproductive/ family health system, and separate the provision of family planning services from demographically driven population policies.

THE NEW VISION: LINK SERVICES AND EDUCATE WOMEN

When a family planning program was first introduced in Nigeria in the late 1970s, the government's mandate was to reduce population growth. Many Nigerians believed that family planning would be used to limit the size and growth of certain ethnic and religious groups. This interpretation embarrassed health and government officials, prompting some to distance themselves from the program. As a result, family planning became culturally, politically, and bureaucratically isolated from other health services. The problem was compounded by a fragmented approach to reproductive health care in Nigeria—a result, in part, of the fact that many reproductive health programs had begun as discrete projects sponsored by various nongovernmental organizations. This set of conditions left large gaps in women's reproductive health knowledge and care.

This had been the situation at Ahmadu Bello University Teaching Hospital prior to the inception of its reproductive health initiative. The hospital had offered a full array of family planning and reproductive health services, but these had been compartmentalized in different programs. It operated separate clinics for general obstetrics/gynecology, family planning, and STIs, each with its own staff. The obstetrics/ gynecology clinic provided basic gynecologic exams, ante- and postnatal care, and postabortion care, including outpatient manual vacuum aspiration (MVA). Staff specializing in cytology performed cancer screenings, but only for individuals who requested them. The family planning clinic operated out of the obstetrics/gynecology clinic three days a week, for three hours after the obstetrics/gynecology clinic closed. Permanent methods of contraception were offered by another set of providers on a separate schedule. The STI clinic was located in a different part of the hospital, and was not linked to the other departments. These arrangements often did not serve patients well. For example, many postabortion patients left the hospital without family planning counseling, or had to make a costly return visit for counseling, as this service was available only three afternoons a week. A woman delivering in the labor ward who indicated that she wished to stop having children would be directed to the delivery nurse, who would refer her to family planning counselors, who would then refer her to providers of surgical contraception.

The effort to integrate family planning and reproductive health services at Ahmadu Bello Hospital began when its doctors and nurses determined that they could no longer provide family planning as an isolated service without considering a woman's overall sexual well-being and awareness. The new vision was to treat women holistically, recognizing their multiple health needs and providing them with reproductive health education, counseling, and care. To accomplish this, the team proposed bringing together the hospital's disparate family planning and reproductive health services into a new, comprehensive reproductive health center. Women who found their way into the facility—whether by way of a pregnancy, an incomplete abortion, or a reproductive tract infection (RTI)—would receive counseling on other aspects of sexual health, including prevention of HIV/AIDS and other STIs, gynecologic cancer screening, infertility, and family planning. Once a client had received this information, she would be referred to all relevant services. She would then have all of her reproductive health needs—no matter how diverse—met by one team of medical providers. This comprehensive approach to family planning/reproductive health care represented a radical departure from business as usual.

Establishing the hospital's reproductive health center entailed securing the support of the hospital administration and retraining providers. Fortuitously, the Nigerian Population Activity Fund Agency (PAFA), a government initiative funded by the World Bank, was simultaneously working to reform the country's reproductive health services in a manner consistent with the hospital's proposal. In 1995 PAFA sponsored a workshop providing didactic and clinical training in modern counseling strategies, family planning, postabortion care, cancer screening, and STI management. Four obstetrician/gynecologists and five nurses from the hospital were selected to participate in the six-week workshop, along with colleagues from hospitals nationwide.

Before this time, many members of the Ahmadu Bello Hospital medical staff had not recognized the benefits of integrating family planning and reproductive health services. However, the doctors and nurses who attended the PAFA workshop returned enthusiastic about the proposed changes. This development—coupled with the fact that PAFA's work was propelled by Ministry of Health directives—persuaded hospital administrators to approve the plan to create a new reproductive health center. The five PAFA-trained nurses were promptly reassigned to the new center, and PAFA-trained staff initiated training sessions for other hospital doctors. These sessions continue to be attended by new physicians joining the hospital staff.

To gain support in the hospital community, leaders of the reproductive health initiative conducted a seminar for administrators, doctors, nurses, medical students, and paramedical staff. Participants discussed patients' reproductive health concerns and the characteristics and shortcomings of strategies that had been employed to address these concerns. The seminar leaders explained the concept of an integrated reproductive health care approach and how the new center would carry it out. One administrator expressed concern that the new approach would increase costs by increasing patient time; however, he also noted that providing services in a coherent manner could reduce patient visits, thereby reducing costs.

Indeed, reinventing reproductive health care at Ahmadu Bello Hospital did not require substantial additional resources. When PAFA was no longer able to provide financial support for the initiative,[1] the experiment proceeded successfully without external funding.

INSIDE THE REPRODUCTIVE HEALTH CENTER

Ahmadu Bello Hospital's reproductive health center opened its doors on 4 July 1995 and remains in operation. The center is permanently staffed by the five PAFA-trained nurses and by pairs of obstetrician/gynecologists—with one PAFA-trained doctor in each pair—who do weekly rotations in the center. Services are provided from 7:30 a.m. to 9:00 p.m. every day except Sunday. Elective antenatal and gynecologic consultations are provided by appointment and are conducted before 2:00 p.m. on designated days, when most of the medical staff are available. Thereafter, patients without appointments are seen on a first-come-first-served basis until 9:00 p.m.

Counseling and reproductive health education are the bedrock of the center's approach to patient care. Every morning nurses lead an hour-long group reproductive health education session, which all patients are encouraged to attend. Conducted in English and the Hausa language, the sessions address sexual health, fertility and fertility regulation, prevention of HIV/AIDS and other STIs, gynecologic exams, and breast cancer screening. In addition, the sessions provide information on harmful traditional practices, advocating against female genital cutting and various food taboos. Individual counseling is provided to all first-time clients, those who desire (or who are deemed by health care providers to need) such counseling, and those whose partners could benefit from this opportunity. Clients can make use of these educational and counseling resources on the day they arrive at the center or at any other time that suits them.

The clinical component of a first-time visit consists of an exam and, if the patient can afford it, cervical smear cytology—regardless of the specific service being sought. During the exam, patients are screened for RTIs using Nigerian national syndromic algorithms.[2] Women presenting with requests as varied as antenatal care, family planning, or treatment of infertility are asked whether they experience such symptoms as pelvic pain, vaginal discharge, or vulval ulcers. A general physical and genital examination is performed to help determine whether an RTI is present. Syndromic treatment is provided and a follow-up appointment is scheduled for a week later. Almost two-thirds of patients treated return to obtain ongoing services of the sort they originally sought (e.g., antenatal care or infertility treatment). Patients with persistent symptoms after initial treatment or with genital ulcers and those referred from other institutions are given relevant laboratory tests.[3]

While this two-stage clinical process ensures that some initially misdiagnosed women eventually receive appropriate treatment, it does have several significant shortcomings. The process relies completely on women returning for follow-up care. In addition, women who do not experience symptoms (a large proportion of the total number infected) receive no treatment when syndromic approaches are used. Finally, uninfected women are often misdiagnosed by syndromic algorithms as having STIs and receive unnecessary treatment. (There are currently no clear answers to these dilemmas in RTI management in resource-poor settings.[4])

Women who are managed syndromically for suspected STIs are not encouraged to notify their partners, because of the uncertainties of syndromic diagnosis and the risks (such as divorce and physical abuse) women may face in disclosing an infection to their partners. Women with laboratory-confirmed STIs, on the other hand, are encouraged to notify their partners, given the need for partner treatment to reduce the cycle of transmission. To date, partner response has been less than 20 percent. Staffing constraints limit provider participation in partner notification and in efforts to ensure compliance with treatment and follow-up.

Clients at Ahmadu Bello Hospital's reproductive health center are offered a Pap smear and are encouraged to seek repeat tests on an annual basis, advice that marks a recent and dramatic shift in reproductive health awareness in this locale. Few women even knew about cervical cancer screening only a few years ago. Because this test costs women about US$3, only about 5 percent of clients avail themselves of it.[5] The hospital's cost-sharing policy has not permitted further concessions in these charges.

The center provides a full range of contraceptive methods, including condoms, injectables, the intrauterine device (IUD), Norplant®, oral contraceptives, and vaginal spermicides, as well as sterilization by laparoscopy and minilaparotomy. Fully informed choice is a prerequisite to the administration of all methods. Following comprehensive contraceptive counseling and method selection, written consent is obtained from clients prior to use of any provider-dependent method, such as the IUD, Norplant, and sterilization.

The center has the capacity to perform in-depth gynecologic and obstetric investigations and interventions, including ultrasound of the pelvis, biopsy of cervical

lesions, MVA for abnormal uterine bleeding, and laparoscopy or laparotomy as indicated. A colposcope has been acquired but is not yet in routine use.

Women who arrive for emergency reproductive health care (e.g., for complications of abortion) also receive other reproductive health services. For example, postabortion
care (now provided in the outpatient complex between 7:30 a.m. and 9:00 p.m. and in
the inpatient gynecology ward at other times) includes family planning counseling and
services. Patients are also provided with pretreatment counseling on the abortion process, treatment options, and recovery. Counselors encourage women to delay resumption of sexual relations until all bleeding has ceased and to use contraception for at least
three months or longer if pregnancy is not immediately desired (Shittu 1998).

Postpartum patients are counseled individually during hospital ward rounds. A
counselor from the center is available twice a day to discuss women's health and self-
care in the postpartum period, family planning options, and breastfeeding issues, with
an emphasis on the benefits of exclusive breastfeeding.

All medical professionals at the reproductive health center are capable of treating a range of reproductive health problems. Doctors provide family planning counseling, and nurses treat STIs. This arrangement promotes efficient use of staff in an
environment where trained medical practitioners are scarce.

INCREASING USE OF SERVICES

In its first few years of operation, the center experienced a substantial increase in its
caseload. While more recent data are not available, an ongoing evaluation suggests
that this trend has continued. A growing number of clients have participated in the
center's reproductive health education sessions and have obtained individual counseling, family planning services, cervical cancer screening, and STI management (see
Table 1). The demand for both endometrial biopsies and Pap smears (which were
infrequently offered before the center opened) more than doubled in three years. The
number of women who received individual reproductive health counseling rose substantially: from 459 in 1994–95 (before the center opened) to 979 in 1997–98. The
number of new RTI patients managed using the syndromic algorithms increased from
0 in 1994–95 to 241 in 1997–98. The number of new contraceptive users nearly
doubled from July 1994 to June 1998, and the number of continuing users increased
by 50 percent in that period.

Use of services at the center increased even though the number of women obtaining antenatal care, previously one of the hospital's primary reproductive health services,
fell or remained the same.[6] This implies that a greater proportion of clients received
comprehensive reproductive health care than would have done so before the integration

Table 1. Services provided to clients at Ahmadu Bello Hospital's reproductive health center

Type of service	1994–95 (before center opened)	1995–96 (after center opened)	1996–97	1997–98
Individual counseling	459	919	809	979
Family planning for new clients	262	302	267	470
Family planning for return clients	1,363	1,731	1,630	1,922
Gynecologic cancer screening (Pap smears)	49	86	103	111
MVA: uterine evacuations	197	146	194	164
MVA: endometrial biopsies	74	120	182	191
Postabortion contraceptive services: number of users (percent of postabortion cases)[a]	15 (8%)	22 (15%)	27 (14%)	28 (17%)
Syndromic RTI management (new clients)	0	61	123	241
RTI treatment based on definitive laboratory tests (new clients)[b]	184	254	253	158
Gynecologic services (new clients)	868	1,052	995	1,033
Antenatal care (new clients)	1,343	435	598	572
Deliveries	906	1,209	1,007	1,248

[a] One reason for the low proportion of postabortion clients who choose to use contraceptives immediately is that many had a spontaneous rather than an induced abortion and desired another pregnancy soon.
[b] Includes women for whom syndromic management was ineffective and who returned for follow-up care (i.e., includes some women also included in the syndromic management category). Reasons for the drop in cases between 1996–97 and 1997–98 are being investigated.

of services within the center. Provision of certain acute care procedures, including uterine evacuations, has declined at Ahmadu Bello Hospital. This is a positive trend, reflecting the dissemination of MVA skills to other public and private medical practitioners in the city through training at the hospital. The wider availability of this safe, efficient, and inexpensive procedure for treating women with bleeding following miscarriage or incomplete abortion has eased the demand for these services at the hospital.

As a tertiary care center, Ahmadu Bello Hospital accepts complicated obstetrics/gynecology cases from the primary and secondary care health facilities in the surrounding region, where the majority of women receive health care. Such referrals have been hampered by the cessation of World Bank funding of PAFA, as some of this funding was being used to enhance referral capacity. Ambulance services in the region are inadequate, thus limiting transport of patients to the hospital for emergency care. Financial and logistic obstacles often prevent relatives of women with obstetric complications from getting these women the medical care they need. Women with obstetric emergencies who do not reach the hospital are likely to suffer serious health consequences, even death. It is not unusual for a patient with obstructed labor or a ruptured uterus to present at the hospital a day or two after being referred.

Increasing women's access to reproductive health care in northern Nigeria requires both removing roadblocks and building new pathways. The latter can be accomplished, in part, by expanding the network of trained reproductive health care workers in the region. To this end, Ahmadu Bello Hospital sponsors reproductive health care training programs for members of the medical community and for caregivers and other individuals in the community at large.

MAGNIFYING EFFECTS THROUGH TRAINING

Ahmadu Bello Hospital's obstetrics/gynecology department is responsible for training nurses and other health care providers, medical undergraduates, and postgraduates from Kaduna State and other parts of the country. Currently 150 physicians and 60 nurses and midwives graduate from the training program each year. All training is based on a holistic approach to reproductive health care. Doctors and nurses learn about postabortion care; nurses and midwives learn how to provide family planning services through a participatory learning process; and community health officers, extension health workers, traditional birth attendants, and even town criers[7] learn to promote child spacing and breastfeeding.

The training program benefits from the hospital's integrated approach to reproductive health care. This approach facilitates practical training in integrated management of clients' reproductive health concerns. It enables the program to cover the full spectrum of reproductive health issues and to address overlapping causative factors and symptoms. All graduates of the program, regardless of their position or place of work, receive comprehensive reproductive health education and enter the clinic environment with a common perspective and consistent priorities.

The hospital has also served as a training site for doctors and midwives affiliated with the Christian Health Association of Nigeria, which includes Catholic hospitals in its network of medical facilities (Baird et al. 1997). More than 40 health care professionals have received this training, which covers diverse areas of reproductive health (some conventional, some controversial), ranging from postabortion care and contraceptive counseling to the syndromic management of STIs. The training provides opportunities to discuss how to integrate services and make use of referral links. This is an important resource, given that—for logistic and, sometimes, policy reasons—not every hospital can provide the full range of reproductive health services. For example,

Table 2. Number of child spacing and family health program clients at five primary health centers

Clients by type of service	1995	1996	1997
New family planning clients	195	347	748
Clients referred to Ahmadu Bello Hospital for cancer screening and other services	2	18	52

some of the Catholic hospitals do not provide family planning services; however, staff at these hospitals have agreed to refer patients interested in contraceptive services to government institutions.

The program of training for religious health systems is being replicated in Ethiopia and Zambia (International Family Health 1999). Ahmadu Bello Hospital is also involved in introducing postabortion and STI (including HIV/AIDS) care into the health care facilities of the Federation of Muslim Women's Associations of Nigeria.

With support from Rotary International, the hospital is working in two nearby service areas to increase community engagement in reproductive health care. Training is being provided to community-based practitioners, including local doctors, nurses, midwives, community health officers, traditional birth attendants, and town criers (Shittu 1999). Practitioners are learning how to counsel women and their families on healthy reproductive behavior and—an essential need in this setting—how to spot pregnancy complications and other problems that warrant emergency referral to Ahmadu Bello Hospital.

Referrals to the hospital for gynecologic cancer screening and other services not provided at primary health centers in the area increased from only two in 1995 to more than 50 in 1997, at least in part owing to this community-based training program (see Table 2). The number of sites providing child spacing counseling and services has also risen substantially, from 16 primary health centers in 1995 to 54 in 1997. Use of family planning services at five primary health centers in the vicinity has increased fourfold since the hospital adopted a client-oriented approach to family planning. The hospital is now working to expand this community engagement program to 15 other states in northern Nigeria.

THREE ISSUES THAT REQUIRE ATTENTION

Ahmadu Bello Hospital's reproductive health care staff is considering how to deal with three complex issues: the particular reproductive health risks faced by pregnant adolescent girls, cost sharing, and unsound and unsanitary practices among traditional healers.

Early marriage is common in Nigeria. In the north, women ages 20–24 years married at a median age of 15 in 1990 (Nigeria Federal Office of Statistics and IRD/Macro International 1992). This cultural practice is seen as necessary to control girls' perceived promiscuity; indeed, it is considered shameful for a girl to menstruate more than once while still residing in her parents' home.

Early marriage and early pregnancy go hand in hand. In 1990 nearly half of adolescent girls in northern Nigeria had begun childbearing (Nigeria Federal Office of Statistics and IRD/Macro International 1992). As a result, rates of pregnancy complications are high. Anemia, pregnancy-induced hypertension, and obstructed labor are common. Some adolescent mothers develop an obstetric fistula (a hole in the wall of the vagina, connecting it to the bladder or rectum) during labor, which can cause incontinence. Girls and women who develop this condition are sometimes abandoned by their husbands and parents and subsequently become destitute or resort to prostitution. An estimated 200,000 Nigerian women have such problems (Chukwudebelu 1995). In 13 percent of cases, fistulas are caused by "gishiri" cuts—vaginal incisions made with razor blades by traditional birth attendants as remedies for various obstetric and gynecologic ailments; these incisions are classified by WHO as Type IV female genital cutting (Tahzib 1983). Obstetric fistulas are usually correctable, and Ahmadu Bello Hospital has gynecologists on staff who are experienced at fistula repair. Most patients, however, cannot afford the cost of the procedure.

Despite the risks of early pregnancy, adolescents and their families rarely seek pregnancy-related care or other reproductive health services. Finding girls at risk may require outreach programs in schools, but these programs will still miss a large percentage of girls. Only 54 percent of Nigerian girls ages 11–15 and 21 percent of girls ages 16–20 were in school in 1990 (Nigeria Federal Office of Statistics and IRD/Macro International 1992). Attempts must be made to reach adolescents—including the substantial numbers of married girls—in other ways. Reaching married girls will be particularly challenging because of their low status and limited mobility.

A second issue of concern is cost sharing. Since the Nigerian economy began declining in the 1980s, public health providers have been forced to pass on to patients a growing portion of the costs of medical services. Medical insurance is not available. Thus, a typical Nigerian woman cannot afford modern health care. A cesarean birth at Ahmadu Bello Hospital, for example, costs US$100—an amount equivalent to about two months' salary for a Nigerian worker earning minimum wage. Since the hospital's reproductive health center opened, the cost of a Pap smear has risen sixfold to US$3. At this price, most women forgo the service.

The costs of modern care predispose women to use traditional healers, even though most women are convinced that modern health care is superior. During the 1970s Ahmadu Bello Hospital doctors performed 4,500 deliveries a year. Now the hospital performs only 1,200 deliveries a year. Two-thirds of all deliveries in Nigeria are performed by individuals lacking appropriate training (traditional birth attendants, relatives, or the woman herself). The use of unsanitary practices and unsound procedures in such deliveries is a matter of grave concern to medical professionals. Such practices include the gishiri cut described above, as well as other forms of female genital cutting that can result in severe complications, including genital infections, septic pregnancies, and vaginal fistulas. Hospital staff take the position that professionals within the formal medical system must cooperate with traditional providers and that the focus should not be on eliminating these providers, but rather on building their capacity to serve the women who come to them, while building the capacity of the formal medical care system to meet women's needs. Traditional healers have been receptive to the hospital's community-based training programs.

THE ICPD AGENDA AT WORK IN AFRICA

Ahmadu Bello Hospital has found a way to bring the ICPD agenda to Zaria. With limited resources, the hospital has adopted an integrated, client-centered approach to family planning and reproductive health care. Doing so has entailed integrating services, reaching out to caregivers outside the formal medical system (including traditional healers), and educating clients so that they can promote their own reproductive health. The effects of this approach are tangible: More women have gained reproductive health awareness, more are promoting their own health through STI treatment and cancer screening, and more are achieving their fertility intentions through contraception. While the hospital continues to face many challenges in providing comprehensive reproductive health care to its clients, its initiative demonstrates that many of the principles and recommendations of the ICPD Programme of Action can be put into practice within the political and economic realities of Africa.

Acknowledgments

The authors acknowledge the commitment of Ahmadu Bello Hospital's chief medical director, A.M. Yakubu, as well as the consultants, resident doctors, and nurses of the obstetrics/gynecology department who work in the reproductive health center. We are particularly grateful to doctors D.P. Haggai, A.T. Olayinka, and A.J. Randawa, and to nurses M. Egbunnu, J.A. Ojo, M. Mukkadas, D. Ehoche, and F. Bello. We thank Laura Herbst, Ipas editorial consultant, for her work on early drafts of this chapter. The assistance provided by Ipas, EngenderHealth, the Population Activity Fund Agency, International Family Health, and Rotary International toward the evolution of the center is also appreciated.

Notes

1   The World Bank withdrew support from PAFA in 1996, in response to Nigeria's deteriorating economic and political situation.

2   Syndromic algorithms are visual flow charts developed to assist clinicians in managing RTIs on the basis of a client's presenting signs and symptoms. The algorithms do not require the use of expensive laboratory tests. Some of the algorithms (e.g., those for vaginal discharge) are limited in their capacity to identify the likely cause of an infection.

3   The hospital's laboratory facilities have the capacity to diagnose bacterial vaginosis, candidiasis, chancroid, gonorrhea, HIV, lymphogranuloma venereum, syphilis (through Venereal Disease Research Laboratory testing), trichomoniasis, and donovanosis. Chlamydia testing is not available.

4   See Chapter 16 for a discussion of the complexities and challenges of managing RTIs in low-resource settings.

5   The minimum wage in Nigeria is US$65 per month.

6   Use of antenatal care dropped precipitously following the introduction in 1995 of patient charges and compulsory blood donation by relatives.

7   Town criers are self-employed individuals who communicate messages of community interest in public places and at social gatherings, sometimes with humor or musical accompaniment, in exchange for tips.

References

Anosike, J.C., C.O. Onwuliri, R.E. Inyang, J.I. Akoh, B.E. Nwoke, C.M. Adeiyongo, S.N. Okoye, and O.B. Akogun. 1993. "Trichomoniasis amongst students of a higher institution in Nigeria," *Applied Parasitology* 34(1): 19–25.

Baird, Traci L., Catherine Plewman, Rakiya Booth, and Ayo M. Tubi. 1997. "Christian hospitals in Nigeria provide postabortion care and STD management," *Dialogue* 1(2): 1–2. Chapel Hill, NC: Ipas.

Chukwudebelu, W.O. 1995. "The epidemiology of vesico-vaginal fistulae in Nigeria," in Clara Ejembi (ed.), *The Vesico-Vaginal Fistulae Scourge: A Preventable Social Tragedy.* Proceedings of the National Workshop on Vesico-Vaginal Fistulae. Zaria: A.B.U. Press, pp 19–22.

Harrison, Kelsey A. 1985. "Child-bearing, health and social priorities: A survey of 22,774 consecutive hospital births in Zaria, Northern Nigeria," *British Journal of Obstetrics and Gynaecology* 92(suppl 5): 1–119.

Henshaw, Stanley K., Susheela Singh, Boniface A. Oye-Adeniran, Isaac F. Adewole, Ngozi Iwere, and Yvette P. Cuca. 1998. "The incidence of induced abortion in Nigeria," *International Family Planning Perspectives* 24(4): 156–164.

International Family Health. 1999. *African Regional Forum of Religious Health Organizations in Reproductive Health,* report of a meeting held in Lusaka, Zambia, 11–17 September.

Nigeria Federal Office of Statistics (FOS) and IRD/Macro International. 1992. *Nigeria Demographic and Health Survey 1990.* Columbia, MD: FOS and IRD.

Shittu, Oladapo. 1998. "An appraisal of post-abortion care needs in healthcare facilities in northern Nigeria," thesis. Liverpool, UK: Liverpool School of Tropical Medicine.

———. 1999. "Nigerian health professional reports on pilot child spacing project," *Fragile Earth,* publication of Rotary International, (March): 7.

Tahzib, F. 1983. "Epidemiological determinants of vesicovaginal fistulae," *British Journal of Obstetrics and Gynaecology* 90(5): 387–391.

UNAIDS/WHO. 1998. "Epidemiological fact sheet: Nigeria." Geneva: UNAIDS/WHO.

Contact information

Oladapo Shittu
Head, Department of Obstetrics
  and Gynecology
Ahmadu Bello University Teaching Hospital
Zaria, Nigeria
telephone: 234-69-332271/3
telephone/fax: 234-69-332542
e-mail: olash@skannet.com

Charlotte Hord
Director of Policy
Ipas
300 Market Street, Suite 200
Chapel Hill, NC 27516 USA
telephone: 919-967-7052
fax: 919-929-0258
e-mail: hordce@ipas.org

13

Improving Postabortion Care in a Public Hospital in Mexico

Ana Langer, Angela Heimburger, Cecilia García-Barrios, and Beverly Winikoff

Despite severe legal restrictions and considerable risks, an estimated 3.4 million illegally induced abortions are performed each year in Latin America.[1] One out of every seven of those abortions—about half a million per year—takes place in Mexico, generally under unsafe conditions (Alan Guttmacher Institute 1994). Although abortion is considered a safe and relatively simple procedure when performed legally and under proper conditions, complications from unsafe or incomplete abortion occur frequently; worse, they often lead to death. Complications from spontaneous and induced abortions constitute the fourth leading cause of maternal mortality not only in Mexico (Secretaría de Salud 1992), but in Latin America as a whole (Alan Guttmacher Institute 1994).

Previous research on abortion in Mexico has concentrated on determining its prevalence, the characteristics of women who have abortions, conditions associated with the decision to continue or terminate a pregnancy, abortion as a cause of maternal death, providers' opinions of women who have abortions, and the abortion experience from women's perspective (Rivas Zivy and Amuchástegui 1996; Romero 1994).

The body of knowledge created by these studies has contributed to the understanding of abortion as a public health problem in Mexico by documenting the discriminatory treatment and low-quality care women receive from health institutions, and the considerable burden of physical and emotional suffering they experience. To address this reality, priority strategies have been identified, including the decriminalization and eventual legalization of induced abortion and the extension and improvement of reproductive health services, including postabortion care, for women suffering from the complications of both induced and spontaneous abortion.[2]

The project described in this chapter sought to achieve the latter goal. We began by assessing postabortion care in a public hospital in the city of Oaxaca, Mexico. On the basis of our findings, we designed, implemented, and evaluated a model to improve the quality of care. According to hospital protocol, no attempt was made to

---

Box 1. Framework for high-quality abortion care

- Appropriate abortion care technology, primarily use of manual vacuum aspiration as an alternative to the more costly and invasive dilation and curettage.
- Technical competence of providers in surgical procedures, infection prevention, and management of complications.
- Availability of essential and appropriate equipment, supplies, and medications, including a wide array of contraceptive methods.
- Nonjudgmental, respectful, supportive, and unbiased interactions between women and providers/staff, which should be conducted in an atmosphere of trust, confidentiality, and privacy.
- Comprehensive, intelligible information and counseling on all aspects of care, including broader reproductive health care, with ample opportunity to express concerns, and ask and resolve questions.
- Access to postabortion family planning, reproductive health care, and appropriate referrals.
- Access to services, including elimination of psychological, sociocultural, administrative, and medical barriers.

Source: Leonard and Winkler 1991.

---

distinguish between women suffering from induced and spontaneous abortions.[3] Instead, we sought to improve the quality of postabortion care provided to each woman suffering complications, regardless of the type of abortion she had experienced.

In developing our assessment and a model of postabortion care, we used the quality-of-care framework for abortion care developed by Ipas[4] (Leonard and Winkler 1991), based on Judith Bruce's framework for quality of care in family planning services (Bruce 1990). This framework is outlined in Box 1. In the context of our project, we categorized quality-of-care elements as follows:

1. Technology, technical capacity, and equipment;
2. Humane treatment and information exchange; and
3. Family planning counseling and services.

THE SETTING

The project was carried out at the Dr. Aurelio Valdivieso General Hospital, the largest public general hospital in the city and southern state of Oaxaca, one of the poorest and most rural states in Mexico. This hospital, as part of the Ministry of Health system, receives uninsured patients with few economic resources; many are indigenous women from surrounding rural areas for whom Spanish is a second language. This public institution also serves as a teaching hospital for the local university and is considered reasonably representative of other public health institutions in Mexico.

In the last several years the demand for services has grown sharply, placing additional pressure on scarce resources and contributing to increasingly rushed, poor-quality care, particularly in the case of postabortion services. According to one physician, "In the 11 years that I have been working at this hospital, I have seen the demand for services triple, even quadruple. Now with the country's economic crisis, people can't afford to go to any other hospital; they all come here instead."

In February 1996, with support from the Population Council, the Valdivieso Hospital initiated steps to improve both the quality and the cost-effectiveness of postabortion care. The hospital was chosen as the project site because of the volume of postabortion admissions (up to four a day), the interest of the hospital authorities in improving quality of care, and the willingness of the professional staff to participate.

In general, a postabortion patient with complications arrives at the hospital's emergency area accompanied by a family member. The timing and nature of the medical care she receives is based on a rapid assessment of the severity of her condition, which may be made successively by the security guard who determines emergency priorities, the nurse who admits her, and other care providers on duty. Within half an hour of admission, medical interns and, occasionally, residents usually perform the initial medical appraisal, which includes a brief interview with the patient about her symptoms and reproductive history and a cursory physical exam. The problem is treated as an emergency requiring immediate treatment, but may be accompanied by implicit or explicit reprimands by hospital staff, who assume that the abortion may have been induced.

The specific quality improvements to be made by the project were based on an initial assessment of quality at the site. This assessment was made using structured interviews with both providers (physicians and nurses) and postabortion patients. We also reviewed patients' medical records and observed the management of postabortion cases from admission to discharge, recording all treatment received and all interactions and verbal exchanges between patients and both hospital staff and medical personnel, as well as contacts with other patients and visitors on the same ward.

Profile of Postabortion Care Patients

The average age of the sample of 339 postabortion patients studied was 26 years. Most (75 percent) were married or in union, and described themselves as living permanently with their partners. About 70 percent were housewives and economically dependent on their partners, about two-thirds of whom had no fixed employment. More than 60 percent of the women were from urban areas, and most had little or no schooling. Among those women who admitted having had an unwanted pregnancy (slightly less than 40 percent), only about 30 percent reported having used a contraceptive method (Langer et al. 1997).

BEFORE THE INTERVENTION

Technology, Technical Capacity, and Equipment

Although manual vacuum aspiration (MVA) is considered to be a simpler, less costly, and safer procedure for treating incomplete abortion than dilation and curettage (D&C), 90 percent of the 136 patients who might have been eligible for MVA nonetheless underwent D&C.[5] The other 10 percent underwent a combination of D&C and MVA. According to standard hospital practice, women who received D&C were given general anesthesia, which contributed to their long hospitalization (18.2 hours postsurgery at the hospital).

Humane Treatment and Information Exchange

Understandably, women arriving at the hospital with an incomplete abortion often feel considerable worry, fear, and/or guilt, in addition to physical pain. Indeed, almost half of the women mentioned that they had been very scared upon arrival at the hospital. Most frequently, they said they were afraid of bleeding, physical pain, and dying, as well as of the surgical procedure itself. Some of the women also feared becoming infertile, receiving poor-quality care, and not knowing what was in store for them. Women in such circumstances need to be seen quickly, treated with respect, given privacy, and provided with information about what to expect. The baseline study found that services were inadequate in all these areas and that staff lacked the skills, time, and, in many cases, concern required for a minimally dignified encounter.

Waiting time. While women were admitted relatively quickly, once they were transferred to the obstetrics/gynecology ward they had to wait an average of 13.3 hours before receiving emergency treatment. Service providers attributed this delay to overcrowding and understaffing. Priority was often given to other obstetric procedures, especially cesarean sections. Comments from the physicians explain their priorities:

> There are patients who are kept waiting up to 48 hours from admission until their surgical problem is resolved. The reason is that if there are no vacant rooms in the morning, they have to wait until the afternoon or evening.

> The main problem is that this is a hospital with a high concentration of acute problems; therefore, in the obstetrics/gynecology ward, priority is given to the pregnant woman who has a problem requiring a cesarean section, which causes a delay in the surgical treatment of the patient who needs a uterine evacuation for whatever reason.

Appropriate pain management. Despite the long, painful wait (93 percent of the patients mentioned having felt great pain), fewer than one in ten women received pain medication before the procedure.

Most providers agreed that inadequate pain management was a problem in the facility, and cited frequent shortages of pain medication as part of the cause. Interviews with patients, however, suggested that the problem extended beyond inadequate supplies. When one of the patients told the attending physician that she was in a lot of pain, the doctor replied, "Right now you don't have any reason to feel pain, because what should have been expelled already has béen."

Privacy. Respect for women's privacy was virtually nonexistent. Many women were examined in the presence of three or more staff members and medical students; seldom were women covered with a sheet or robe while being examined; and the examining room had no door, so that passers-by had full view of the uncovered patient. Providers cited lack of hospital gowns, blankets, and dividing curtains as part of the cause of these problems.

Respectful communication. The time physicians spent with patients was fleeting and often poor in quality. In general, doctors and nurses acted as if the patient were not present in the room. Only 26 percent of doctors introduced themselves to the patient, and only 59 percent addressed the patient by name. Less than half of the patients (46 percent) received an explanation of their condition prior to surgery. The few explanations that were given regarding the patient's diagnosis and treatment were equally brief and not very clear; for example, "Señora, you have had an abortion and we're going to perform a sharp curettage." In addition, some comments made by physicians actually terrified the women. One woman recalled a physician's crude reference to making "just one little cut": "Afterward he said it was a joke, but it scared me because I thought they were going to operate without any anesthesia."

As one doctor commented in a preintervention interview: "There is no communication with the patient, telling her 'Look, your problem is this, so we're going to clean your womb.'" Another added: "I don't have the exact numbers or percentages of how many don't know, but there are cases where the patient arrives completely ignorant of what will be done to her."

Not surprisingly, most of the patients did not understand either their diagnosis or treatment: "They only told me it was an abortion; I didn't really understand." Another patient shuddered as she remembered: "The doctor said, 'We're going to give you a good scraping.' It sounded like something that would hurt a lot."

Even during the extended postprocedure period (an average of 18.2 hours), while women were recovering from the anesthesia and waiting to be released, they received very little information about the procedure itself, the subsequent self-care regimen, or warning signs of possible complications (Langer et al. 1997).

The ward seemed to be operating almost as if the postabortion patients were unwelcome intruders. Asked about the failure to offer patients adequate information about their diagnosis and treatment, providers blamed rigid hospital routines and lack of time. One nurse explained:

> More often than not, the ones who take care of the abortions are not the staff doctors. The medical residents . . . have to do everything. If they have an abortion patient there, another here, and another one over there at the same time, they have to register all the clinical histories, then they don't have time to be with the patient.

One physician put it more directly: "If one has to see ten patients in half an hour, then it's difficult to spend a sufficient amount of time with every patient."

Part of this lack of communication may, however, be attributable to the providers' own attitudes toward patients. According to one nurse: "The majority [of the patients] come from a very low [socioeconomic status]; [they] always show up very inhibited and unwilling to collaborate." Many providers are particularly prejudiced against women they believe have induced an abortion themselves. Most of the physicians claim that they "don't get involved enough to find out if the abortion was induced or not, so as not to cause problems for the patient or the institution," and that their main concern is to deal with emergency complications. However, others were more open in their criticism. As one doctor declared, "The sin carries its own penance."

Family Planning Counseling and Services

Postabortion clients are often desperate to avoid another pregnancy. Hence, family planning is a critical component of postabortion care. Before the intervention, only 42 percent of patients received any counseling on ways to prevent additional unwanted pregnancies. Scant information was provided about the benefits of family planning in general, the existence of various methods, or the advantages and disadvantages of each. Among the 55 patients who received some counseling, fewer than one in five felt confident enough to ask questions about family planning during the session. Only 25 percent of those patients felt that the amount of time devoted to counseling was sufficient. Seventy percent of patients left the hospital without a contraceptive method. Condoms were generally not provided and supplies of injectables were in chronically short supply, so that women's choices were usually limited to oral contraceptives (when available), the intrauterine device (IUD), or tubal ligation.

The picture was no less worrisome with regard to the 39 women who received a contraceptive method. According to medical records, 19 postabortion patients received a hormonal injection, 13 had an IUD inserted, and seven were sterilized; however, these numbers did not fully correspond to the methods for which women had expressed a preference during the interviews, either because those methods were not available prior to hospital discharge, or because one of the providers convinced them that another method would be more appropriate for them at that time (Langer et al. 1997). Furthermore, six women who reported not having had an IUD inserted or a tubal ligation performed were found to have these procedures noted in their clinical chart, strongly suggesting that they were performed without the woman's knowledge.

Our intervention thus faced the twin challenge of promoting greater access to postabortion family planning and seeking to halt violations of patients' rights within the family planning service.

THE INTERVENTION: IMPROVING THE QUALITY OF POSTABORTION CARE

The Oaxaca hospital staff members were presented with the baseline findings outlined above during two brainstorming workshops. Many offered suggestions for improving services in spite of the perceived shortage of time and resources. In collaboration with hospital staff, an intervention and training program for the hospital was designed, beginning with a series of "quality circles." The objective of these meetings was to identify ways to improve quality, using the seven elements of quality of care outlined in Box 1.

The quality circle meetings consisted of an exchange of ideas in a setting in which every participant's input was valued and taken into account. This process was unusual, in that health care workers (staff physicians, residents, interns, registered nurses, nurses' aides, and social workers) are seldom given the opportunity to interact on an equal basis regardless of their rank. In addition, staff were offered the opportunity to make decisions about the intervention rather than simply carry out orders after changes in procedures had already been made.

Several priorities were established. Some required outside training and others required modification of hospital logistics and procedures. The intervention plan included most of the elements of the quality-of-care framework, as outlined below.

Technology, Technical Capacity, and Equipment

A decision was made to provide MVA training to all attending medical personnel so that the technique could be used instead of D&C wherever appropriate. Hospital physicians and administrators prepared a protocol for the treatment and care of patients with incomplete abortion. The main modification stipulated that if a patient's uterus was estimated to be smaller than 12 cm she would undergo uterine evacuation using MVA with local anesthesia and would be given analgesics before and after the procedure.

The hospital designated several physicians to become master trainers in MVA and sponsored their participation in an intensive training program, which included demonstrations followed by supervised practice and monitoring. The master trainer course used Ipas equipment (i.e., cannulas, dilators, vacuum syringes) and training materials. The latter addressed issues relevant to the improvement of technical competence as well as postabortion contraceptive counseling and the more humane treatment of postabortion patients. Master trainers were then to instruct their junior colleagues and residents and provide supervision and follow-up training.

There was some initial resistance to MVA among physicians. As one senior physician commented:

> In general I'm very reserved about employing apparently new procedures, given that sometimes they are not procedures that are appropriate for our way of seeing the world, of working, of practicing medicine here at this level, nor of solving the medical problems of our patients.

Another staff physician was concerned that MVA would not be accepted by the patient population:

> If I tell the patient and her relatives that she'll be leaving the hospital soon, they'll think "They won't give her the right treatment then, that's for sure."

Humane Treatment and Information Exchange

Staff agreed on the need to reduce waiting time, improve pain management, and improve interpersonal relations. This last step included emphasizing patient privacy and dignity, providing sensitive support for patients' needs, avoiding punitive attitudes, and delivering appropriate information throughout the period of diagnosis, treatment, and recovery.

To reduce waiting time, it was determined that all operating rooms would function 24 hours a day, seven days a week, to provide timely attention to postabortion patients arriving at the hospital at night and on the weekends. Shortened waiting times would also reduce the amount of time women spent in pain.

All staff were invited to participate in a two-day, 14-hour workshop on interpersonal relations. The intent of this workshop was to sensitize providers to the psychosocial realities of the abortion experience, modify providers' often negative attitudes toward postabortion patients, and emphasize the importance of compassion, human warmth, and two-way communication. Physicians, residents, nurses, assistant nurses, and social workers participated. Each workshop consisted of four modules: (1) initial contact with the patient; (2) anxiety and information management; (3) how to accompany and counsel the patient from admission through discharge; and (4) roles of health staff. Experts in Gestalt therapy techniques led the participating obstetrics/gynecology staff in sessions using interactive talks, role-playing, meditation, relaxation exercises, and imagery techniques to recreate the abortion experience through the patients' eyes and thereby enhance providers' empathy.

As a result of this workshop and the quality circle meetings, staff agreed to several concrete procedural changes to protect women's privacy and dignity. For example, staff agreed to provide sheets to cover patients and to eliminate shaving of pubic hair from preoperative procedures.

Written materials were developed to reiterate the most important points covered in the workshops. Copies of a poster entitled "Quality and Warmth in the Care of Postabortion Patients" were distributed for display to remind medical staff of information that should be provided to all postabortion patients and the humane and comprehensive manner in which it should be delivered (see Box 2).

In addition to the poster, an illustrated brochure entitled "Your Health Comes First" was developed to give to patients before they left the hospital. The brochure served as written counseling guidelines for nurses and other staff members and as a take-home reminder for the patient about potential complications (e.g., prolonged or heavier bleeding), self-care during recovery (e.g., the importance of having access to a trusted friend or relative in case she feels depressed, which is common following abortion), and the date of the patient's scheduled follow-up appointment.

Family Planning Counseling and Services

Within the range of broader reproductive health services called for by the quality-of-care framework, priority was placed on postabortion contraceptive counseling and the provision of methods to women who chose to use them. Upon request by the hospital nurses and social workers, Ipas provided training in postabortion family planning counseling. The training emphasized that, at a minimum, all postabortion patients should be provided with information on: (1) the possibility and dangers of getting pregnant before their next menstrual period; (2) the mechanisms of action, advantages, and disadvantages of safe and effective methods to avoid or postpone pregnancy; and (3) the availability and accessibility of immediate and future family planning services based on an assessment of women's needs and their fully informed consent (Leonard and Ladipo 1994). This last component was intended to bring attention to the importance of voluntarism in contraceptive use and to explore why some sexually active women who did not want to become pregnant would still choose not to use contraception. Providers were not trained to tailor contraceptive counseling for women who lost a wanted pregnancy and were eager to get pregnant again.

Box 2. Poster for providers entitled "Quality and Warmth in the Care of Postabortion Patients"

1. Remember that your patient needs you in these difficult moments.
2. Ask her name and tell her yours.
3. Ask how she feels.
4. Show interest in her and listen attentively to her.
5. Take into consideration your patient's modesty. If there is no private space, leave while she undresses.
6. Before examining her, cover her with a sheet.
7. Give her detailed information about the treatment itself and what is happening to her.
8. Offer her emotional support.
9. Answer her questions and help her express her fears.
10. Try to alleviate your patient's pain by treating her as soon as possible.
11. Inform her of the procedure step-by-step, and tell her about her state of recovery.
12. Give her counseling about family planning, cervical and breast cancer screening, and STIs, including AIDS.
13. Before hospital discharge, make sure that she knows how to recognize warning signs and where to go should they occur.
14. Convince her of the importance of a follow-up visit and give her an appointment or refer her to the corresponding health center.
15. Make sure you answer any remaining questions that she might have.
16. Say a friendly goodbye.

In order to broaden contraceptive choice by ensuring a more readily available supply of hormonal contraceptives and condoms, hospital administrators asked the central level of the Ministry of Health to provide a more steady supply.

Along with instructions for posthospitalization self-care, the patient brochure included information about fertility, contraception, and reproductive health. For example, it explained the nearly immediate return to fertility, described the contraceptive methods available to avoid pregnancy, and encouraged women to involve their partners in any contraceptive decisionmaking. Broader reproductive health issues were also touched on: The brochure mentioned some of the symptoms of sexually transmitted infections and the importance of seeking treatment for both partners, and it encouraged women to get Pap smears for cervical cancer screening and to perform breast self-examinations.

RESULTS OF THE INTERVENTION

After the intervention, we conducted a follow-up assessment of postabortion care quality that was, again, based on review of medical records and observations of and interviews with providers and women seeking care for complications of abortion.

Technology, Technical Capacity, and Equipment

After the intervention, staff began performing MVA more readily, and the number of patients treated with MVA and local anesthesia jumped from less than one percent to 78 percent (see Table 1). In a postintervention interview, one of the physicians commented on acceptance of the new technique: "The residents take their [MVA] equipment with them when they go out to the field—that's by way of saying that not only do they accept it but they also incorporate it as part of their routine and, little by little, disseminate it." Because the complication rate with D&C was already quite low at this hospital, no significant reduction in complications was observed. Nonetheless, greater use of MVA yielded other benefits by contributing to reductions in waiting times—both before and after the procedure—as discussed further below. One nurse commented: "MVA is a less traumatic technique, less aggressive for the patient. . . . Since they are no longer administered general anesthesia, they are not exposed to the risks [that its use] implies."

Humane Treatment and Information Exchange

Waiting time. While the time spent waiting to be admitted to the hospital did not change, the average time spent between hospital admission and surgery declined slightly—but significantly—from 13.3 to 10.5 hours, primarily as a result of changes in hospital routine and providers' attitudes. This was particularly important because it meant that women in pain did not have to wait as long for surgery. Some of the factors that contributed to this decrease were the use of all obstetrics/gynecology operating rooms 24 hours a day (so that women who arrived at night no longer had to wait until the next morning for their procedure); the type of anesthesia used (a cervical block, the administration of which does not require an anesthesiologist); and the cooperation of the staff. One physician commented:

> When the MVA program was implemented, things changed. The operating rooms were opened on a permanent basis in order to have all the materials and personnel available to provide the fastest possible care to the woman to keep her from suffering any longer.

In addition, average postprocedure inpatient time diminished by more than one-third, from 18.2 to 11.6 hours. As a result of the intervention, women spent an average of 11 hours less (a 36 percent reduction) in the hospital overall. These reductions in postprocedure and overall hospitalization time are both statistically significant.

Appropriate pain management. Reports of pain during the procedure actually increased with the shift from D&C to MVA, largely because MVA patients do not receive general anesthesia and are alert throughout the procedure. As one nurse commented, "Now the patients come out of the operating room without as much sedation so they recover faster and can be discharged sooner." Because acute pain is common

Table 1. Postabortion care, pre- and postintervention

Component of postabortion care	Preintervention % (no. of women)[a]	Postintervention % (no. of women)[a]
Procedure used for uterine evacuation		
MVA (%)	0.0 (144)	78.1* (178)
D&C (%)	89.6 (144)	20.8* (178)
Combination D&C and MVA (%)	10.4 (144)	1.1* (178)
Waiting time		
Before uterine evacuation (average in hours)	13.3 (132)	10.5* (207)
After uterine evacuation (average in hours)	18.2 (132)	11.6* (207)
Total length of stay in hospital (average in hours)	29.5 (132)	18.9* (207)
Pain management		
General anesthesia during the procedure (%)	91.2 (136)	29.7* (209)
Moderate to intense pain after the procedure (%)	9.8 (136)	19.8* (207)
Privacy		
Fewer than four people present during initial exam (%)	84.1 (129)	89.9 (198)
Respectful communication		
Patient knew who attending physician was (%)	17.4 (132)	74.4* (199)
Physician introduced him/herself (%)	26.1 (23)	51.0* (147)
Physician addressed patient by name (%)	59.1 (22)	84.8* (145)
Physician explained diagnosis before the procedure (%)	45.5 (22)	92.4* (131)
Patient received information about		
Warning signs of possible complications (%)	3.0 (132)	50.7* (207)
When to resume normal activities (%)	7.6 (132)	27.1* (207)
When to resume sexual relations (%)	14.4 (132)	38.8* (206)
Immediate return to fertility (%)	19.1 (131)	54.4* (204)
Patient satisfied with information received (%)	17.6 (132)	72.5* (207)
Contraceptive counseling		
Patient received some counseling (%)	42.4 (132)	85.5* (207)
Patients counseled by attending physician (%)	8.9 (56)	45.8* (177)
Patients felt confident enough to ask contraceptive questions (%)	18.2 (55)	28.4* (176)
Amount of counseling time was sufficient (%)	25.0 (56)	58.0* (174)
Satisfaction with information received (%)	74.5 (55)	94.2* (173)
Satisfaction with the way treated (%)	89.1 (55)	97.1* (175)
Contraception		
Any method provided (%)	29.5 (132)	59.7* (206)
Methods prescribed:		
Hormonal injectables (%)	48.7 (39)	51.2 (123)
IUDs (%)	33.3 (39)	16.3 (123)
Tubal ligations (%)	17.9 (39)	10.6 (123)
Oral contraceptives (%)	0.0 (39)	13.0 (123)

Note: For more detailed information, see Langer et al. 1999.
* $p < 0.05$, after adjusting for differences in level of schooling, parity, and desire for future pregnancy.
[a] Represents total number of women for whom information is available; variation is due to medical eligibility criteria or missing cases.

and nearly inevitable unless good local anesthesia is provided, these results may suggest that the use of anesthesia during the MVA procedure and subsequent administration of analgesics were not adequate. Some of the physicians interviewed believed that the pain could be attributed to an insufficient waiting period between application of the paracervical anesthetic and the beginning of the surgical procedure. It is also possible that analgesics are in short supply at the hospital and cannot be offered to all women preoperatively; some physicians may provide medication only to women in severe pain or may administer it only after the procedure is completed. Finally, physicians may wrongly interpret women's stoicism as an absence of pain—despite the project's efforts to modify this perception. While there was an increase in pain experienced following the procedure, only one in five women report more than mild pain during this period. Improved pain management is an important area for further investigation, and some work on this issue is underway.

The patients reported sensing the emotional support of the nurses when they experienced this pain, and this helped distract them so that time passed more quickly. One patient recalled: "I was complaining because it hurt, so the nurse came closer to me and started talking, started reminding me of other things, of my child, of my husband. . . ." The physicians, on the other hand, did not seem to be aware that women often experienced a great deal of pain during the procedure. As one physician commented: "Later on they say that they had a lot of pain, or that they had even been screaming. But in general they seem to be pretty calm."

Privacy. The physicians reported that they had become more sensitive to patients' needs for privacy and were interested in changing their attitudes. One doctor said, "We try at least to provide [the patients with] sheets . . ." while another doctor advised, "There's no need to rattle off [unnecessary or inappropriate] commentaries when the patient is being examined." In addition, staff instituted simple practices to protect the modesty and privacy of the patient. For example, a door was installed to replace the curtain on the outside of the examining room, and all postabortion patients were covered with a robe or sheet during the initial medical exam.

Despite these small measures, the intervention failed to promote adequate respect for the patient's privacy and sense of modesty. In part, this is because the hospital is a teaching facility for the state-run medical school, and the curriculum requires that medical students observe and practice all procedures. One nurse stated: "There are usually students present; sometimes the cleaning staff might even come in. That's why there's not total privacy during the initial medical evaluation." However, the nurses also expressed the opinion that the residents and interns were simply not concerned about respecting the patient's modesty.

Respectful communication. There was a notable shift toward greater compassion for the patient. Some providers expressed satisfaction with the new skills and perspectives they had acquired during the workshop. As one nurse said:

> *I learned that we as well as the doctors should put ourselves in the patients' shoes in order to understand all their needs, that apart from the physical ones are also emotional. . . . The course reminded me of a lot of things I had forgotten that I can use now to help the patient better. . . . [We] always use the pretext of not having enough time or having too many patients, but I think if we set our minds to it, with just five minutes during the time the procedure is being performed, we can talk with the patient."*

A physician's comments reflected a similar change in attitude: "Any woman, independent of her socioeconomic status, deserves to be treated well; at the very least, everybody has the right to simply be treated in a nice way."

Communication with women during the procedure improved significantly. Doctors and nurses came to share the belief that the patient should be amply informed about all aspects of her postabortion care, and that it was their responsibility to do so. Once inside the operating room, the physician tended to stay at the patient's side, and would even accompany the patient and talk with her while she was being transferred to the operating room from the waiting area. More than half (51 percent) of the attending physicians introduced themselves, compared to 26 percent before the intervention, and 85 percent addressed the patient by name, compared to 59 percent preintervention. Consequently, the proportion of women who knew which doctor had performed the procedure increased more than fourfold to 74 percent. In general, doctors and nurses took greater care and showed more kindness when situating the patient on the operating table and preparing her for the procedure. They also used this point of contact with the patient to explain the procedure—before it took place—to nearly all patients (92 percent, compared to 46 percent preintervention). All of these improvements in communication were statistically significant. An example of a providers' remarks to a patient after the intervention follows:

> *You're going to stay in the hospital because unfortunately you had a miscarriage. That means you've lost the baby. What you have now is an incomplete abortion, and what we're going to do is to clean out your womb. We're going to give you a few small shots so that you won't feel anything, and then we're going to do a little scraping on the inside. It is a minor surgical procedure, which is not dangerous but does require hospitalization. You might even possibly be ready to go home by 8 p.m. tonight, but you probably won't be discharged until tomorrow.*

While still far from perfect, the information was generally more precise and easier to understand than that provided before the intervention. As a result, more patients remembered the exact words health personnel had used to explain the diagnosis, treatment, and possible complications. Some physicians and residents provided this information, but the nurses played the greatest role. One nurse told us:

> *I asked [the patient] if she knew what they were going to do. She said she did, so I just wanted to confirm. 'Did they tell you that they were going to give [your womb] a little cleaning?' Because that's the way you've got to explain to them, that they're going to clean the womb using MVA. That's part of the routine now; I include it in my talks with patients without even thinking about it.*

A patient was also more likely to receive an explanation of what she might feel during the procedure, and the nurses were more likely to approach the patient to comfort her, sometimes on their own, sometimes following the resident's lead. One patient described her experience:

> *They took me directly to the operating room, and started explaining things to me. The doctor explained everything really well and boosted my morale. She told me, "This is the only pain that you're going to feel" as they gave me the anesthesia. Later I started to feel the room going around, but I heard the voice of the doctor telling me to calm down, everything would be all right.*

Postprocedure information and counseling also improved, with the majority of patients receiving spoken information and/or the illustrated brochure. Twenty-seven percent of postintervention patients received information on when to resume normal activities (e.g., strenuous household chores) compared to 8 percent before the intervention. Approximately three times as many patients received counseling on postabortion sexual activity (39 percent compared to 14 percent), and 54 percent received information on the nearly immediate return to fertility (compared to 19 percent preintervention). The percentage of women who showed an understanding about monitoring and responding to possible complications after leaving the hospital also increased. All of these improvements in postprocedure information and counseling are statistically significant.

Despite these improvements, postprocedure counseling is still far from adequate: Half of the women still did not receive any type of spoken information about postabortion care. There are several possible reasons for this. First, the distribution of written materials, rather than direct contact with the providers, may have provided necessary information for many women. Second, as expressed in the testimonies below, women are hesitant to engage the physician and do not always air their concerns:

> *I just assumed they were not going to tell me anything.*
>
> *They're going to say that I'm nosy.*

If I do ask, [the doctor's] going to scold me.

I was too embarrassed, I couldn't. I didn't feel confident enough.

Some women would wait for the nurse to ask questions. Others would read the brochure themselves and make it a topic of conversation among fellow patients on the ward. In these informal talks, the patients' questions and worries arose and were often discussed more openly than was the case during exchanges with the nursing staff.

Physicians, especially residents, recognize the difficulties they sometimes have when trying to understand and be understood by their patients. One doctor explained: "It seems as if we're speaking two different languages, because we explain things and they just don't understand." They suggested that ideally a specially trained staff member, preferably a psychologist, should be added to the medical team in order to tend specifically to patients' emotional needs.

Despite the lack of spoken communication with many patients, nearly three-quarters (73 percent, compared to 18 percent before the intervention) said they were satisfied with the information they received. This result was statistically significant. Family planning counseling also improved significantly, as outlined further below.

Family Planning Counseling and Services

Contraceptive counseling became a fairly standard component of postabortion care. Furthermore, the attending physician counseled almost half of the women directly. One of the staff obstetricians recognized this improvement: "Before, very little counseling was given, and really it was just a lot of propaganda in relation to contraceptive methods. At the present time we insist more on the counseling part."

Counseling sessions became increasingly interactive, and more women (28 percent, compared to 18 percent before the intervention) felt confident enough to ask questions about contraceptive methods. Twice as many patients (58 percent, compared to 25 percent before the intervention) felt that the amount of time devoted to counseling was sufficient, and more patients were satisfied with the information they received (94 percent compared to 75 percent) and the manner in which they were treated during contraceptive counseling (97 percent compared to 89 percent). All of these improvements are statistically significant. One patient's comments reflect this change:

> *The nurse told me that there are many methods to keep me from getting pregnant, and that if later on I decide to have another baby, I can stop using it. If not, I can choose [a permanent method]. She told me about a tubal ligation, monthly injections, the IUD, and pills, but said that it depends on the couple, on what we think, on what we decide.*

The effect of these changes was evident: The number of women who left the hospital with a contraceptive method doubled, from 30 percent to 60 percent. This result is statistically significant. Most women expressed a desire to prevent another pregnancy immediately, while the greatest concern of others was to end their child-bearing altogether. The Ministry of Health had begun to maintain the supply of hormonal contraceptives and condoms, in addition to the steady supply of IUDs already available. The proportion of patients who chose a tubal ligation decreased from 18 percent before the intervention to 11 percent postintervention, although the difference was not statistically significant. At the same time, awareness of and respect for patients' right to decide not to use a method was growing. As one provider said:

> I believe there should be no [obligation] for a [postabortion patient to accept] a contraceptive method prior to her discharge.

Family planning counseling was a new addition to the hospital's postabortion care service. As a result—and because no effort was made to distinguish between spontaneous and induced abortion cases during the intervention—this counseling was not explicitly tailored to the needs of women who might be eager to try to conceive again in the short term. In future interventions, all women should be asked about their fertility desires and pregnancy prevention needs, so that contraceptive advice can be provided based on these needs.

Improving quality and cost-effectiveness simultaneously. A cost analysis was undertaken as a corollary to the study. Its results indicate that the per patient costs of postabortion care services decreased from the equivalent in pesos of US$264 to US$180, as a result of the substitution of MVA for D&C (Brambila et al. 1999). Thus, efforts to improve quality of postabortion care that involve the substitution of more appropriate technologies can also improve their cost-effectiveness. Even if some elements of the effort to improve quality require more provider time and other resources than was the case before, costs per patient can be reduced. In the present case, the only cost that increased was that associated with the slight increase in nurses' time required to provide postabortion family planning counseling.

LESSONS LEARNED

Unsafe abortion is a critical public health problem in Latin America (Paxman et al. 1993), as well as in many other regions. Improving the quality of postabortion care is one feasible and effective way to improve outcomes among women who have experienced unsafe abortion and to create greater sensitivity to its health and human costs. This study and similar studies in Latin America and other parts of the developing world (Benson et al. 1998; Chambers and Saldaña-Rivera 1996; Díaz et al. 1999; Fuentes-Valázquez, Billings, and Cardona-Pérez 1998; Huntington and Nawar 1998; Solo et al. 1999) yield several important lessons:

- It is possible to improve the quality of postabortion care programs in hospitals, despite limited funding, staff, and medical supplies. Requirements include a commitment to training staff on a continuous basis, maintaining and replacing equipment, and ensuring a ready stock of supplies (e.g., analgesics and contraceptives). Indeed, quality improvement programs that include replacement of D&C with MVA can reduce the costs of postabortion care.

- A special focus on the improvement of interpersonal relationships can favorably modify the attitudes and practices of clinicians even with respect to sensitive matters like abortion. One practice our intervention was not able to modify, however, was pain management—perhaps because of a lack of analgesics in the hospital, which may have prompted providers to restrict use to the most "severe" cases. It may also reflect providers' entrenched punitive attitudes or their reluctance to recognize women's pain. Future efforts should emphasize the proper administration of pre- and postoperative analgesics and a sufficient waiting period between the application of local anesthesia and the MVA procedure.

- Efforts to improve communication must attend to the kind of information relayed, and how it is conveyed. Improving provider–patient interaction requires more than visual contact, a reassuring word or smile, and active listening. The provider and the patient must engage in a true, two-way dialogue.

- It is important to provide appropriate contraceptive counseling and a variety of method choices to postabortion patients. Providers have an obligation to treat the problem at hand first and later provide complete and truthful information about the array of available methods and to secure the woman's fully informed and free consent in advance of method provision. Ideally, providers should base their counseling on each woman's reproductive intentions, ascertaining whether or not the previous pregnancy was wanted but could not be sustained, or whether there is truly an unmet need for contraception that should be addressed in order to avoid a recurrence of unwanted pregnancy. Good provider training would cover all possible scenarios.

- While the intervention described in this chapter focused on improving the quality of postabortion care, including family planning counseling, postabortion care should include or refer women for other reproductive health and social services, such as management of sexually transmitted infections and gender violence counseling, if appropriate. In addition, postabortion care services ideally should encompass infertility counseling for women who suffer repeat spontaneous abortions.

Based on the success of this intervention in Oaxaca and with additional funding from the European Union, the Ministry of Health—with technical assistance from the Population Council and Ipas—is upgrading the Valdivieso Hospital in Oaxaca to a Regional Training Center of Excellence and improving upon and extending this model of care to two other states in Mexico. In addition, the Mexican Institute of Social Security has implemented various programs to introduce MVA into its clinics and otherwise improve the quality of postabortion care for women insured under this plan. As these improvements are increasingly institutionalized, Mexico will have taken an important step toward providing the kind of comprehensive reproductive health care to women that reflects the spirit of the 1994 International Conference on Population and Development.

Acknowledgments

The authors thank the European Union for its generous funding of the intervention. We also acknowledge the technical assistance provided by Ipas, and the collaboration of our colleagues at the Dr. Aurelio Valdivieso General Hospital, especially former director Arturo Molina, as well as Vilma Barahona, Francisca Ramírez, Beatriz Casas, and Felipe Pérez Zainos.

Notes

Some of the findings included in this chapter were also presented at various stages and discussed previously in Langer et al. 1997 and Langer et al. 1999.

1   The exception is Cuba, where abortion is legal and is generally performed under safe conditions.

2   When abortion is decriminalized, the criminal penalties associated with provision and procurement are removed. When it is legalized, it is validated or sanctioned under the law. Decriminalization is often referred to as the liberalization of abortion laws, and can sometimes be viewed as a step toward the legalization of abortion under all circumstances in countries where its practice is legally restricted.

3   This is the case partly because there are few reliable measures to accurately differentiate between induced and spontaneous abortions and partly to avoid implicating women in any illegal activity.

4   Ipas is a nonprofit agency that works globally to improve women's lives by focusing on reproductive health. Strategic initiatives include increasing women's access to high-quality elective abortion services and postabortion care and improving practice by putting appropriate reproductive health technologies in the hands of skilled providers.

5   MVA technology for uterine evacuation consists of a handheld vacuum syringe and flexible plastic cannula inserted into the cervical os with the application of a paracervical block or with no anesthesia, depending on the site/practitioner. The contents of the uterus are removed through the cannula using the manual syringe as a vacuum source. D&C is a surgical procedure that involves scraping the surface lining of the uterine wall with sharp curettes. In Mexico, general anesthesia is used. The stated advantages of MVA over D&C are that "suction curettage is more rapid (3 minute average),

less cervical dilation is necessary (thus, lessening the likelihood of cervical tears), fewer failed abortions result, less anesthesia and analgesia are required, blood loss is less, infection is less common, and there is less trauma to the uterus" (Benson and Pernoll 1994, p. 740).

References

Alan Guttmacher Institute. 1994. *Clandestine Abortion: A Latin American Reality*. New York: Alan Guttmacher Institute.

Benson, Jane, Victor Huapaya, Marian Abernathy, and John Nagahata. 1998. "Provider practices and patient perspectives in an integrated postabortion care model in Peru," paper presented at Global Meeting on Postabortion Care: Advances and Challenges in Operations Research, Population Council, New York, 19–21 January.

Benson, Ralph C. and Martin L. Pernoll. 1994. *Benson and Pernoll's Handbook of Obstetrics and Gynecology*, 9th ed. Singapore: McGraw-Hill, Health Professions Division.

Brambila, Carlos, Ana Langer, Cecilia García-Barrios, and Angela Heimburger. 1999. "Estimating costs of postabortion services at Dr. Aurelio Valdivieso General Hospital, Oaxaca, Mexico," in Dale Huntington and Nancy J. Piet-Pelon (eds.), *Postabortion Care: Lessons from Operations Research*. New York: Population Council, pp. 108–124.

Bruce, Judith. 1990. "Fundamental elements of the quality of care: A simple framework," *Studies in Family Planning* 21(2): 61–91.

Chambers, M. Virginia and Andrea Saldaña-Rivera. 1996. "Resumen de experiencias programáticas con la atención postaborto en México" [Summary of programmatic experiences in postabortion care in Mexico]. Mexico City: Ipas.

Díaz, Juan, Mariel Loayza, Yamile Torres de Yépez, Oscar Lora, Fernando Alvarez, and Virginia Camacho. 1999. "Improving the quality of services and contraceptive acceptance in the postabortion period in three public-sector hospitals in Bolivia," in Dale Huntington and Nancy J. Piet-Pelon (eds.), *Postabortion Care: Lessons from Operations Research*. New York: Population Council, pp. 61–79.

Fuentes-Valázquez, Jaime A., Deborah L. Billings, and Jorge Arturo Cardona-Pérez. 1998. "Women's experience of pain during postabortion care in Mexico," paper presented at Global Meeting on Postabortion Care: Advances and Challenges in Operations Research, Population Council, New York, 19–21 January.

Huntington, Dale and Laila Nawar. 1998. "Introducing improved postabortion care in Egypt: Moving from a pilot study to large-scale expansion," paper presented at Global Meeting on Postabortion Care: Advances and Challenges in Operations Research, Population Council, New York, 19–21 January.

Langer, Ana, Cecilia García-Barrios, Angela Heimburger, Lourdes Campero, Karen Stein, Beverly Winikoff, and Vilma Barahona. 1999. "Improving postabortion care with limited resources in a public hospital in Oaxaca, Mexico," in Dale Huntington and Nancy J. Piet-Pelon (eds.), *Postabortion Care: Lessons from Operations Research*. New York: Population Council, pp. 80–107.

Langer, Ana, Cecilia García-Barrios, Angela Heimburger, Karen Stein, Beverly Winikoff, Vilma Barahona, Beatriz Casas, and Francisca Ramírez. 1997. "Improving post-abortion care in a public hospital in Oaxaca, Mexico," *Reproductive Health Matters* 9: 20–28.

Leonard, Ann H. and O.A. Ladipo. 1994. "Post-abortion family planning: Factors in individual choice of contraceptive methods," *Advances in Abortion Care* 4(2). Carrboro, NC: Ipas.

Leonard, Ann H. and Judith Winkler. 1991. "A quality of care framework for abortion care," *Advances in Abortion Care* 1(1). Carrboro, NC: Ipas.

Paxman, John, Alberto Rizo, L. Brown, and J. Benson. 1993. "La epidemia clandestina: La práctica del aborto ilegal en América Latina" [Clandestine epidemic: The practice of illegal abortion in Latin America], *Perspectivas Internacionales en Planificación Familiar* [International family planning perspectives], special edition.

Rivas Zivy, Maria and Ana Amuchástegui. 1996. *Voces e Historias Sobre el Aborto* [Voices and stories about abortion]. Mexico City: EDAMEX and Population Council.

Romero, Mariana. 1994. "El aborto entre adolescentes" [Abortion among adolescents], in Adriana Ortiz Ortega (ed.), *Razones y Pasiones en Torno al Aborto* [Reasons and passions related to abortion]. Mexico City: EDAMEX and Population Council, pp. 242–245.

Secretaría de Salud. 1992. *La mujer adolescente, adulta, anciana y su salud* [Adolescents, adults, and older women and their health], report of the Dirección General de Salud Materno Infantil, Programa Nacional "Mujer, Salud y Desarrollo." Mexico City: Secretaría de Salud.

Solo, Julie, Deborah L. Billings, Colette Aloo-Obunga, Achola Ominde, and Margaret Makumi. 1999. "Creating linkages between incomplete abortion treatment and family planning services in Kenya," in Dale Huntington and Nancy J. Piet-Pelon (eds.), *Postabortion Care: Lessons from Operations Research*. New York: Population Council, pp. 38–60.

Contact information

Ana Langer
Director, Latin America and the Caribbean Regional Office
Population Council
Escondida 110, Col. Villa Coyoacán
México D.F. 04000 Mexico
telephone: 52-5554-0388
fax: 52-5554-1226
e-mail: alanger@popcouncil.org.mx

14

Addressing Gender Violence in a Reproductive and Sexual Health Program in Venezuela

Alessandra C. Guedes, Lynne Stevens, Judith F. Helzner, and Susana Medina

Gender-based violence is endemic in Venezuela, as it is in many other countries. Despite this fact, few organizations within the country address the problem. Family planning organizations have largely ignored it, because they see it as outside the purview of their mission. In the capital city of Caracas, only one organization, a feminist nongovernmental organization (NGO) called AVESA (for Asociación Venezolana para una Educación Sexual Alternativa, or Venezuelan Association for Alternative Sexual Education) had a well-established program to combat gender-based violence and assist victims. In concert with a broad Latin American feminist movement, AVESA has argued that violence is a sexual and reproductive health issue—and that bodily integrity is a human right. This is the story of how the staff at the Asociación Civil de Planificación Familiar (PLAFAM)—the International Planned Parenthood Federation/Western Hemisphere Region (IPPF/WHR) affiliate in Venezuela—came to share that vision, to recognize the effect that women's social context has on its clients' sexual and reproductive health, and to meet the needs of victims of violence. Although PLAFAM has already learned many lessons about integrating work on gender-based violence into its sexual and reproductive health programs, the ongoing project described in this chapter has little precedent. As such, it proceeds, in part, by trial and error.

GENDER-BASED VIOLENCE IN VENEZUELA

In Venezuela, as elsewhere, there are few reliable data on the overall prevalence of gender-based violence. Available data come mostly from the small number of cases reported to the authorities or, occasionally, to NGOs. Because such data are not always reliably gathered and because gender-based violence tends to be greatly underreported, these statistics are not likely to present an accurate picture of the true scope of the problem. Nonetheless, they suggest that gender-based violence is commonplace. In Caracas, 40 percent of women who seek hospital emergency services report having been beaten by their partners; 89 percent of violence victims had been treated previously for problems related to violence (Davies 1998). The Justice of Peace,[1] which handles cases involving disputes between families or neighbors, receives ten complaints of violence every day in Caracas; 97 percent of its caseload involves domestic violence perpetrated against women and children (Calzadilla 1998). The abuse is not limited to battering. In Venezuela an average of 12 women report being raped every day; 72 percent of these women are under the age of 19, and most are raped by someone they know (AVESA 1998a). Because the majority of victims do not dare report the abuse to authorities, these figures represent only a fraction of the true prevalence of violence against women.

The existence of such violence is minimized, rationalized, and denied by individuals from every social class. Yelling, slapping, and hitting a partner with an object are often called "lovers' troubles" (AVESA 1998b). Aggressors who are detained by police are generally released without any sanctions, allowing the pattern of violence to continue unchecked.

WHERE PLAFAM BEGAN

Throughout the 1970s and 1980s, PLAFAM offered medical services, including family planning, gynecological services, antenatal care, testing for sexually transmitted infections (STIs), basic infertility services, and ambulatory surgery such as tubal ligation. By the mid-1990s, it was operating three clinics (one expressly for adolescents, and two outside of Caracas). By 1995 PLAFAM was conducting about 1,000 family planning visits each month, primarily from its central clinic in Caracas. Counseling activities were introduced in 1986, but addressed only family planning.

Staff realized that they were seeing women who were the victims of violence, usually at the hands of their partners. For many years, most staff did not see a connection between violence and sexual and reproductive health. Some wanted to help but lacked the skills to do so. Fearful of what could emerge if they initiated a discussion of violence, they likened the experience to opening Pandora's box. As one staff member put it: "The organization had no mechanism that helped me to help a woman who had been abused. I did not know what to do." When a client was bold or desperate enough to initiate a discussion of the topic, she was referred to AVESA for psychological and legal counseling. This precarious arrangement, by which a staff member at

PLAFAM would telephone AVESA to alert staff there that a client was being referred, did not allow for continuity of care or appropriate follow-up by PLAFAM. The staff member would provide the client with AVESA's address, telephone number, and the name of a contact. Clients who decided to use AVESA's services negotiated fees on a sliding scale, with a maximum fee of approximately US$7. Because of time constraints and safety concerns associated with contacting victims of violence, staff were not always able to follow up to determine whether the woman had reached AVESA or whether the services she received had been helpful.

In July 1997 PLAFAM'S executive director and its information, education, and communication (IEC) director attended a two-day IPPF/WHR workshop in New York designed to sensitize affiliate leaders to the prevalence of violence and to delineate its connection to sexual and reproductive health. The workshop included exercises, role-plays, and didactic material that examined how such violence affects victims, why it is not discussed, how to introduce the topic to staff, and possible programmatic responses.

CONFRONTING "LOVERS' QUARRELS": SENSITIZING STAFF

Upon returning to Venezuela, PLAFAM's leaders decided to find a way to address violence in their services. They showed PLAFAM staff *The Tribunal of Vienna,* a documentary film of the testimony of victims of violence who spoke at the International Conference on Human Rights in 1993. The documentary, along with the ensuing discussion, illustrated the overwhelming frequency and devastating impact of violence against women. It also helped staff realize that this issue hit close to home and involved not only the clients they treated professionally but also many individuals they knew socially, including members of their own families. They talked about the use of the "lovers' quarrel" euphemism as a way to ignore and excuse a serious problem. They also explored the ways that the fear of violence affects a woman's health and impedes her ability to use contraception or protect herself from STIs. Staff, who had sent a representative to the 1994 International Conference on Population and Development in Cairo and discussed its outcomes and their relevance to PLAFAM's mission, agreed that they needed to help clients who were experiencing violence.

PLAFAM adopted three key strategies: (1) increasing staff awareness of violence and developing their skills to identify, assess, counsel, and appropriately refer violence victims; (2) developing and procuring materials for clients on violence and sources of support; and (3) collaborating with existing community alliances that engage in advocacy against violence. Each of these activities is described below.

The initiative began in September 1997 with a two-day awareness workshop for every employee, including clerical and technical staff, janitors, and receptionists in addition to administrators, clinicians, and counselors. The rationale for involving all employees was twofold. First, PLAFAM recognized that if the project was to succeed, all staff would need to be aware and convinced of the relevance of violence to sexual and reproductive health, the organization's main mission. Second, many types of staff would need to be involved in identifying and assisting victims for maximum project effectiveness. The workshop was led by the IEC director, a consultant on gender, and a Venezuelan feminist with expertise in group dynamics and violence issues. The objectives were to enable staff to (1) gain a conceptual understanding of gender violence; (2) understand the personal and interpersonal effects of gender violence; and (3) design a plan of action compatible with PLAFAM's mission and resources.

Participants began to understand the effect of violence on women's reproductive and sexual health. They also learned that when clinic staff pose questions about violence in a sensitive and nonjudgmental manner, many clients will talk about their experiences. Moreover, they realized that as the only health care agency many women visit, PLAFAM was in a unique position to assist women who were experiencing violence. As they began to rethink the ways they could help these women, the participants' apprehensions diminished. As one counselor explained: "I knew something about gender-based violence, but before the workshop I felt anxiety whenever the topic arose."

HELPING WITHOUT FIXING: REORIENTING STAFF

The next stage of staff development emphasized allowing staff to determine how they would use this new knowledge in their work. It moved beyond sensitization to assisting providers in defining their roles, teaching them how to identify victims' symptoms, and finding ways to lift the barriers to clients' disclosure. Staff worked on techniques to initiate discussion with clients, and also began to explore how working with victims of violence might affect them personally.

A three-day skills training workshop for all clinicians, counselors, administrators, and receptionists was held in June 1998. Staff responded positively to the initial exercises, which focused on internal and external barriers to integrating violence into their work. However, by the second day of training, the providers began to realize that they were being asked to make radical changes to the way they worked, from actively doing or giving something concrete to clients (e.g., a physical exam or a contraceptive) to what they perceived as more passive engagement of clients (e.g., offering support, listening nonjudgmentally, and providing referrals to qualified professionals). Participants became anxious and overwhelmed. They expressed concern that if they raised the topic of violence they would upset the client without being able to provide her with tangible ways to handle her psychological pain and "fix" the trauma. Participants also expressed anxiety that clients would require more than they would be able to provide. Furthermore, participants worried that they were being required to add an additional assignment to their already busy schedule and that they would fail.

On the third day, the participants engaged in role-plays. As "clients," they were better able to appreciate both the hesitation about and the relief of disclosing violence, and saw how helpful it was to have someone listen carefully and communicate a sense of caring and concern. As "staff," they could feel the client's palpable relief at disclosure and her appreciation for being listened to and cared for. Staff, initially concerned that they could not fix clients' dilemmas, found that disclosure and emotional support were useful and helpful in and of themselves.

Even with training, staff capacity would be inadequate to deal with the many requirements of clients who revealed violence. As a result, PLAFAM recruited a project coordinator (a psychologist), who was to oversee the project in all clinic sites, and two part-time psychologists, who were responsible for conducting in-depth follow-up assessments of clients who disclosed violence, providing counseling in individual and group settings, and convening support groups to help staff deal with difficult cases and respond to the feelings that emerged as they listened to women's painful stories. Because none of the psychologists had prior direct experience with gender-based violence counseling, PLAFAM arranged training in collaboration with AVESA that included three-month part-time internships at AVESA.

REORIENTING SERVICES TO ADDRESS VIOLENCE IN CLIENTS' INTIMATE RELATIONSHIPS

In addition to helping clients who were experiencing gender-based violence, PLAFAM staff wanted to educate all of its clients about violence. To alert clients that PLAFAM was a safe place to talk about a previously taboo topic, staff used a range of print materials, including:

- Posters on the clinic walls telling clients that violence is common but unacceptable and informing them that help is available at PLAFAM.
- A booklet of examples of acts that constitute physical, psychological, and sexual violence and information on where clients can go for legal, medical, and psychological help.
- Two-sided bookmarks, with information on violence on one side and referral numbers on the other.

These materials were placed in the waiting room, consulting rooms, and bathroom. Staff felt that the materials would help some clients feel more comfortable discussing violence with their counselor. If some women were not ready to explore the issue during the clinic visit, they could keep the bookmark until they felt ready to make a call or visit one of the referral facilities. Clients could also take the literature with them and pass it on to a friend or relative.

SCREENING FOR VIOLENCE

Attention to the topic of violence begins as soon as a new client checks in for her appointment.[2] To help prepare her for the sensitive questions that will follow, the receptionist describes PLAFAM's services, including those related to violence.[3] A counselor (most likely a social worker or educator) then takes the client to a private office and follows a general protocol that was developed during the three-day skills training workshop to introduce the topic of violence and screen the client. Although a special form was developed for this purpose, it was found to be too time-consuming and repetitive, and was never used. In the early stages of the project, counselors thus used their own discretion in introducing the topic of gender violence and asking related questions. Later in the project a more systematic and specific protocol was adopted, which requires:

- Investing extra effort in establishing rapport while asking preliminary general questions.
- Explaining that PLAFAM is concerned about the high incidence of abuse and the lack of safe, supportive places where women can discuss this problem— and that, for this reason, counselors ask all new clients the same set of questions. The client may decline to be screened.
- Asking the client four direct questions to assess whether she has experienced emotional, physical, and sexual violence, including sexual violence in childhood (the process used to develop this tool is described later in this chapter). The counselor asks about specific behaviors because many women do not view such behaviors as abusive or label themselves as victims of abuse.
- Observing other clues (e.g., affective change, nonverbal communication) that suggest the client is extremely anxious about the topic.
- Documenting the client's answers and other observations in her chart.
- Asking two questions to assess a victim's current safety and, if needed, taking appropriate steps, such as assisting with the development of a safety plan.

If a woman answers "yes" to any of the questions about exposure to violence, the counselor's job is to listen, provide emotional support, and inform the woman about the availability of a voluntary in-depth consultation with the staff psychologist, who can better identify her needs and help her determine the best course of action. A client who chooses to have an in-depth consultation is sent directly to the psychologist before undergoing her clinical exam. If a woman is distressed and a psychologist is not available, the counselor provides the client with emotional support before she continues on to her clinical exam. (PLAFAM recently hired two additional psychologists to ensure that women who wish to see a psychologist will, in most instances, be able to do so immediately.)

The psychologist conducts an in-depth evaluation and a more thorough risk assessment[4] to document the client's history of violence and to assess the seriousness of her symptoms, her current vulnerability, and whether and how the violence is affecting her children. On the basis of this information, the psychologist identifies the types of services the client may need. If the psychologist determines that a client is in imminent danger, she will try to help her formulate a safety plan, if that is the client's choice. Safety strategies can include memorizing important phone numbers, opening a bank account in the woman's own name, rehearsing an escape plan, and/or leaving extra money, copies of important documents, and a change of clothes with a trusted friend or relative.

Onsite referrals may include: (1) follow-up individual counseling; (2) further assessment by the psychologist, if necessary; or (3) if the client has been recently battered, a consultation and exam with the PLAFAM physician, who will document her physical injuries, sometimes using a "body map."[5] The psychologist may also make outside referrals to social, psychological, and legal agencies listed in the resource directory (see below) and call agency staff to inform them of the referral. After the psychological assessment, the client may choose to complete her visit and obtain the services for which she originally came, generally on the same day. If the woman has run out of time or is too distraught to undergo her medical consultation, her visit may be rescheduled.

Clinicians, too, have been trained to recognize symptoms of violence by observing marks on the body, to be responsive if a client chooses to disclose that she is being abused, and to provide related counseling. If a client has already discussed the issue of violence with a counselor and/or psychologist, her chart provides the clinician with this information. A client who states during the initial interview that she has not experienced violence may choose subsequently to disclose its occurrence to the clinician. This may happen because the clinician has asked the client about it in response to psychological or physical symptoms, or it may occur in response to the concerns noted on the chart by the counselor. Alternatively, the client may feel able to disclose it spontaneously with this particular person at this point in her visit. Then, if the client chooses, she is referred to the psychologist for the in-depth assessment and appropriate referrals. Depending on the client's emotional state, the clinical exam is completed, interrupted and continued later, or rescheduled for another day.

OFF-SITE REFERRALS

To provide clients with safe and useful referrals, PLAFAM set out to learn about other agencies involved in work related to violence. The agency hired a consulting psychologist to develop a directory of psychological, social, and legal organizations in or near Caracas for women exposed to violence. The psychologist created a questionnaire to evaluate the type and quality of assistance each organization offered. Eight key organizations were asked 17 questions about the populations they served, the services they provided, and whether and how they handled the referrals they received. She also identified other organizations that provide services to victims of violence. The results were compiled into the *Institutional Directory of Gender-based Violence Service Providers*. The directory has three sections: The first defines violence, violence prevention, and gender; the second describes in detail 25 institutions to which referrals can be made for various legal, social, and other services; and the last is an index that can be used to cross-reference referrals. PLAFAM gives each of its counselors a copy of the directory and instructions on how to use it.

JOINING THE ANTI-VIOLENCE ADVOCACY COMMUNITY

Venezuela had never had a law regarding gender-based violence. PLAFAM joined an alliance of feminist NGOs working to sensitize Venezuelan parliamentarians about gender-based violence and the need for a law that addressed it. PLAFAM had some experience with advocacy, particularly in the area of adolescent sexual health. While the feminist groups thought it was unusual for a reproductive health NGO to become involved in the topic of violence, PLAFAM was welcomed, in part because of its efforts to sensitize the feminist community to the connection between gender violence and sexual and reproductive health. To promote the law on violence, which had been stalled in the National Congress for years, PLAFAM, in collaboration with other NGOs, engaged in advocacy activities such as developing mass-media campaigns (using television, radio, and print media); distributing flyers in public places, including subway stations; and co-organizing demonstrations outside and inside the National Congress. All of these activities were focused on increasing public awareness about gender violence with messages about its pervasiveness and unacceptability and promoting rapid passage of the anti-violence bill.

In 1999, a law was passed outlawing both violence against women and violence within families. This was a major victory for PLAFAM and the advocacy alliance the agency had joined. To publicize the law, PLAFAM is distributing flyers in its waiting room that describe women's rights under the law, and potential avenues of action and redress.

PLAFAM'S NEW PROGRAM IN PRACTICE

When PLAFAM staff began screening women for violence, they had many questions. Would clients readily disclose their experiences with violence? Would they resent the invasion of their privacy? Would the counselors feel overwhelmed? Would the service make a difference in women's lives?

It did not take long for the staff to feel the effects of the new initiative. The very first client interviewed disclosed a history of incest, was given the opportunity to explore its impact with the counselor, and expressed appreciation for being asked about abuse. Efforts to measure progress more systematically were initially hampered by the evolving nature of the assessment tools. As noted earlier, the screening form initially developed was never integrated into the screening protocol. Whether and how the counselors introduced the topic of gender violence and asked related questions was left to their discretion. Without a concise and standardized set of questions, the process of screening was challenging and difficult to document.

In an effort to standardize the screening process and to reduce the time required for this task, four IPPF/WHR affiliates and the IPPF/WHR regional office jointly created an abridged screening form that contained four questions addressing psychological/emotional violence, physical violence, sexual violence, and sexual violence in childhood (see Box 1). If a woman responds affirmatively to these questions, two additional questions are asked to assess her current safety: "Are you afraid of your partner or another person close to you?" and "Will you be safe when you return home from PLAFAM?" Based largely on previously validated screening tools, this abridged form has been adapted to the Venezuelan context and is currently being tested.[6] The form requires between four and ten minutes to administer, depending on the client's responses.

The prevalence of gender violence detected among women with this form is striking: Over one-third (38 percent) of new clients were identified as victims of violence, compared to only 7 percent when the counselors relied on unsystematic screening. At the central clinic, where the most complete data are available, 161 clients were determined to be victims of gender violence between September and November 1999 (see Table 1).[7] The majority of cases involved psychological violence (61 percent), followed by childhood sexual abuse (44 percent), physical violence (42 percent), and sexual violence (34 percent).

There are several likely reasons for the increase in the prevalence of violence detected with the new screening form. First and foremost, all new clients are screened using the form. In addition, the more systematic approach, coupled with counselors' greater reported comfort with the process, may contribute to a higher response rate among those screened. Another contributing factor may be the approval and increased public awareness

---

Box 1. Abridged screening form for victims of gender violence

Case number: Date: Name of counselor:

Introduction. You know, at PLAFAM we offer education and services about domestic violence, violence in the workplace, and violence in childhood. There are many types of violence that affect a great number of women, and many women living in violent situations have found it helpful to receive assistance for themselves and their children. We at PLAFAM are concerned about the well-being of our clients and we always ask these questions in a confidential manner.

1. Psychological/emotional violence in the family. Have you ever felt hurt emotionally or psychologically by your partner or another person important to you? (For example, constant insults, humiliation at home or in public, destruction of objects you felt close to, ridicule, rejection, manipulation, threats, isolation from friends or family members, and so forth.)

❑ Yes   ❑ No   Who _____

When _____ How _____

2. Physical violence. Has your partner or another person important to you ever caused you physical harm? (For example, hitting, cutting, or burning you?)

❑ Yes   ❑ No   Who _____

When _____ How _____

3. Sexual violence. Were you ever forced to have sexual contact or intercourse?

❑ Yes   ❑ No   Who _____

When _____ How _____

4. Sexual violence in childhood. When you were a child, were you ever touched in a way that made you feel uncomfortable?

❑ Yes   ❑ No   Who _____

When _____ How _____

---

of the new law against domestic violence, which was passed shortly before the new screening form was instituted. The increased public discussion that resulted from the advocacy campaign undertaken by PLAFAM and feminist NGOs and the passage of the law may have made the topic more "discussable."

While clients' responses to PLAFAM's new services have not been systematically assessed, several smaller-scale efforts to document women's views have yielded preliminary feedback. When women have voiced complaints, they have stemmed primarily from their frustration with the legal system, which tends not to respond as quickly as they expect. The vast majority of reactions, however, have been positive:

> *I had never had the help of a psychologist. If I had not come here, I don't know what I would have done, where I would have gone. I could have even taken my life; it was a matter of disappearing.*

Table 1. Number and percentage[a] of clients identified as victims of gender-based violence in PLAFAM's central clinic, Caracas, Venezuela, September–November 1999

Total no. of new clients (%)	No. of clients identified as victims of gender-based violence (%)	Cases of psychological violence (%)	Cases of physical violence (%)	Cases of sexual violence (%)	Cases with a history of childhood sexual abuse (%)
429 (100)	161 (38)	99 (61)	68 (42)	55 (34)	71 (44)

[a] Percentages of types of violence total more than 100 percent because some women experience multiple types of violence.

I feel much better now [that] I confront things [including my abuser]. . . . I invite my friends to come to PLAFAM, too. If I had known about this before, imagine how many problems I could have avoided. The thing is that we are not going to talk about our problems to anyone because we think that there's nobody to help but we can always find a friendly hand.

Before coming to this clinic, I felt like anyone could step over me. Now I feel safe. . . . Staff provided me with a lot of support. [Now] nobody can do to me what they did when I was a little girl. I don't feel bad saying that I went through . . . this bad experience.

In addition, many clients have taken the educational materials to use or pass on to others. As word of the services spreads, some women have started to come to PLAFAM specifically for services related to violence.

Staff at the clinics have been sensitized so effectively to this issue that the cleaning woman, the watchman, and the receptionist have all referred women themselves. Counselors derive a great sense of satisfaction:

In the beginning, it was very complicated for me to ask people [about violence] because I thought, "What are they going to say?"; maybe they don't want someone meddling in their lives. Well, to my surprise, it's been the opposite. It turns out that women are waiting for someone to ask them about this topic. It's incredible but I believe that when we ask, women think: "Finally someone is giving me the chance to talk about this suffering." I think this is an accomplishment.

It's really incredible to be able to help somebody who arrives for a cytology appointment and leaves here thanking us because in addition to that, we've been able to help her with her relationships.

To me, this has been one of PLAFAM's initiatives that has more closely met the real needs of clients. . . . [Violence] affects most of the population that attends the clinic.

The issue of violence is something that is very close to women's hearts and the fact that we talk about it here is wonderful.

As staff became aware of the prevalence and consequences of violence, they also began to understand its link with sexual and reproductive health. The voluntary or coercive nature of sex may surface in a discussion with a woman choosing a contraceptive method, a teenager with an unplanned pregnancy, or a client with multiple episodes of STIs. A doctor who sees marks on a woman's body no longer ignores what such bruises imply. Now, PLAFAM staff "see" the problem and know what to do next: ask, assess, counsel, and refer.

In spite of the dedication of some physicians, most remain reluctant to screen women themselves because they believe that gender-based violence is in the domain of psychologists. PLAFAM has continued to sensitize physicians to the importance of their role, but their full engagement remains a challenge.

Following up on outside referrals to determine whether or not they have taken place, as well as whether or not they were helpful, has also proven difficult. Telephoning clients is not feasible, because receiving a follow-up phone call would endanger some women, and many do not have a phone. Staff had requested that the referral organizations keep track of women referred by PLAFAM so they could determine, at a minimum, whether women had proceeded with the referral. Unfortunately, this has not worked as smoothly as hoped, as outside referral organizations are not always willing or able to comply. As a result, the staff are devising new monitoring procedures, which may include the use of referral coupons—slips of paper that are given to clients to hand to the referral site during check-in and later collected by PLAFAM staff.

Keeping the information in the referral directory current and accessible also requires ongoing attention. PLAFAM is presently updating the directory and creating a condensed version that will be a more user-friendly "rapid resource" for counselors. The original directory, although useful, was too lengthy, making it difficult for providers to quickly find the appropriate referral for each client. Finally, PLAFAM continues to struggle with the scarcity of referral organizations—particularly shelters and safe houses—that provide services to victims of gender violence in Venezuela.

EXPANDING SERVICES

Given the demonstrated need for and acceptability of PLAFAM's violence intervention, the agency is exploring various ways to expand its services, including:

- Providing violence-related screening and counseling for returning clients as well as new ones. PLAFAM plans to implement this gradually and with careful monitoring so as not to overload existing staff or decrease the quality of services provided.

- Implementing onsite follow-up support and self-help groups for victims at all three clinic sites.
- Providing assistance and referrals for perpetrators of gender-based violence who seek help.

Two additional psychologists and two part-time lawyers have been hired to make this expanded mission possible. This staff recruitment was made possible by the generous financial support PLAFAM now receives for its gender-based violence work. The association is also seeking ways to enhance the long-term financial viability of the project, as well as evaluating the effects of the first phase of its gender violence work before it expands into a wider range of services. In the interest of sustainability, PLAFAM has developed consultancy agreements with municipalities and NGOs that may play greater roles in providing violence services in the future. PLAFAM has also been asked to conduct information, education, and communication activities with the Caracas public defender's office, and is encouraging other public-sector organizations to assume greater responsibility in this area.

The volume of clients at PLAFAM clinics may also require attention as this project evolves. A woman who comes for a Pap smear and discloses violence may end up in a lengthy counseling session and decide to postpone her clinical exam to another day. Conversely, a client who comes expecting to speak only with a counselor or nurse (e.g., for a condom refill) may unexpectedly be referred to the physician for an examination of physical injuries. So far, the clinic has remained flexible. However, it may become increasingly difficult to maintain this flexibility as the demand for services grows and staff time is stretched to capacity. In addition, providing counseling services on an individual level may not be the most effective or cost-effective method to assist victims of violence. PLAFAM is therefore exploring the potential contributions of community volunteers, self-help groups, group counseling sessions, and other strategies.

DOCUMENTATION AND DATA COLLECTION

As discussed previously, PLAFAM is still refining its data collection procedures in order to facilitate follow-up on referrals and to track service needs and performance.

Efforts are being made to incorporate information about violence into the institution's management information system. There is a plan to incorporate violence-related data into an existing software system (called CMX). Currently, the system is being tested in a few Latin American countries. During this process, CMX's ability to protect client confidentiality and to manage violence-related data will be assessed.[8]

Given the pilot nature of this project, it is critical to monitor and evaluate the effectiveness of the interventions in a way that is both methodologically satisfactory and substantively thoughtful. Toward this end, PLAFAM, in concert with IPPF/WHR affiliates in the Dominican Republic and Peru, has developed tools to evaluate certain aspects of its gender violence work. These tools include an institutional assessment questionnaire to measure the degree to which gender violence has been integrated into existing services; a knowledge, attitudes, and practices questionnaire to assess providers; and an observation and interview guide for assessing physical characteristics of the clinics, including whether private space is available for counseling. These IPPF/WHR affiliates also hope to create tools, such as exit and in-depth interviews, to evaluate client perspectives on violence services, and to develop case studies of women referred to other organizations to evaluate the nature and quality of their services.

Over the next year, PLAFAM and IPPF/WHR will use these tools to assess the longer-term effects of the project on both the agency and its beneficiaries.

CONCLUSION

As governments in many countries gradually assume responsibility for providing contraceptive services, NGOs continue to play a role in advocating for the support of sexual and reproductive rights, creating new service options, and broadening attention to the context of women's lives. While the gender violence project described in this chapter is at an early stage, several important lessons are already clear.

Many women want to talk about the violence they have experienced, even when they have never done so before. While many providers were initially skeptical about routine screening for gender-based violence, and particularly about asking women direct questions on the subject, PLAFAM's experience confirms the experience reported elsewhere: Women will take advantage of the opportunity to discuss their experiences with violence if invited to in a caring and confidential manner. Even the question concerning childhood sexual abuse, which was heatedly debated during the development of the screening form, has not been perceived by women as too invasive.

Routine gender violence screening in the context of sexual and reproductive health programs raises a number of ethical questions. Is it advisable to screen when the full range of services victims might need is not readily available? Does the screening ultimately have a positive effect on these women's lives? Does it put women in danger? Readers are advised to consult Heise, Ellsberg, and Gottemoeller (1999), relevant chapters in Burns et al. (1997), Shrader and Sagot (2000), and IPPF/WHR (2000, 2001) for detailed information on the critical elements that should be in place before violence screening programs are initiated.

Having a chance to talk and feel supported is itself a valuable experience for most victims of violence. One of the providers' main concerns was that there was little that they could offer to victims. They had been trained to fix problems and did not perceive acknowledging violence and validating a woman's experience with violence as interventions. Helping providers to see such services in this light requires a major change in perspective. This is particularly true among physicians, who often consider gender-based violence concerns to be outside their purview.

Staff can overcome their own anxieties about responding to victims of violence. They can be trained to provide screening, counseling, and referrals, as long as they are supported in doing so through training, proper protocols and tools, and supervisory support. The collaborative development of these tools has been invaluable in supporting staff and clarifying their roles. Sensitive, caring providers can be trained to screen and counsel women even if they hold no formal training in psychology or social services.

Finding support for women who have experienced violence is a challenge. Referral systems for gender-based violence are extremely limited in many settings. This work thus requires an understanding of the capacity of other organizations and the creation of strong alliances in order to meet client needs for legal assistance and other services. PLAFAM is working with a range of other private and public organizations to expand the range of available services, thus helping to ensure the future viability of the project and enabling the association to focus on the areas in which it has greatest expertise.

Addressing gender-based violence within the context of sexual and reproductive health is complex but possible. A violence project may require conventional family planning programs to revise client-flow patterns, introduce new tools and data systems and adapt existing ones, provide emotional support mechanisms for staff, interact with an array of community and governmental agencies, and become familiar with the legal framework affecting both victims and providers. Although these can be time-consuming and complex tasks, family planning programs must recognize that unless a woman's experience with gender-based violence is taken into consideration, even conventional family planning services may not be successful. How, for example, can a provider counsel a client on the best contraceptive method or on HIV prevention strategies if he or she is not aware of the level of negotiating power the client holds? Given the fact that sexual and reproductive health workers are often the only health care providers to whom women have access, it would be ideal if they could systematically screen all clients and provide them with the appropriate psychological, medical, social, and legal services either in-house or through nearby organizations. If this is not feasible, there are a number of steps that both providers and organizations can take. They can ensure a client's privacy and respect her confidentiality, validate her experience with violence, facilitate links to other services that are not available in-house, inform a client of her legal rights, respect her choices and autonomy, inform her of the existence of emergency contraception, and further educate themselves about gender-based violence and its relationship to sexual and reproductive health. Most importantly, providers and organizations can consider a client's experience with violence when providing family planning counseling and STI/HIV prevention and testing.

Ultimately, screening for violence allows for thorough and context-sensitive counseling for other reproductive health matters such as contraception, STI prevention, and unwanted pregnancy. Indeed, by recognizing and responding to the violence that is a part of many women's lives, PLAFAM has taken steps toward transforming family planning clinics into programs for sexual and reproductive health. Its experience will undoubtedly prove useful for other family planning programs seeking to help victims of violence around the globe.

Acknowledgments

We thank Sarah Bott, Loryan Calzadilla, and Gisela Diaz for their assistance. This project could not have been carried out without their efforts. We are also grateful to the Bill and Melinda Gates Foundation, the John D. and Catherine T. MacArthur Foundation, the European Commission, and the Ford Foundation for their support of this project.

Notes

1   The Justice of Peace is a legal organization run by communities in conjunction with the municipal civil courts.

2   Because PLAFAM had no way of knowing what sort of response to expect from clients, it had no way of anticipating the demands clients might place on staff and the disruption such demands might cause to client flow. It was therefore decided that counselors would begin by screening only new clients for violence.

3   The initial counseling service is free. Thereafter, counseling fees are negotiated on a sliding scale, with a maximum fee of approximately US$5.

4   To assist with and standardize the consultation, an in-depth assessment form was developed to help the psychologist secure a thorough documentation of the client's experience. In addition, a danger assessment form, developed in the United States by Jacquelyn Campbell at Johns Hopkins University, was adapted to help counselors evaluate women's current risk.

5   A body map is a diagram of a woman's body, both front and back, on which the health care provider can document injuries. It permits visual confirmation by women with limited literacy, who can point to body parts that have been injured without using embarrassing or unknown terms, and is also helpful in legal proceedings. Not all providers recognized the value of this tool, so it was not used in all cases.

6   It is expected that after validation, other family planning associations might choose to incorporate these questions into their clinical history forms—a step toward institutionalizing attention to gender violence.

7   The data for January–August 1999 were collected using the original protocol (which was applied inconsistently, asked different questions, and detected a prevalence of only 7 percent), and were recorded in a manner that did not reflect multiple types of violence. The data are thus not comparable and are not included in Table 1.

8   IPPF/WHR anticipates that as CMX becomes fully available, it will enable all the region's affiliates to collect and manage data related to gender-based violence.

References

AVESA. 1998a. "Hoja de datos" [Fact sheet] no. 5. Caracas: AVESA.

———. 1998b. "Informe de Venezuela sobre situación de la violencia de género contra las mujeres" [Venezuela report on gender violence against women]. Caracas: AVESA.

Burns, A. August, Ronnie Lovich, Jane Maxwell, and Katharine Shapiro. 1997. *Where Women Have No Doctor: A Health Guide for Women.* Berkeley, CA: Hesperian Foundation.

Calzadilla, Tamoa. 1998. "1998 se lleva consigo la impunidad por acoso y maltrato a la mujer" [1998 takes with it freedom from punishment for those who harass and abuse women], *El Nacional,* 24 November, Section C, p. 1.

Davies, Vanessa. 1998. "Violencia en la TV y consumo de alcohol propician maltrato doméstico en Caracas" [Violence on TV and alcohol consumption lead to domestic violence in Caracas], *El Nacional,* 12 March, Section C, p. 2.

Heise, Lori, Mary Ellsberg, and Megan Gottemoeller. 1999. "Ending violence against women," *Population Reports,* Series L, no. 11.

International Planned Parenthood Federation/Western Hemisphere Region (IPPF/WHR). 2000. "Integrating gender-based violence into sexual and reproductive health," *Basta!* newsletter (summer). New York: IPPF/WHR.

———. 2001. "Providers' attitudes and behavior toward gender-based violence," *Basta!* newsletter (winter). New York: IPPF/WHR.

Shrader, E. and M. Sagot. 2000. *Domestic Violence: Women's Way Out,* Occasional Publication no. 2. Washington, DC: Pan American Health Organization.

Contact information

Alessandra C. Guedes
International Planned Parenthood Federation/Western Hemisphere Region
120 Wall Street, 9th Floor
New York, NY 10005 USA
telephone: 212-248-6400
fax: 212-248-4221
e-mail: info@ippfwhr.org

Readers may also consult the section on gender-based violence on IPPF/WHR's Web site at www.ippfwhr.org

15

Sexual Risk, Sexually Transmitted Infections, and Contraceptive Options: Empowering Women in Mexico with Information and Choice

Christiana Coggins and Angela Heimburger

Sexually transmitted infections (STIs), including HIV/AIDS, cause substantial morbidity and mortality worldwide. Because family planning programs serve sexually active women—a population vulnerable to STIs—and because contraceptive methods affect STI risk and sequelae, such programs are a logical entry point for helping women to prevent initial acquisition of these infections, as well as their spread. Women—whether or not they are seeking to regulate their fertility—need information about methods that will help protect them against STIs. Women seeking intrauterine devices (IUDs) or women whose providers recommend IUDs must be adequately screened for STIs, because introducing an IUD through an infected cervix can result in upper genital tract infection, including pelvic inflammatory disease (CONASIDA and SSA 1996–97).[1] Pelvic inflammatory disease can lead to ectopic pregnancy, infertility, chronic abdominal pain, and recurrent infection (Cates 1998).

In recent years, the international reproductive health community has discovered that screening IUD users for STIs is a daunting task. In some settings, screening is not attempted at all; in others, clinicians who try to screen for STIs do not have access to laboratory diagnostic facilities and must rely on clinical assessment. Moreover, cervical STIs, such as chlamydia and gonorrhea, are asymptomatic in over half of women. Thus, most infected women would be missed through such clinical assessments.

Syndromic algorithms (flow charts that guide the clinician through a series of decisions and lead to a conclusion about the presence or absence of infection) have been developed to standardize management and treatment of STIs in low-resource settings that do not have access to laboratory diagnostic capability. Along with risk scores, clinicians use these tools to assess whether women have an infection on the basis of their symptoms (e.g., complaint of vaginal discharge), signs (e.g., cervical mucopus), and responses to questions on risk based on sexual history. Both algorithms and risk scores have been shown to have very low predictive value for cervical infection in populations of women attending family planning or antenatal clinics (Dallabetta, Gerbase, and Holmes 1998; Haberland et al. 1999; Sloan et al. 2000). This means that infected women cannot be reliably identified using these tools and, conversely, that most of the women who are identified as infected in reality are not. Additionally, few providers have the time or skill to explore questions about women's sexual partners and practices, and many women are reluctant to provide such sensitive and potentially embarrassing information to clinic personnel.

This dilemma is of more than marginal interest in Mexico, where the IUD is the most commonly used reversible contraceptive; more than one in five contraceptive users in Mexico is given this method (Pathfinder International 1996). More than 70 percent of modern method users in Mexico obtain their method in a government institution, and at the largest public-sector provider, the Instituto Mexicano de Seguro Social (IMSS), more than one-third of clients (35 percent) who come for family planning methods have an IUD inserted (Vernon and Palma 1998). In most of these public-sector settings, screening for cervical infection before IUD insertion, if done at all, is limited mainly to clinical assessment or, occasionally, assessment using syndromic algorithms and risk scores. While official data on chlamydia and gonorrhea prevalence are not collected, studies have found these rates to range from 2 percent to 16 percent (Acosta-Cázares, Ruiz-Maya, and de la Peña 1996; Echániz-Avilés et al. 1992; Uribe-Salas et al. 1997). In short, as a matter of routine clinical practice, IUDs are inserted every day into an unknown number of women who harbor unidentified but active cervical infections.

PROJECT GOALS

Given the inadequacy of STI screening protocols and the need to develop and validate alternative procedures, the study team carried out an experiment to assess the value of information in helping women themselves choose a contraceptive method appropriate to their life situations. Specifically, the team hypothesized that women might be somewhat better than clinicians at determining whether they are appropriate IUD candidates when given adequate information for decisionmaking. In developing the information for women, project staff incorporated information from two exploratory background studies (one of IMSS service-delivery conditions, the other an ethnographic analysis of belief systems about reproductive tract infections [RTIs]) undertaken by collaborating agencies. These studies are described in Boxes 1 and 2.

Box 1. How standard services are provided in IMSS

Colleagues at AVSC (now known as EngenderHealth) assessed institutional capacity, service-delivery practices, and client knowledge and attitudes at three IMSS clinics in and near Mexico City.

Service-delivery practices. According to clinical observations, provision of information about family planning and STIs was inconsistent:
- While most providers gave some sort of family planning information, the quality and content of the information varied.
- Certain important information about IUDs was not systematically covered, including method effectiveness and warning signs for complications.
- Information, education, and communication materials that integrate family planning and RTI/STI information were rare, and discussion of these issues with clients was even rarer.

Clinical screening. While IMSS doctors are required to provide both IUD and STI services, the clinics assessed had no established RTI/STI risk-assessment protocol. In practice:
- Doctors did not routinely screen IUD clients either for risk or for clinical evidence of STIs.
- STI risk assessment usually meant asking a client her age and marital status, but not asking about her or her partner's current or prior history of STIs, symptoms, or number of partners.
- Providers were conscientious in reviewing medical histories and carrying out speculum exams.
- Providers were unlikely to carry out pelvic exams.
- Because of the complexity of chlamydia testing, the clinics usually referred clients to a nearby hospital for diagnosis or confirmation of the presumed diagnosis.
- In interviews, some providers identified a general physical exam as a routine procedure for IUD candidates; however, such an exam was seldom performed during clinic observation.

Source: AVSC International and IMSS 1999.

The work was carried out by the Population Council and the Instituto Nacional de Salud Pública (INSP) at IMSS Clinic Number 31, which serves the Iztapalapa neighborhood of Mexico City.[2] Iztapalapa is an urban community in which most workers are employed in the formal wage-earning sector and are therefore entitled to IMSS services. This high-volume clinic also attends walk-ins who are not formally entitled to IMSS services. Women who came to the IMSS family planning clinic requesting a method were randomized into two groups. The clinician-screened (control) group underwent routine clinical procedures, relying on a physician's judgment regarding appropriate contraceptive method choice. In addition to receiving routine care, women in the self-screening (experimental) group attended a carefully prepared, 20-minute, one-on-one information session with visual aids on available methods and the risks and characteristics of STIs. They were then asked to select a method for themselves, considering the information they had just received. Cervical and vaginal samples were taken from women in both groups and analyzed for chlamydia and gonorrhea infection, and investigators determined which infected women were inappropriately assigned or chose for themselves the IUD as a contraceptive method.

Box 2. How women talk about STIs

The Instituto Mexicano de Investigación de Familia y Población (IMIFAP), which is affiliated with the International Center for Research on Women, worked at the community level to learn about how women and men describe and classify RTIs. IMIFAP researchers used "free-listing" and "pile-sort" techniques in community-based surveys and focus-group discussions to explore the terminology women used to talk about RTIs and STIs, the signs they recognized, their perceptions of causal factors, and the treatment they sought. IMIFAP conducted this research among potential family planning clients in two communities served by IMSS clinics in Atlacomulco, in the state of Mexico, and in Mexico City, the population of interest. In Mexico City, women did not use the terms STIs or RTIs to describe their infections. Rather, they usually used the term "vaginal infections," which are considered to be "a woman's disease" but also sexually transmissible. A "lack of hygiene" was the most frequently mentioned cause of vaginal infections. It is possible, however, that women are more aware of the possible role of sexual transmission than they are willing to voice, as the precipitating factor—marital infidelity—is much harder to face. In terms of health-seeking behavior, it was clear that some pain or discomfort is considered "normal," and consequently symptoms are not always seen as indicative of infection. Treatment-seeking behavior includes taking home remedies and/or seeing the doctor. The most widely recognized family planning method by far was the IUD. Most women considered the IUD safe, practical, and economical; the disadvantages they saw were increased blood flow during menstruation and intense cramping. The condom was not a commonly used method among the women surveyed, although it was recognized as a safe, accessible, easy, and cheap method to prevent pregnancy. However, the women also indicated that sex does not "feel the same" with a condom, and that men often refuse to use one (Collado et al. 1999).

CLINIC NUMBER 31: ROUTINE PRACTICE

Accounts of routine clinical practice as observed by project nurses at Clinic Number 31 were consistent with AVSC's (now known as EngenderHealth) general findings (see Box 1). According to routine clinical procedure, a woman who requests a reversible contraceptive method is directed to the family planning clinic, where a social worker asks standard medical history questions: her age, obstetric and gynecologic history, method requested, and marital status. No questions are asked about her sexual behavior. The only question occasionally asked about her partner is whether or not he is circumcised.

The woman waits in a crowded reception area until she is called by a nurse and ushered into the physician's consultation room. The provider ascertains that the woman has come to get a family planning method, and then gives her some information about the reversible methods available at the clinic (IUD and pills), or mentions sterilization if the woman indicates that she wants a permanent method. In the case of the IUD, the provider superficially reviews the technical aspects of the method (e.g., briefly explaining how long it can stay in place, how it is inserted, and its contraceptive effectiveness). He then conducts a brief visual inspection of the cervix in the presence of the nurse. Rarely does the physician explain to the woman what he is doing.

There appears to be a strong bias among health professionals—and the system within which they operate—toward physician-controlled methods with the highest effectiveness rates, such as the IUD and female sterilization. Anecdotal evidence suggests that some physicians perceive considerable institutional pressure, driven by government policies, to fulfill monthly IUD insertion quotas. Providers also tend to steer clients away from barrier methods, which they see as an unreliable means of contraception because their effectiveness is dependent on a client's behavior.

According to comments made by the project nurses, when a woman expressly solicits pills the physician questions her preference and reiterates the effectiveness of the IUD, trying to persuade her to adopt it if she has no medical contraindications based on the cursory clinical assessment. Only when the doctor is not able to convince the client to accept an IUD does he prescribe oral contraceptives and explain their use. However, he rarely, if ever, explains what side effects may result or what to do if the client misses a dose.

Women who request condoms are typically counseled by nurses. Because staff consider condoms to be a method of disease prevention but not effective contraception, the nurses request that the woman return to the clinic to receive a more effective contraceptive such as the IUD. Clients are occasionally counseled about condom use for protection against both pregnancy and infection, but only if they do not have a regular sexual partner or have infrequent sexual relations.

Once an IUD has been inserted, the doctor simply tells the woman to get dressed while he makes notes in her file. The doctor normally does not make any reference either to the sorts of problems the woman might encounter or to warning signs of possible infection. The physician then indicates that the woman should have her IUD checked occasionally and get an annual Pap smear.

Routine clinical procedure changes little when a client presents with visible signs of an infection, such as purulent discharge or a friable cervix.[3] There are no official guidelines regarding the timing of IUD insertion or treatment if an infection is present, although international medical guidelines indicate that any diagnosed STI should be treated before IUD insertion. In clinical practice in public settings, where time is short and lines are long, the family planning physician will most often insert the IUD and simultaneously prescribe treatment based on a presumptive clinical diagnosis. He does not, however, actually provide the necessary medication. On occasion the physician might refer the woman to a family doctor within the same institution, if she is insured, or more likely to an outside laboratory for testing, and wait for her to return with the laboratory results. Because of time constraints and the perceived likelihood that a client will not return for a follow-up appointment even if she tests positive, the physician very rarely treats a suspected infection before inserting the IUD.

As in most service-delivery settings around the world, counseling about infections or how to prevent them is virtually never part of the clinical encounter. As a general rule, physicians do not broach the subject of sexuality or risk-taking behavior during their brief sessions with clients, probably because of a combination of limited time, pressure to provide the most effective contraceptive, and an aversion to speaking with clients about an embarrassing topic. Nurses reported that providers might offer a client condoms only if they suspect that she is "promiscuous" and only after questioning her—often in a patronizing, scolding manner—about her sexual behavior. Likewise, a clinician might suggest—but rarely distribute—condoms as a measure to prevent infection transmission for IUD or pill users who are already protected against pregnancy but present with a cervico-vaginal infection. Nurses also reported that if a man came to the clinic to procure condoms, he would receive them only if could convince the provider that he had an infection. Even in this case, the provider would insist that the man bring his partner for a subsequent visit so that she could receive a more effective contraceptive method.

FINDING THE RIGHT WORDS AND MESSAGES

To design the counseling guide that became the basis for the self-screening education session provided to individual women in the experimental group, the project staff reviewed the pertinent literature and existing counseling instruments, and drew lessons from IMIFAP's community study (see Box 2). Two components of reproductive health were linked in developing the intervention: contraception and STI management. Hence, it was decided that information should be provided on the temporary contraceptive methods available at the IMSS clinic—the IUD, pills, and condoms—including information on efficacy, mechanisms of action, contraindications, and advantages and disadvantages. In addition, general information was provided on STI risk factors, signs, symptoms, and consequences. On the basis of qualitative community studies, the project staff also decided to dispel some myths about the causes of sexual infections, including poor hygiene, "getting wet" (e.g., understood to be accidentally splashing oneself with dirty laundry water or dishwater or getting soaked in the rain), and going to public baths. The language was modeled after popular expressions and the message was tailored to maintain its impact while holding the listener's attention. For example, the counseling guide refers to STIs interchangeably as "STIs" and as "vaginal infections" because, though not strictly correct, "vaginal infections" is the term that most women use and understand; by using both terms, the project staff sought to familiarize women with the term that most doctors use.

The information script underwent many revisions. The challenge was to strike a balance between providing enough information to allow the woman to make an educated decision and not overwhelming her with less critical and potentially confusing facts; to present the advantages and disadvantages of each contraceptive method objectively; and to alert the woman to the risk factors for acquiring an STI without raising needless worries about the possibility that her partner might be sexually unfaithful. At the same time, project staff wanted to educate women so that they would pay more attention to their bodies and their intuition and be better informed about how to care for themselves. The staff also hoped that this knowledge would give some women a necessary tool with which to confront concerns about their partners' sexual behavior and protect themselves from both infection and unwanted pregnancy.

Often the balance was found in word choice and phrasing rather than in compromising the content of the information provided. For example, in an early version of the guide, the fact that one can never be sure of a partner's sexual fidelity was emphasized, as was the idea that any suspicion of outside sexual activity warrants testing for STIs. Not only did this message promote universal lab testing for STIs—an unrealistic option for the IMSS system—it also created needless anxiety. Moreover, it ignored the fact that women, too, have extramarital relations. The text was modified to define the risk factor as follows: If the woman or her partner had unprotected sexual relations with more than one partner, she or he might be at increased risk of exposure to infection. In addition, the message stated that many STIs, if detected early, could be easily and successfully treated and cured, and subsequent infection could be prevented through the use of condoms.

The script consciously avoided moralistic messages about STIs and sexual behavior to avoid blaming women. Instead, it presented concise, well-balanced information about the pros and cons of all available methods and the corresponding risks of STI transmission in order to empower a woman to make the best, most informed decision to meet her own needs.

TRAINING PROVIDERS TO TRANSMIT AN EXPANDED MESSAGE

In November and December 1996, the Population Council recruited and trained two project nurses to conduct the informational session for the self-screening group of women. Because these registered nurses had worked on other projects run by the INSP, they had a good working knowledge of the subject matter and were aware of the importance of adhering to the protocol. Project staff provided the nurses with background material on STIs, contraceptive methods, and counseling techniques. The nurses then participated in a two-day formal training session that explained in detail the project's background, purpose, and design. A gynecologist presented technical sessions on specific contraceptive methods and STIs.

During those two days, a reproductive health social worker led question-and-answer sessions on counseling techniques, using simulated role-plays. Some of these techniques focused on how to establish rapport with and inspire confidence in clients and to anticipate objections or difficult questions. The information script was used to familiarize the nurses with the dynamics of intimate, one-on-one counseling.

During these training sessions, questions arose about the norms and practices of the IMSS clinic: What type of contraceptive pills did they normally furnish? What percentage and segment of the general public had IMSS benefits? Would a psychologist be available to see women who received positive STI results or had mental health needs? The nurses were asked to keep track of all questions that arose once they started seeing clients so that they could continue to receive appropriate materials to prepare them for future questions.

As the pilot-test of the intervention drew nearer, project staff decided to incorporate additional training in safe-sex demonstrations. The director of a local AIDS organization (Fundación Méxicana para la Lucha contra SIDA) gave a brief workshop on counseling techniques and condom use for prevention of STI transmission. The trainer's easygoing style and humorous anecdotes based on years of experience gave the nurses the confidence to ask questions and shed some of their own inhibitions. They learned how to put condoms on a penis model and how to prepare women to handle difficult situations when women's partners refused to use condoms or accused the women of being "promiscuous."

PILOT-TESTING THE INTERVENTION

The two nurses participating in the study expressed uncertainty about the intervention during the pilot-test phase. As with any new project, they were initially uncertain of their ability and authority and were met with some reticence and skepticism on the part of the clinic staff. In addition, clinic staff were distracted by the presence of outsiders in the clinic and skeptical of patients' ability to perform self-screening. Some clients who had attended the clinic previously wanted to know why they were being given this information now. The nurses explained the need to expand on the information usually given because, although clients thought they had correct information, their understanding was often inaccurate. Initially, the nurses were also uncomfortable demonstrating condom use, as doing so attracted a lot of attention, not only from the women being counseled, but also from curious onlookers in the clinic.

The pilot-test provided an opportunity for the team to revise logistical aspects of the project and for the nurses to settle into their role. While the nurses continued to seek answers to new questions as they arose, to refer patients to physicians for questions of a technical nature, and to consult the project staff for further clarification, they became more confident of their own expertise. The novelty of condom demonstration also wore off. Gradually, the nurses came to appreciate the importance of their role in providing adequate reproductive health counseling.

VISUAL AIDS

Initially, the project planned for nurses in the self-screening group to use only a type-written information guide, which would serve as a reference during the individual client-education sessions. After the pilot-test phase, however, project staff developed and tested a 14-page laminated color companion guide to visually reinforce the 20-minute session (see Box 3). The study nurses reported that when the companion guide was used, women paid greater attention and were more likely to ask questions. At one point, the project team considered distributing flyers that women could take home, but the idea was abandoned because doing so might discourage an immediate question-and-answer exchange. In addition, the project team realized that distributing flyers could not easily be sustained by the clinic in the long run.

THE INTERVENTION: GIVING WOMEN INFORMATION TO MAKE THEIR OWN DECISIONS

The full-scale experiment began in March 1997. After being screened[4] and listening to a brief description of the project given by the social worker, women were asked to give their consent for participation. An important aspect of the study design was that participants consented to a two-visit protocol, because best practices suggest that a woman should wait for her test results and return to the clinic for her final method one to two weeks later, rather than run the risk of inserting an IUD in a woman with an asymptomatic infection. Before the end of the first visit, all women received a brief safe-sex talk along with a sufficient supply of condoms for use until the following visit.

Women who volunteered for the study were randomized to either the clinician-screened (control) or self-screening group. Following normal clinic practice, women in the clinician-screened group were sent to wait for a consultation with the physician, while women in the self-screening group were given the one-on-one education session (see Box 3). Women in the self-screening group were then asked to indicate on a confidential form which method they would like. They were not asked to disclose why they had made their selection. Following the information session, they, like women

Box 3. Translation of the companion guide used during the information session

It's great that you're interested in using a family planning method! We're going to give you information on the three contraceptive methods offered here at the clinic—condoms, pills, and the IUD—so that you can choose the most appropriate method for you and your partner.

Condoms

Advantages
- They protect against HIV/AIDS and vaginal infections that are sexually transmitted.
- There are no negative health effects.
- They are easy to obtain.
- They prevent pregnancy when used correctly.

Disadvantages
- If condoms are not removed carefully, the semen may stay inside the vagina and you can get pregnant.
- The decision to use a condom depends almost entirely upon the man.
- If they are not put on carefully and correctly, occasionally they can break or slip off.

The condom is the only contraceptive method that prevents vaginal infections that are transmitted sexually.

Pill (prevents ovulation)

Advantages
- It is a very effective method for avoiding pregnancy.
- It will not adversely affect your health.
- It reduces menstrual pain and discomfort.

Disadvantages
- If the pill is not taken daily, it is likely that the method will not work and you will become pregnant.
- It is not recommended if you have certain health problems.

Contraceptive pills do *not* protect you from STIs.

IUD (inserted inside the uterus, where it blocks the union of egg and sperm)

Advantages
- It is a very effective method for preventing pregnancy.
- It can stay inside the uterus for up to ten years without your having to worry about it.
- You can ask to have the IUD removed at any time you wish.

Disadvantages
- It can cause irregular or prolonged menstruation.
- If you have a vaginal infection, it is very important that it be treated before inserting the IUD. Otherwise it is possible for the infection to spread and produce complications.

The IUD does *not* protect you from STIs. If the IUD is inserted when you already have an STI, the infection can spread and produce serious inflammation.

Some "vaginal infections," otherwise known as STIs, are chlamydia, gonorrhea, and trichomoniasis.

How are STIs transmitted? By having sexual relations with an infected person. Beware! The infections are not always noticeable. How are they *not* transmitted? You cannot get an STI by "getting wet," using public restrooms or baths, because of poor hygiene, or by not going to see the doctor.

What behaviors increase the risk of STIs? When a woman and/or her partner has sexual relations with other people and does *not* take precautions against these infections by using condoms. If you think you might have an STI, it is very important that you not accept an IUD before having a proper diagnostic exam and receiving proper treatment.

(continued)

(continued from previous page)

What are some of the possible complications of STIs? Some vaginal infections, when left untreated, can ascend to the uterus and the fallopian tubes, causing pain and fever. This complication can eventually leave a woman sterile. This is a major risk when an IUD is inserted in a woman who has an untreated infection.

How are STIs recognized? Symptoms in women include abnormal discharge, itching, burning when urinating, desire to urinate frequently, vaginal ulcers or lesions, and discomfort when having sexual relations. However, many women who have an STI do *not* have any symptoms. The only sure way to know whether you have an infection is with a laboratory analysis of vaginal secretions. In this clinic we will take a sample from you and perform the tests.

Recommendations. With the results of the vaginal secretion analyses, the physician will tell you whether or not you have an infection and whether or not you and your partner need treatment. At that time, you and your physician will decide which contraceptive method is the most suitable for you.

in the clinician-screened group, received a consultation and physical exam with the physician.

Women in both groups provided samples for diagnostic tests to detect gonorrhea and chlamydia. Following the clinical encounter, the clinicians seeing women in both groups were asked to indicate on a form whether or not they considered particular women to be appropriate candidates for an IUD. The laboratory test results were available one to two weeks after the initial clinical visit and served as the "gold standard" against which to evaluate and compare the decisions of clinicians versus those of the women themselves about their appropriateness as IUD candidates.

When women returned to the clinic for their second visit, those whose lab results indicated infection[5] were directed to the doctor, who would dispense the appropriate medication if he had samples on hand. Otherwise, he would write a prescription for the patient and her partner, and give her a follow-up appointment for re-evaluation once treatment was completed. In all cases, infected women were advised to abstain from sexual relations or use a condom at each act of intercourse during treatment. Those who had requested an IUD were told they would need to treat the infection first and return for a third visit for the IUD insertion.

Of the 2,107 women who were tested for chlamydia and gonorrhea, 44 were positive. Two of the infected women claimed that they would not be able to return to the clinic for a third visit (when treatment would be completed) and insisted on having an IUD inserted on the second visit (when treatment was dispensed and initiated). An exception was made for these women, who received their IUDs and were prescribed antibiotics at the same time. They were also asked to sign an informed consent form. The remaining 42 infected women returned for a third visit to receive a contraceptive method after the full course of antibiotics. At that time, a second vaginal sample was taken to ensure that the infection had in fact cleared. However, none of the women returned for a fourth visit to receive the results of the second lab test.

RESULTS

Women who participated in the information session were far less likely to select the IUD than women who were dependent on the clinician's judgment (58 percent compared to 90 percent, p<0.001).[6] The study team's original hypothesis that women would be somewhat better than clinicians at deciding whether their individual risk of infection made the IUD an inappropriate method was far too modest. In fact, women were much better at making that decision: 52 percent of the infected women in the self-screening group correctly chose not to use the IUD, contrasting sharply with the clinician-screened group in which only 5 percent of infected women were screened out of IUD use (Lazcano et al. 2000). Hence, infected women were much less likely to opt for an IUD when they screened themselves than when physicians screened them.

Within the self-screening group, infected women were significantly less likely to opt for an IUD than women who were not infected (48 percent versus 58 percent, p<0.001). Clearly, a substantial proportion of uninfected women also decided not to select the IUD when provided with information and a choice of methods. The fact that a significantly larger proportion of infected women than uninfected women selected an alternative to the IUD suggests that the information provided was especially relevant to infected women.

Women's Experience of the Counseling Session

Through a focus-group discussion with the project nurses, the study team attempted to analyze the value of the intervention to women who participated. The nurses felt that there were more advantages than drawbacks. "Those patients who showed a lot of interest and asked a lot of questions thanked us afterward for having explained all the methods so well and especially the STIs." Many participants were grateful for the opportunity to ask questions and wondered why this was not the norm in all clinics. Several women planned to send their friends and family members to participate in the project. As one of the nurses said:

> It's a good opportunity to talk about diseases because the majority of people totally ignore the fact that they might have an infection. They think "Oh, I have a little bit of discharge; who knows what that's all about?" And then they treat it with anything—an herb, an ointment, and all the rest—just to stop [the symptoms] and go on about their business. . . . Once the participants receive the intervention, they realize that they could have an infection.

When asked whether they felt that women had understood the information they received, the nurses replied that in general the women seemed to understand. The women's questions pointed primarily to a need for clarification of the characteristics of the IUD, pills, and condoms: "They ask us how an IUD is inserted and about pills—a lot of women who come here know nothing about pills." According to another nurse, "A lot of women come with questions in spite of the fact that they are using a method, but often they don't know how it works inside their bodies." One nurse said, "A lot of women come in with ideas of things their family members or friends have said—I mean, wrong ideas, like that the IUD is an abortifacient or that it will leave them sterile. The information [we give them] helps to clear up these doubts."

Participants' main concern was that this information had not been available earlier. Many expressed hope that it would always be available, and to all women. Others mentioned that the information should be provided to men as well, as they are typically the source of STIs. When asked whether a woman should be accompanied to the session by her partner, women responded emphatically that men should be invited to participate but seen separately, as a woman would be unable to give an honest answer to the question of which method is appropriate for her if the partner was present.

The need for multiple follow-up visits was the primary drawback of the intervention for many women. As mentioned earlier, none of the 42 infected women who received treatment returned for the results of their retest, which was conducted to ensure that the infection had cleared. Several women also noted that their partners would probably refuse to take any treatment for infection.

In the two cases of women who were infected and did not return on their own, the nurses found that they had given false contact information. A final problem noted by the nurses was that uninsured patients coming to the clinic were often unable, in the few cases where it was necessary, to purchase the medication needed for treatment of infections—even at the reduced prices available at the IMSS clinic or nearby pharmacies.

According to the nurses, the time required to attend the information session was of concern to a few women, who did not have the time to wait. A small proportion of participants, most of whom were mothers with small children, seemed to be in a hurry during the session and did not pay much attention. For those women, the nurses tried to speed up the session by providing a shorter discussion of each topic.

Nurses' Experience

The nurses felt that the information they gave, in some cases, ran counter to that provided by doctors: Whereas the nurses emphasized condoms as an effective way to prevent infection and pregnancy, doctors would encourage women to choose the IUD, or less often pills, as the surest way to prevent pregnancy. The nurses worried about appearing to contradict the doctor and feared that such a conflict of information might be confusing to the client. One nurse explained: "The companion guide put a lot of emphasis on the fact that the condom protects you against STIs; but here the providers promote the IUD and the pill instead of condoms." Also, condoms, while freely available during the intervention, are not routinely available at the family planning clinic. One of the nurses lamented, "Some people just came here for condoms and nothing else, but we can't assure them that we will keep giving them out [once the project is over]."

The nurses emphasized the importance of having a private location for the education session, where the participants would not feel inhibited about asking questions. In fact, the space available for the sessions during the project was sectioned off with a temporary partition and was open on one side to passers-by who would occasionally stop to listen. In general, the noise in the area made it necessary for the nurses to speak loudly. Even though the nurses were able to carry out the intervention successfully under these conditions, which would be similar to those in any public-sector clinic, they strongly recommended that an enclosed space with a door be made available in the future.

The project did not attempt to overcome some of the physicians' more "medicalized" approaches to family planning, stereotypically condescending attitudes, and often patronizing and moralizing prescriptions for clients in matters of sexuality and sexual health. For example, nurses believed that one of the clinic doctors felt pressure to fulfill an institutional quota to insert a certain number of IUDs per week. He would frequently try to persuade women who chose not to use an IUD to reconsider their decision. This highlights the fact that an approach that depends on women's ability to weigh options and make their own decisions will not reach its full potential in contexts where no parallel efforts are made to change provider behavior. Indeed, several women who indicated a preference for pills or condoms were given an IUD by the doctor anyway.

CONCLUSIONS

The study results show that the information describing family planning methods and STI risk factors significantly affected women's choice of contraceptive method. The intervention reduced selection of the IUD as a contraceptive method in general and increased selection of condoms, particularly among infected women.[7] Furthermore, the quantitative results indicate that the information provided substantially reduced inappropriate IUD selection by infected clients.[8]

Clinicians' inability to identify family planning clients with chlamydial and gono-coccal infections may be a consequence of several factors: emphasis on contraception and lack of training in reproductive health issues, including STIs and RTIs; lack of awareness of the magnitude of the problem; limited time spent with each client; ab-sence of clinical signs that correctly identify most cases of infection, and most indi-viduals without infection; and the strong promotion of IUDs in the Mexican public health sector. Since these factors will probably not change significantly in the near future, it is even more urgent that women play a greater role in assessing their own risk. Ideally, however, clients and providers should decide together which contracep-tive method is most appropriate; for this to occur, providers must be able to ask about and discuss STI risk in a supportive and nonjudgmental manner.

Giving women the information and opportunity to assess their own risk of STI infection and actively participate in the choice of a contraceptive method should re-duce inappropriate IUD insertion, while not excluding the IUD from the range of methods available. This is an imperfect but preferable alternative to current practices that are dependent on clinicians' judgment alone. In addition, it increases women's participation in their own reproductive health care.

NEXT STEPS: EXPANDING THE EXPERIMENT

Expanding this experiment to test this approach further in settings with different pro-files (e.g., where the institutionalized preference for IUD provision is weaker, but where other biases may exist) will be invaluable. While the study results are statistically signifi-cant, they cannot be considered representative of settings outside Mexico City's public-sector health system. Questions remain about the replicability of this model, even in the same setting, given the need to train and employ staff who may not be convinced of its relevance and the need to maintain the content and quality of information provided to patients over time with little supervision. It is also unclear whether one-on-one infor-mation sessions are feasible and affordable in all settings. For these reasons, the study team pilot-tested the use of a videotaped information session in the clinic waiting room and auditorium to determine whether this less expensive and more easily standardized mechanism could have similar effects on clients' method choice. More extensive evalu-ation is needed to assess this alternative system of information delivery.

LESSONS LEARNED

- *Women want information but are rarely given it.* Many study participants were grateful for the opportunity to ask questions and wondered why they were not given this opportunity in all clinics.

- *Information about partner relations, sexual risk, and method characteristics is powerful.* Women, when properly informed, generally make better decisions about their own risks and the appropriate response than do physicians on their behalf.
- *Men should receive information too, but separately from women.* Many women felt that information on behavioral risk should be provided to men as well, since they are typically the source of STIs. However women felt strongly that men should be seen separately, so that women could disclose their questions and worries without a partner present.
- *Clinic staff need adequate training, supervision, and support.* Even experienced clinic staff are often in need of special training. The nursing staff were often asked questions by clients, especially at the start of the project, to which they could not provide answers without consulting with a physician. In addition to adequate training, staff need appropriate training materials, protocols, and supportive supervision in order to do their jobs well. Finally, clinic staff need a means to register and respond to clients' complaints (e.g., inadequacy of materials, lack of privacy for counseling, and so forth).
- *Medical staff need to be made aware of women's right to choose and to be more respectful and less condescending toward them.* Medical staff should be evaluated on these fundamental aspects of the provision of high-quality care. Indeed, the study team found that while a number of women decided against IUD use, they were given the IUD by the doctor anyway.

Clearly there is a need both to retrain providers and to stimulate greater participation of women in reproductive health decisionmaking. Providers should be supported in efforts to temper institutionally driven method priorities in favor of women's own participation in choice and must be willing to change their own, in some cases predetermined, decision as to what method is best suited for each woman.

Acknowledgments

Population Council staff from New York and Mexico, together with colleagues from INSP, conducted this project with generous support from the Andrew W. Mellon Foundation. We are grateful for the invaluable assistance of our Mexican partner organizations: IMSS and INSP. We also acknowledge support from our U.S. partner organizations in implementing this study: EngenderHealth, the International Center for Research on Women, its partner organization IMIFAP, and the Pacific Institute for Women's Health.

Notes

1   The use of nonsterile techniques during insertion may represent an additional, independent mode of introducing infection into a woman's uterus. Infection control procedures are, therefore, an important part of IUD insertion training.

2   The research team comprised Eduardo Lazcano-Ponce and Carlos Conde-Glez of INSP; Nancy
     Sloan, Beverly Winikoff, Ana Langer, Christiana Coggins, and Angela Heimburger of the Population
     Council; and Jorge Salmeron of IMSS.

3   A cervix is termed "friable" if it bleeds easily when touched during a pelvic exam or cervical
     specimen collection.

4   Women were excluded from the study if they were pregnant, were using an IUD at the time of the
     visit, had been sterilized or were coming to the clinic for that purpose, had taken certain antibiotics
     that interfere with diagnostic testing in the previous ten days, and/or had used a vaginal douche in
     the previous 24 hours.

5   The project design called for actively tracking down clients who had positive test results but failed
     to report for their second visit. Social workers at the clinic made discreet phone calls and/or house
     visits in an attempt to locate infected women.

6   For more detail on the study design and results, see Lazcano et al. 2000.

7   Although using the pill rather than an IUD will not protect a woman from future risk of STIs, it
     does protect her from the risk of pelvic inflammatory disease resulting from IUD insertion in the
     presence of a cervical infection.

8   The fact that within the self-screening group more infected than uninfected women opted for
     alternatives to the IUD suggests that being given information on methods, and not simply a
     choice of methods, was influential.

References

Acosta-Cázares, B., Lilia Ruiz-Maya, and J. Escobedo de la Peña. 1996. "Prevalence and risk factors for
     Chlamydia trachomatis infection in low-income rural and suburban populations of Mexico," *Sexu-
     ally Transmitted Diseases* 23(4): 283–288.
AVSC International and Instituto Mexicano de Seguro Social (IMSS). 1999. *Factors Affecting the Safe
     Provision of IUDs: A Service Delivery Perspective from Mexico.* New York: AVSC International.
Cates, Willard, Jr. 1998. "Reproductive tract infections," in Robert A. Hatcher, James Trussell, Felicia
     Stewart, Willard Cates, Jr., Gary K. Stewart, Felicia Guest, and Deborah Kowal (eds.), *Contracep-
     tive Technology,* 17th ed. New York: Ardent Media, pp. 179–210.
Collado, Maria Elena, Nilly Grosbeisen Gurvich, Gery Ryan, Susan Pick, and Joanne Spicehandler.
     1999. "Understanding reproductive tract infections from women's perspectives: A study in urban
     and rural Mexico," draft summary report presented at the Factors Affecting the Safe Provision of
     IUDS in Resource-poor Settings Meeting, Washington, DC, 1 June.
CONASIDA (National Council on AIDS) and SSA (Ministry of Health). 1996–97. Document on
     AIDS/STIs, 2(4). Mexico City: CONASIDA and SSA.
Dallabetta, Gina A., Antonio C. Gerbase, and King K. Holmes. 1998. "Problems, solutions, and chal-
     lenges in syndromic management of sexually transmitted diseases," *Sexually Transmitted Infections*
     74(suppl 1): S1–S11.
Echániz-Avilés, Gabriela, Eileen Calderón-Jaimes, Noemi Carnalla-Barajas, Arneeli Soto-Noguerón,
     Aurelio Cruz-Valdez, and Rodolfo Gatica-Marquina. 1992. "Prevalencia de infección cervicovaginal
     por *Chlamydia trachomatis* in población femenina de la ciudad de Cuernavaca, Morelos" [Preva-
     lence of cervicovaginal infection with *Chlamydia trachomatis* in the female population of the city
     of Cuernavaca, Morelos], *Salud Public de Mexico* 34(3): 301–307.
Haberland, Nicole, Beverly Winikoff, Nancy Sloan, Christiana Coggins, and Christopher Elias. 1999.
     "Case finding and case management of chlamydia and gonorrhea infections among women: What
     we do and do not know," The Robert H. Ebert Program on Critical Issues in Reproductive Health.
     New York: Population Council.

Lazcano Ponce, Eduardo C., Nancy L. Sloan, Beverly Winikoff, Ana Langer, Christiana Coggins, Angela Heimburger, Carlos J. Conde-Glez, and Jorge Salmeron. 2000. "The power of information and contraceptive choice in a family planning setting in Mexico," *Sexually Transmitted Infections* 76(4): 277–281.

Pathfinder International. 1996. "Indicadores básicos sobre planificación familiar en la fase intermedia de la SDES" [Basic family planning indicators in the intermediate phase of the SDES (service delivery expansion support)], working paper series no. 2. Mexico City: Pathfinder International.

Sloan, Nancy L., Beverly Winikoff, Nicole Haberland, Christiana Coggins, and Christopher Elias. 2000. "Screening and syndromic approaches to identify gonorrhea and chlamydial infection among women," *Studies in Family Planning* 31(1): 55–68.

Uribe-Salas, Felipe, Mauricio Hernández-Avila, Carlos J. Conde-Glez, Luis Juárez-Figueroa, Bethania Allen, Rosalio Anaya-Ocampo, Carlos del Río-Chiriboga, Patricia Uribe-Zúñiga, and Barbara de Zalduondo. 1997. "Low prevalences of HIV infection and sexually transmitted disease among female commercial sex workers in Mexico City," *American Journal of Public Health* 87(6): 1012–1015.

Vernon, Ricardo and Yolanda Palma (eds.). 1998. "Resultados de investigación para mejorar los servicios de planificación familiar," INOPAL III. Mexico City: Population Council.

Contact information

Ana Langer
Director, Latin America and the Caribbean Regional Office
Population Council
Escondida 110, Col. Villa Coyoacán
México, D.F. 04000 Mexico
telephone: 52-5554-0388
fax: 52-5554-1226
e-mail: alanger@popcouncil.org.mx

16

Pitfalls and Possibilities: Managing RTIs in Family Planning and General Reproductive Health Services

Nicole Haberland, B. Ndugga Maggwa,
Christopher Elias, and Diana Measham

Clinicians and policymakers have increasingly recognized that family planning and general reproductive health services should pay greater attention to reproductive tract infections (RTIs). This recognition stems from several interrelated factors. First, RTIs account for a substantial burden of disease in the developing world. Second, there is an urgent need to curb the AIDS epidemic, as well as growing recognition of the role that other RTIs play in augmenting HIV transmission. Third, both family planning and RTI services require access to sexually active populations, overlapping supplies and equipment (e.g., condoms, speculums), and similar provider knowledge and counseling skills. Fourth, contraceptives interact with RTIs—they can either protect people from infection (i.e., barrier methods) or exacerbate infection (i.e., intrauterine devices); thus RTI presence and risk should be taken into account in contraceptive method selection. Fifth, while women's health activists have long called for attention to women's reproductive health concerns beyond family planning, the 1994 International Conference on Population and Development and the 1995 World Conference on Women in Beijing reinforced this at the level of international policy by advocating a more holistic approach to reproductive health service delivery, including attention to RTIs.

Reproductive tract infections are typically classified into three types: (1) sexually transmitted infections (STIs), such as chlamydia, gonorrhea, syphilis, trichomoniasis, and HIV; (2) endogenous infections resulting from an overgrowth of organisms normally present in the reproductive tract, such as bacterial vaginosis and yeast infection (including candidiasis); and (3) iatrogenic infections related to medical procedures such as abortion and IUD insertion. All cause significant morbidity and/or mortality among women and represent a substantial burden of disease.

Table 1. Estimated prevalence (%) of the four major curable STIs among men and women, 1995

Region	Syphilis		Gonorrhea		Chlamydia		Trichomoniasis	
	Males	Females	Males	Females	Males	Females	Males	Females
Latin America and the Caribbean	0.6	0.7	0.6	1.1	2.5	4.0	0.8	8.1
Sub-Saharan Africa	3.1	3.9	2.0	2.8	4.8	7.1	1.4	14.1
North Africa and the Middle East	0.4	0.5	0.2	0.4	1.2	1.7	0.3	3.3
East Asia and Pacific	0.1	0.1	0.1	0.1	0.4	0.7	0.1	1.4
South and Southeast Asia	1.4	1.8	1.0	1.4	3.7	4.9	1.0	9.7

Source: Gerbase et al. 1998.

THE SCOPE AND CONSEQUENCES OF RTIs

HIV is the reproductive tract infection with the gravest consequences. At the end of 2000, some 36.1 million men, women, and children were infected with HIV. Sub-Saharan Africa bears the largest burden: 70 percent of adults and 80 percent of children with HIV/AIDS live in this region (UNAIDS/WHO 2000).

Other viral STIs for which there are currently no cures include herpes and human papillomavirus. These infections are believed to be common in developing countries, although population-based prevalence data are limited (Bosch et al. 1995; O'Farrell 1999).

Syphilis, gonorrhea, chlamydia, and trichomoniasis are considered the four major curable STIs with an estimated 333 million cases among men and women ages 15–49 in 1995 (Gerbase et al. 1998). Among these, trichomoniasis is thought to have the highest incidence at 170 million new cases in 1995, compared to 89, 62, and 12 million new cases of chlamydia, gonorrhea, and syphilis, respectively. The prevalence of these infections is highest in sub-Saharan Africa, and, in the case of chlamydia, gonorrhea, and trichomoniasis, is substantially higher among women (see Table 1 for prevalence rates by STI, gender, and region) (Gerbase et al. 1998).

These four STIs increase the risk of sexual transmission of HIV. Syphilis can have other serious consequences, including death of the fetus and newborn among infected pregnant women. Gonorrhea and chlamydia can also result in grave complications when not treated in a timely fashion, potentially causing pelvic inflammatory disease and its sequelae: ectopic pregnancy and related maternal mortality; infertility; and chronic pelvic pain. They can also cause ophthalmia neonatorum (eye infections) in the newborns of infected pregnant women, which can lead to blindness if left un-

Table 2. Illustrative prevalence rates (%) for bacterial vaginosis and candidiasis

Study	Bacterial vaginosis	Candidiasis
Pregnant women making their first antenatal visit at an antenatal clinic in Libreville, Gabon (Bourgeois et al. 1998)	—	31
Women presenting with genitourinary complaints at a central hospital in Malawi (Costello Daly et al. 1998)	23	28
Women attending family planning (FP) clinics in Dar es Salaam, Tanzania (Kapiga et al. 1998)	—	8
Symptomatic, nonpregnant women attending an outpatient clinic and symptomatic pregnant women attending routine antenatal care services in Mwanza, Tanzania (Mayaud et al. 1998a)	Nonpregnant: 37 Pregnant: 21	Nonpregnant: 38 Pregnant: 38
Women attending an antenatal clinic in Mwanza, Tanzania (Mayaud et al. 1998b)	24	39
Symptomatic women at a primary health center and FP clinic in Morocco (Ryan et al. 1998)	Primary health center: 24 FP clinic: 19	—
Women attending the gynecology and FP clinics of a hospital in Lima, Peru (Sánchez et al. 1998)	30	—
Women attending FP services in rural South Africa (Schneider et al. 1998)	29	—
Maternal and child health/FP clients at FP and antenatal clinics in Nakuru, Kenya (Solo et al. 1999)	FP clinics: 33 Antenatal clinics: 30	FP clinics: 17 Antenatal clinics: 34

Note: Most of the studies cited above were published in the 1998 supplement to *Sexually Transmitted Infections.*

treated. Finally, there is some evidence that both gonorrhea and chlamydia can increase the risk of postpartum infections (Plummer et al. 1987). While trichomoniasis has less severe complications, it can facilitate HIV transmission and may cause considerable symptomatic morbidity related to vaginal discharge and irritation, soreness, or itching. It has also been associated with low birthweight and premature delivery among pregnant women (Cates 1998).

The prevalence of endogenous infections such as bacterial vaginosis and candidiasis is less well documented. Table 2 shows illustrative rates from several studies in

Africa and Latin America among both symptomatic populations and routine family planning and antenatal care clients. Among women, the prevalence of bacterial vaginosis and candidiasis tends to be substantially higher than that of chlamydia and gonorrhea.

Bacterial vaginosis is a disturbance of the vaginal ecology characterized by an overgrowth of endogenous organisms that replace the protective microbial flora of the vagina. It is sometimes considered a sexually associated condition, because sex (or associated health behaviors such as douching) may predispose some women to its occurrence. It is not, however, an STI per se, and treatment of the male partner does not prevent reinfection. Bacterial vaginosis may cause vaginal irritation and is associated with increased risk of preterm delivery and low birthweight. Significantly, it has recently been found to be associated with increased risk of pelvic inflammatory disease (Peipert et al. 1997), as well as increased risk of HIV transmission (Taha et al. 1998). Candidiasis may cause burning and severe vaginal itching, and one study has shown an association between symptomatic candida and increased risk of HIV transmission (Martin et al. 1998).

HOW CAN FAMILY PLANNING AND GENERAL REPRODUCTIVE HEALTH SERVICES ADDRESS RTIs?

There are several ways to incorporate attention to RTIs into family planning and routine reproductive health services. One is primary prevention, which takes different forms depending on the type of RTI targeted. For example, iatrogenic RTIs can be prevented through enhanced infection control and prevention measures that include training clinic staff and ensuring proper maintenance of equipment.

Prevention of STIs can take the form of counseling and informing clients regarding STI transmission and prevention (including the use of barrier methods), increasing women's ability to negotiate condom use, promoting a reduction in the number of sexual partners, and so on.[1] Some clients may also wish to consider dual protection (the use of male or female condoms together with another contraceptive), because condoms are not as effective at preventing pregnancy as some other contraceptive methods, whereas the most effective pregnancy prevention methods do not provide protection against STIs; an alternative is condoms with emergency contraception as a backup. Similarly, providers can prevent pelvic inflammatory disease by ensuring that IUDs are appropriately provided to women (i.e., that they are not given to women with chlamydia and gonorrhea before these infections are treated).[2] (Some argue that the presence of gonorrhea or chlamydia should exclude a woman from IUD use because, even if treated, the fact that she has one of these infections indicates that she may be at risk of acquiring a new STI.)

Prevention of endogenous infections is less well understood. However, it is clear that douching (especially with substances other than plain water) and traditional practices, such as inserting herbs or powders into the vagina, should be discouraged (van de Wijgert et al. 2000).[3] There are no data on the role of menstrual hygiene in endogenous infections. Nevertheless, in places where use of disposable menstrual protection (such as cotton wads or tampons) is not feasible, the cloths women reuse should be boiled, if possible—especially if some or all of the cloth is inserted into the vagina. Family planning and other reproductive health services can help educate women about these issues.

Reproductive health and family planning programs can also be involved in the diagnosis and treatment of RTIs in order to better meet their clients' broader reproductive health needs, as well as to provide contraceptive services more appropriately. Their role in this area is posing considerable challenges for a number of reasons. First, a high proportion of women with RTIs do not exhibit signs or symptoms. Of the primary curable RTIs, only syphilis causes potentially distinguishable ulcers in its primary stage, although these ulcers are often painless and not noticed. Gonorrhea and chlamydia infect the cervix and are also frequently asymptomatic among women— they may or may not cause endocervical or vaginal discharge that in turn may or may not be noticed by the woman or a health care provider during a pelvic examination. HIV infection can be asymptomatic for months or years. While the organisms responsible for bacterial vaginosis, candidiasis, and trichomoniasis commonly cause abnormal vaginal discharge, a considerable proportion of women with these infections also do not exhibit signs or symptoms. In addition, many women who do have symptoms will not seek care because they are embarrassed, do not recognize the symptoms as serious, or consider them a burden that must be borne. Even diagnosing women who present with a primary complaint of vaginal discharge is complicated, as described below. While simple diagnostic tests exist for some RTIs, the diagnosis of others is complex, particularly in low-resource settings.

The standard tests for the more easily diagnosed RTIs are outlined in Table 3. While these tests can be conducted in some peripheral laboratories, such as those attached to health centers and district hospitals (van Dyck et al. 1996), they require trained personnel, microscopes, and other materials that are not always available in low-resource settings and are usually absent from lower-level health service delivery points.

The primary test for HIV is the enzyme-linked immunosorbent assay (ELISA),[4] which screens for HIV antibodies in the blood. Because ELISA requires skilled technical staff, a steady power supply, specific equipment, and regular equipment maintenance, it is less feasible for smaller or more isolated laboratories, hospitals, and clinics (UNAIDS 1997). Simple and rapid (simple/rapid) HIV screening assays that do not require special

Table 3. Standard diagnostic tests for bacterial vaginosis, candidiasis, syphilis, and trichomoniasis

RTI	Standard diagnostic test
Bacterial vaginosis	Diagnosed by detecting at least three of the following four characteristics in a vaginal discharge specimen: a thin, homogenous discharge; a positive Gram's stain (a vaginal specimen is smeared onto a slide and stained with different solutions that distinguish cells by color) or saline wet mount (either examined for clue cells); amine (fishy) odor when combined with 10 percent KOH (potassium hydroxide) (whiff test); and vaginal pH greater than 4.5 (measured by smearing vaginal fluid onto a dipstick with a swab).
Candidiasis	Diagnosed with either a 10 percent KOH wet mount (a wet preparation of vaginal specimen on a slide to which a drop or two of KOH is added and examined for yeast cells under a microscope) or Gram's stain.
Syphilis	Diagnosed with an assessment of genital ulcer symptoms or by serological (blood) screening using simple tests such as rapid plasma reagin (RPR, which uses plastic-coated cards on which the antigen–antibody reaction is visible to the naked eye) or the Venereal Disease Research Laboratory test (VDRL, a slide test antigen to measure antibodies; the reaction is visible under a microscope). Positive serological screening tests should be confirmed using a more specific treponemal test (*Treponema pallidum* is the organism that causes syphilis).
Trichomoniasis	Diagnosed with a saline wet mount (the infecting agent, in the case of trichomoniasis, is a protozoa that is easily recognizable when vaginal fluid is suspended in saline and examined under a microscope) or Gram's stain. Trichomonads are relatively easy to identify on a wet mount because they are still alive and motile.

Source: Larsen, Hunter, and McGrew 1991; Spiegel 1991; van Dyck et al. 1996.

equipment or highly trained staff are also available. Typically, a dot or line visible to the naked eye indicates a positive result. However, a positive result from an ELISA or simple/rapid test does not definitively indicate that the person has HIV; a supplemental test is necessary to confirm diagnosis. Western blot has been the standard confirmatory test, but it is complicated and expensive. Alternatively, carefully selected combinations of screening tests (ELISA and/or simple/rapid assays) have performed as well as the ELISA/Western blot combination (UNAIDS 1997; WHO/UNAIDS 1997). UNAIDS and WHO thus recommend testing strategies (tailored to the prevalence of infection and whether or not the person exhibits symptoms) that entail two or three sequential ELISA and/or simple/rapid assays, and, when there is a discrepancy in the results, a confirmatory assay such as Western blot (WHO/UNAIDS 1997).

Negative results derived from any of these diagnostic strategies do not rule out HIV infection, because there is a "window period" of about 3–8 weeks between HIV infection and the time when antibodies become detectable. During this "window

---

Box 1. Voluntary HIV counseling and testing

People infected with HIV can remain asymptomatic for many years (AIDS onset can range from six months to 10 years or more after exposure), yet they can transmit HIV to others as soon as they become infected. The only way for a person to know whether he or she is infected is to take an HIV test. Even then, negative test results do not necessarily indicate that an individual does not have HIV, because of the "window period" between infection and the time when antibodies become detectable. Providers trained in pre- and post-HIV test counseling can play an important role in helping uninfected and infected individuals (including individuals with currently undetectable infections) reduce risky behavior to protect themselves and prevent transmission to others, make informed childbearing and infant care decisions, keep healthy, better manage opportunistic infections, and access support programs. High-quality voluntary HIV counseling and testing can be an effective strategy for reducing HIV sexual risk behaviors among adults. A recent multi-center study showed that individuals undergoing voluntary testing and counseling exhibited changes in risk behaviors, such as an increase in condom use and reduction in the number of sex partners (Coates et al. 2000).

For these reasons, there is a strong argument for establishing the technical capacity to conduct HIV testing and counseling in family planning clinics. Both family planning services and HIV counseling and testing services require access to sexually active populations, a supply of condoms, and similar basic technical capacity, knowledge, and counseling skills among providers. The human and other resource requirements for incorporating HIV counseling and testing into family planning and reproductive health services are generally lacking, but are not impossible to put in place. Much remains to be learned about how to do so, and relevant research is underway. In Asia, for example, research is focused on the requirements for introducing voluntary counseling and testing in antenatal clinics, as part of an overall perinatal HIV prevention strategy. In Africa, research is focused on counseling and testing in antenatal clinics, among adolescents, and in public-sector primary health care facilities.

---

period" an individual infected with HIV can transmit the virus. The implications of this for HIV counseling and testing are highlighted in Box 1.

The diagnosis of chlamydia and gonorrhea is more complicated, as it requires more expensive and sophisticated laboratory tests. Such diagnostic capabilities might be found in regional or provincial hospitals, but in many settings are available only in central labs in capital cities or in university hospitals (van Dyck et al. 1996). Gonorrhea is definitively diagnosed with culture, which requires a culture medium; an incubator; a humid, enriched CO_2 environment; careful handling in transport to a lab if an incubator is not available locally; and a trained technician. Chlamydia culture is similarly complex and requires scarce cell-culture facilities. Other tests used for chlamydia, such as direct fluorescent antibody (DFA), ELISA, and DNA amplification methods such as polymerase chain reaction (PCR) and ligase chain reaction (LCR),[5] require state-of-the-art laboratory facilities.

Because of the lack of simple, accurate, low-cost tools to diagnose many RTIs, WHO developed syndromic algorithms to assist clinicians in deciding, on the basis of a client's symptoms and clinical signs, what infection she or he might have and what medications could be used to treat the major pathogens responsible for that syndrome. Syndromes for which such nonlaboratory management strategies have been developed include urethral discharge and testicular pain and swelling in men, genital ulcers in both men and women, and abdominal pain and abnormal vaginal discharge in women.

Some of these syndromic management tools are effective. For example, the WHO algorithm for urethral discharge in men, which is recommended when no microscopy is available, is highly accurate (Djajakusumah et al. 1998).[6] However, the algorithms for vaginal discharge in women, which seek to manage bacterial vaginosis, candidiasis, chlamydia, gonorrhea, and trichomoniasis, have been problematic. Primary attention has been focused on determining and improving the efficacy of these tools for managing chlamydia and gonorrhea, given their severe sequelae and the lack of simple lab tests for their diagnosis. Studies among family planning and antenatal care clients consistently show that these algorithms perform poorly for these infections (Dallabetta, Gerbase, and Holmes 1998; Sloan et al. 2000). Poor performance can mean that the tools failed to identify a substantial proportion of women with infection (i.e., the algorithms had low sensitivity) or that the tools identified too many women as infected, when in fact they were not (i.e., they had a low positive predictive value). As one article concludes, "the application of the algorithm was only modestly better than random treatment" (Dallabetta, Gerbase, and Holmes 1998, p. S4). This is of concern, since mislabeling a woman as having an STI when she does not, and providing her with unnecessary treatment, has consequences in terms of drug resistance; it may also put her at risk of partner accusations, abuse, or divorce. In addition, if a test cannot identify a substantial majority of women with infection, and those whom it does identify as infected are not, serious questions of cost and efficacy arise.

A meta-analysis of 32 studies (Sloan et al. 2000) found that in populations with moderate prevalence (defined as less than 20 percent chlamydia or gonorrhea prevalence, as would be found in most family planning program populations), algorithms based on signs and symptoms identified approximately 28 and 42 percent of all infections, with and without speculum exams, respectively, missing between 58 and 72 percent of infected women. Of the women identified as infected with chlamydia or gonorrhea, less than 12 percent actually had these infections (i.e., at least 88 percent of the women identified as having chlamydia or gonorrhea were misdiagnosed).

One of the inherent drawbacks of the syndromic approach is that, by definition, it will miss all asymptomatic cases. As noted above, the proportion of asymptomatic cases is not inconsequential. Indeed the majority of women with chlamydia or gonorrhea do not exhibit symptoms, and a substantial proportion of women with trichomoniasis and bacterial vaginosis are also asymptomatic. Moreover, even women with symptoms often dismiss them as "normal" and do not seek treatment. These same women may regularly attend family planning or pregnancy-related services. Thus there has been interest in identifying cases of infection among general family planning and antenatal clinic populations (case finding) in addition to managing women who present with symptoms.

Efforts to improve the efficacy of these algorithms have led to the inclusion of social and behavioral risk factors to supplement physical signs and symptoms, as well as to the development of risk scores. This has been done with two objectives. The first is to help distinguish symptomatic women who have a higher likelihood of cervical infection (chlamydia or gonorrhea) as opposed to vaginal infection (such as bacterial vaginosis, candidiasis, or trichomoniasis) and who should be given medication for treatment of chlamydia and gonorrhea. The second is to use risk assessment as a screening tool to find infections among women who are asymptomatic and/or not presenting with the primary complaint of vaginal discharge.

These enhancements have not yielded the desired results (Dallabetta, Gerbase, and Holmes 1998; Sloan et al. 2000). In the meta-analysis by Sloan et al., risk scores (which are derived by assigning weights to specific signs, symptoms, and risk factors) performed better than syndromic algorithms with or without speculum exams and better than syndromic algorithms that incorporate risk factors (i.e., individual or behavioral risk factors, such as age, more than one sexual partner, and so on) in moderate-prevalence populations.[7] However, even risk scores were able to identify only slightly over half (54 percent) of women infected with chlamydia and/or gonorrhea, and 82 percent of the women identified as infected did not, in fact, have these infections (Sloan et al. 2000).[8]

Less research has been done to assess the performance of the vaginal discharge algorithm in managing bacterial vaginosis, candidiasis, and trichomoniasis. Asymptomatic bacterial vaginosis and yeast infection (i.e., the infection is visible on a wet mount or by Gram's stain, but the woman has no complaints) are usually not treated. This is because both conditions are transient—they come and go—and their sequelae are not considered serious. Given the association of bacterial vaginosis with pelvic inflammatory disease and recent evidence that both symptomatic and asymptomatic bacterial vaginosis, and possibly symptomatic candidiasis, may also be associated with increased transmission of HIV, an amplified focus that includes these infections appears warranted.

Finally, most of the experiments to test the algorithms apply them under ideal conditions: Clinicians are well trained in their use and carefully monitored. Case studies of clinics in East and Southern Africa found that in at least some settings, providers were not following the diagnostic algorithms correctly and did not carry out a full risk assessment, despite the emphasis on STI management in training, and algorithms displayed on the walls (Maggwa and Askew 1997).

CASE EXAMPLES FROM ZIMBABWE AND VIETNAM

We now review experiments to manage RTIs in maternal and child health/family planning (MCH/FP) clinics in two very different settings: Zimbabwe and Vietnam. Specifically, we offer lessons from studies in three clinics of the Zimbabwe National Family Planning Council (ZNFPC) (Maggwa et al. 1999) and in the MCH/FP Center in Hue, a city in central Vietnam (Lien et al. 1998). A substantial proportion of women attending clinics in both settings suffer from RTIs according to standard, definitive laboratory tests: 35 percent in Zimbabwe and 21 percent in Vietnam (see Table 4). While higher prevalence rates are found in Zimbabwe, the most common infections in both settings are candidiasis and bacterial vaginosis, which are endogenous, non–sexually transmitted infections. Trichomoniasis is the most common STI in both settings, followed by syphilis, chlamydia, and gonorrhea.

A substantial proportion of clients presenting to the Zimbabwe clinics had come with the primary complaint of RTI symptoms (25 percent). More than a third (35 percent) had come for an annual checkup, while 27 percent had come for resupply of their contraceptive method.[9] The MCH/FP Center in Hue provides a broad range of reproductive health services, including family planning, abortion and menstrual regulation, and gynecologic, antenatal, and delivery care. Most of the clients (87 percent) had come to the clinic because of gynecologic problems (primarily complaints about vaginal discharge), with small proportions coming for family planning (6 percent) and abortion services (2 percent).

BEFORE THE INTERVENTION

The clinics evaluated in Zimbabwe were generally well-equipped, with working toilets, water supply, an energy source, and a separate counseling/exam room; some had microscopes. However, services and information related directly to RTI management were deficient. Client record forms did not provide any guidance to service providers as to what questions to ask when they took histories or performed STI/HIV risk assessments, nor did they provide space to record the answers to such questions (e.g., number of partners in last three months) or the results of clinical exams (e.g., presence/absence of vaginal discharge) that would help in identifying and managing clients at increased risk for STIs/HIV. Indeed, very few of the service providers (three out of 19) asked women about their, or their partners', sexual behavior.

Pelvic exams were conducted moderately well. Providers generally explained the procedure to women; inspected the thighs, pubic area, and external genitalia for ulcers; separated the labia for proper inspection; and performed a speculum exam. However, most providers did not ask clients to pass urine before the exam, did not carry

Table 4. Prevalence (%) of reproductive tract infections, ZNFPC clinics and Hue MCH/FP Center

RTI	Zimbabwe (3 clinics)	Vietnam (MCH/FP Center)
Candidiasis	17.3	12.0
Bacterial vaginosis	9.0	6.3
Trichomoniasis	4.1	2.8
Syphilis	3.9	1.2
Chlamydia	2.9	0.8
Gonorrhea	1.8	0.2
Any RTI	35.0	21.0

out a bimanual exam, and did not take a Pap smear—essential components of pelvic exam protocols in Zimbabwe.

While staff used algorithms to manage clients presenting to the clinics with complaints of RTI symptoms, the tools used were not those approved by the national sexually transmitted infection project of the Zimbabwe Ministry of Health and Child Welfare. As noted earlier, the algorithms for vaginal discharge perform poorly for diagnosing chlamydia and gonorrhea, especially in low-risk populations, even when developed specifically for the setting and applied consistently and properly. Finally, many of the drugs recommended for the treatment of RTIs by the national algorithms were not in stock.

In the Hue clinic, standard practice—consisting of a service provider's assessment following a pelvic exam—was compared with definitive laboratory diagnosis. Clinicians conducted a thorough pelvic exam and recorded whether they thought an RTI was present, and, if so, whether they thought it was vaginal, cervical, and/or pelvic in nature. According to the clinicians' judgment, 60 percent of the women had an RTI. The clinicians thought 43 percent of women had a vaginal infection, 44 percent had a cervical infection, and 2 percent had a pelvic infection. These figures are significantly higher than the RTI prevalence rates found upon laboratory diagnosis (see Table 4). The discrepancy is particularly striking in the case of cervical infections (chlamydia and gonorrhea), for which actual prevalence was 1 percent. "There was thus a greater than 40-fold overdiagnosis and treatment of cervical infections among these experienced clinicians" (Lien et al. 1998, p. 12).

AN INTERVENTION IN ZIMBABWE: GOALS AND ACHIEVEMENTS

To help improve the capacity of ZNFPC, project staff trained ZNFPC providers on the syndromic management of RTIs, developed an RTI checklist, and attempted to ensure the availability of RTI drugs.

Staff Training

Service providers, their supervisors, ZNFPC trainers, and program managers attended a one-week refresher course on the syndromic management of RTIs. The workshop covered presenting symptoms and signs, complications, risk factors, and the management of common RTIs. More specifically, the course sought to refine providers' skills in taking histories, assessing STI/HIV risk, performing clinical examinations, and using the approved syndromic management algorithms for common RTIs. (See Figure 1 for a diagram of the Zimbabwe national algorithm for vaginal discharge.) The national algorithms for management of RTIs were introduced, reviewed, and practiced through role-plays, and later in participants' own clinics under the supervision of a trainer. In addition, to ensure that the skills learned were being used, the trainers visited the providers at their clinics and observed them applying the algorithms at regular intervals throughout the evaluation period. The role-plays and practical training sessions were also used to improve RTI/HIV counseling skills.

Most of the service providers who attended this training had not previously attended a refresher course that included management of RTIs. They reported that the course improved their skills and helped them standardize RTI management.

RTI Checklist

Many service providers cited the lack of a systematic reminder or guide as one of the reasons they did not undertake STI/HIV risk assessment and counseling. To respond to this need, an integrated checklist was developed to replace the client record form, and staff were trained in its use. The six-page checklist combined the routine information collected from clients for the purpose of providing high-quality family planning counseling with interview and exam information essential for the identification and management of clients with or at risk for STIs. The checklist included eight sections:
- Clinic and personal information, including marital status, education, and age at first marriage.
- Reason for clinic visit, obstetric and gynecologic history, and current symptoms, including lower abdominal pain, abnormal discharge, or pain during intercourse.
- General medical and contraceptive history.
- Clinical exam results, diagnosis, and treatment, including whether the clinician observes any ulcers or discharge on pelvic exam, cervical discharge on speculum exam, or adnexal tenderness on bimanual exam. This section also includes a space in which to record the syndromic diagnosis and treatment, as well as the family planning method provided.

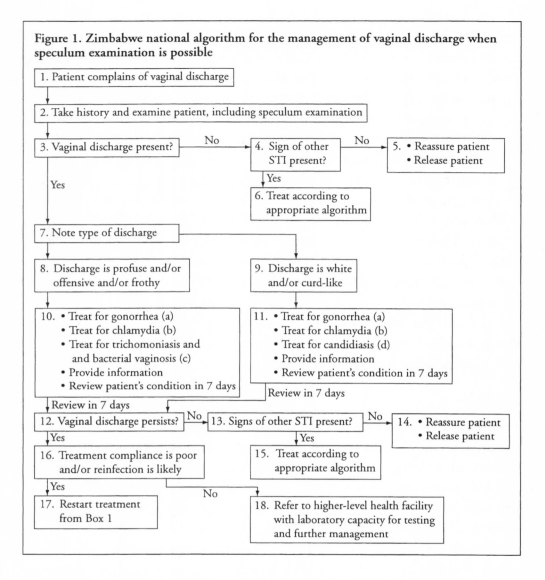

Figure 1. Zimbabwe national algorithm for the management of vaginal discharge when speculum examination is possible

1. Patient complains of vaginal discharge

2. Take history and examine patient, including speculum examination

3. Vaginal discharge present? — No → 4. Sign of other STI present? — No → 5. • Reassure patient • Release patient

Yes (from 3)

Yes (from 4) → 6. Treat according to appropriate algorithm

7. Note type of discharge

8. Discharge is profuse and/or offensive and/or frothy

9. Discharge is white and/or curd-like

10. • Treat for gonorrhea (a) • Treat for chlamydia (b) • Treat for trichomoniasis and and bacterial vaginosis (c) • Provide information • Review patient's condition in 7 days

11. • Treat for gonorrhea (a) • Treat for chlamydia (b) • Treat for candidiasis (d) • Provide information • Review patient's condition in 7 days

Review in 7 days

12. Vaginal discharge persists? — No → 13. Signs of other STI present? — No → 14. • Reassure patient • Release patient

Yes (from 12)

Yes (from 13) → 15. Treat according to appropriate algorithm

16. Treatment compliance is poor and/or reinfection is likely

Yes → 17. Restart treatment from Box 1

No → 18. Refer to higher-level health facility with laboratory capacity for testing and further management

- Counseling for STIs/HIV. Guidance is provided on the types of information that should be given to all family planning clients and to clients suspected of having an STI. For example, the checklist requires that all family planning clients be counseled about STI/HIV risk factors, modes of transmission, symptoms and signs, complications, dual methods of protection, and condom use. The checklist also requires the provider to record whether these messages were relayed.
- Laboratory tests, including specimens taken and test results (the provider completes this section at a later time).
- Follow-up information to be filled in when the client returns for her next appointment. This includes whether the client was clinically cured if she was

suspected of having an STI, and, if not, any change in treatment the provider advises.

- STI/HIV risk assessment checklist. The 23 items on the list include questions regarding the sexual behavior, STI symptoms, condom use, and risk/protective behaviors of the client and the client's partner(s).

Drug Availability

ZNFPC, with assistance from the U.S. Agency for International Development, negotiated an arrangement with the national STI project, the World Bank, and the Department for International Development to include the clinics in an ongoing project that supplies RTI drugs to health facilities. ZNFPC would now regularly receive all necessary drugs for RTIs directly from the central medical stores on a quarterly basis. Clinic statistics on medication use were used to determine each clinic's requirements.

EFFECTIVENESS OF THE INTERVENTION IN ZIMBABWE

RTI Management

Providers affiliated with ZNFPC clinics now give clients a systematic exam and counseling session. The integrated checklist is used both as a provider's guide and as the client's record form. Since the checklist was introduced, consultations for new family planning clients have lasted an average of 27 minutes, up from 20 minutes previously. While making STI screening and counseling part and parcel of the client record form has increased the time required for initial counseling and exams, each client is asked the same comprehensive set of questions, managed in the same manner, and counseled on sexual and other behaviors that put them at risk for STIs, the symptoms of STIs and HIV/AIDS, how to protect themselves from infection, and how to use a condom. Clients who are suspected of having an STI are informed about the importance of completing drug therapy, the need to protect their partners during the course of treatment, how to protect their partners during the infectious period, the need to inform their partners and ensure that they obtain treatment, and the importance of returning for a follow-up exam.

All women are given pelvic, breast, and general physical exams. Since the standardized checklist was introduced, more staff check uterine size and assess the client for the presence of abdominal tenderness, rebound tenderness, vaginal or cervical discharge, genital ulcers, changes in the color and friability of the cervix, and adnexal masses and tenderness. The presence or absence of these variables is noted on the checklist/client record.

The clinicians also carry out an STI/HIV risk assessment. As noted above, they ask all clients a series of questions, including:

- Does your employment or the activity from which you derive most of your income involve traveling and/or staying away from home frequently? (The same question is asked about the client's partner.)
- Some men have sex with more than one woman. Do you think that your spouse (partner) has sex with other women?
- Have you experienced ———— (specific RTI symptoms are inserted, such as "purulent vaginal discharge" and "painful sexual intercourse") in the past 12 months? (A similar question is asked about possible symptoms experienced by the client's partner[s] in the past four weeks.)
- Have you had more than one sexual partner in the past three months?
- Did you receive or give money or other types of gifts the last time you had sex?
- Have you used any intravaginal preparations for the purpose of constricting and/or drying the vagina to prepare yourself for sexual intercourse in the past three months?

At first, providers felt uncomfortable with the checklist. In an initial postintervention interview, less than a third (29 percent) thought it was "fine." Most thought it was either too long (43 percent), too cumbersome (7 percent), too complicated (7 percent), or not useful (7 percent). However, after clinicians had used the checklist for several months, their feelings changed dramatically: 86 percent thought that it was easy to use and had greatly improved the quality of their work.

Using information obtained through the checklist, staff apply the national syndromic algorithms to determine the likely cause of infection, decide on treatment, and provide appropriate counseling. For example, if a woman has vaginal discharge, clinicians are expected to use the presence or absence of other factors, such as adnexal tenderness and the woman's response to the risk assessment questions, to determine whether she has a vaginal or a cervical infection. The client is then given the medication specified by the national algorithms. She is asked to return on a specified date for a follow-up visit after completing her initial course of treatment.[10]

Using the national algorithms, clinicians identified RTI syndromes in 41 percent of clients. Lower abdominal pain (27 percent) and vaginal discharge (22 percent) were the most common syndromes. However, application of the guidelines was uneven. While 33 percent of clients had clinical evidence of vaginal discharge, only about half of these women were diagnosed as having vaginal discharge syndrome and treated according to the national algorithms. The algorithms recommend that clients complaining of lower abdominal pain be treated for pelvic inflammatory disease, yet while 43 percent of clients had this complaint, again only about half were diagnosed and treated accordingly. These findings suggest that clinical indicators do not always guide clinicians' diagnosis and treatment decisions. Moreover, they suggest that clinicians do not always follow the national algorithms even when extra efforts are made in the form of training, protocols, supplies, and improved drug availability.

But how did the clinicians perform compared to definitive laboratory diagnosis? Perhaps their divergence from the national guidelines, for whatever reason, was warranted. To answer this question, researchers assessed the sensitivity (proportion of women with infections identified as infected) and positive predictive values (proportion of those identified as infected who actually have an infection) of the tools for managing clients with cervical and vaginal infections. Researchers differentiated between "all clients" and "RTI clients" (clients specifically attending the clinic with an RTI-related complaint), because the prevalence of infection among clients who come with the primary complaint of RTI symptoms is typically higher than among all clients; the more prevalent the infection, the less likely that a screening tool or diagnostic test will result in substantial overdiagnosis (i.e., the higher its positive predictive value).

The analysis showed that syndromic case management was not effective when applied by clinicians in these family planning clinics (see Table 5). The providers were able to identify only one-third of the women who had a laboratory-diagnosed cervical infection. Their ability to identify cases of infection improved somewhat when only those women who had attended the clinics with RTI-related complaints were considered. However, approximately 90 percent of women identified as having a cervical infection did not in fact have such an infection. The clinicians performed somewhat better in identifying women with laboratory-diagnosed vaginal infection (bacterial vaginosis, candidiasis, and trichomoniasis). While the proportion of women with vaginal infections identified by clinicians using the algorithms was similar to that for cervical infections, vaginal infections were less frequently overdiagnosed. Nevertheless, overdiagnosis was quite high—two-thirds of the women identified as having a vaginal infection did not, in fact, have such an infection.

To determine whether the algorithms would work if they had been applied properly and consistently, application of the algorithms was simulated (i.e., it was assumed that all clients with the indicative symptoms and signs were managed according to the algorithms) and compared to definitive laboratory diagnosis. Even under these ideal simulated conditions, the performance of the algorithms was poor. Table 6 presents the results.

These data indicate that the algorithms are ineffective for managing RTI clients in family planning clinics in Zimbabwe for two reasons: (1) clinicians do not consistently use the information obtained during consultations to manage clients with signs and symp-

Table 5. Effectiveness of syndromic case management when applied by clinicians, ZNFPC clinics

	Percentage of infected women accurately diagnosed (sensitivity)		Percentage of uninfected women misdiagnosed (false-positive rate[a])	
	All clients[b]	RTI clients only[c]	All clients[b]	RTI clients only[c]
Cervical infections	36	59	93	90
Vaginal infections	37	51	71	65

[a] False-positive rate = 100 − positive predictive value.
[b] All clients attending the family planning clinic, regardless of reason for visit.
[c] Clients attending the clinic with an RTI-related complaint.

Table 6. Effectiveness of simulated application of the syndromic algorithm for managing vaginal discharge, ZNFPC clinics

	Percentage of infected women accurately diagnosed (sensitivity)		Percentage of uninfected women misdiagnosed (false-positive rate[a])	
	All clients[b]	RTI clients only[c]	All clients[b]	RTI clients only[c]
Cervical infections	33	55	92	89
Vaginal infections	24	40	62	59

[a] False-positive rate = 100 − positive predictive value.
[b] All clients attending the family planning clinic, regardless of reason for visit.
[c] Clients attending the clinic with an RTI-related complaint.

toms suggestive of an RTI; and (2) the symptoms and signs of vaginal discharge and lower abdominal pain are not good predictors of either cervical or vaginal infections.

As noted earlier, the project had implemented a two-visit approach (as recommended by the Zimbabwe national algorithm) in the hope that women initially misdiagnosed by the algorithm would return for their follow-up visit with persistent symptoms/signs and would receive alternative treatment. This approach, however, relies completely on clients' returning for a second visit; less than 20 percent of clients returned for this follow-up visit.

EFFECTIVENESS OF SYNDROMIC MANAGEMENT IN VIETNAM

In Hue, the vast majority of women had come to the clinic with the primary complaint of vaginal discharge. In this instance, the WHO flow chart for managing symptomatic vaginal discharge in settings where simple light microscopy is available was applied (via simulated application). This algorithm requires providers to ask several risk-assessment questions, examine for the presence of cervical discharge, and observe organisms, such as yeast or clue cells, under a microscope.

The algorithm performed well for the diagnosis of bacterial vaginosis, candidiasis, and trichomoniasis. While clinicians presumptively diagnosed 45 percent of the women with vaginal infection (using current standard practice), use of the algorithm decreased the level of overdiagnosis and closely approximated definitive laboratory diagnosis. This is largely a result of the use of simple microscopic tests such as wet mounts and Gram's stain. Center staff were able to accurately detect most cases of bacterial vaginosis and candidiasis. The results for trichomoniasis were less striking, because center staff found it difficult to read trichomoniasis specimens under a microscope.[11]

In the case of cervical infection (chlamydia and gonorrhea), the algorithm did not offer any advantages over current clinical practice, generating a 49 percent prevalence rate as compared to the clinicians' 48 percent, and 1 percent based on laboratory diagnosis. Even when only very specific cervical discharge syndromes were used, there was still substantial overdiagnosis: 98 percent of the women identified as having cervical infection using the algorithm did not have chlamydia or gonorrhea.

LESSONS FOR REPRODUCTIVE HEALTH AND FAMILY PLANNING SERVICES

In this section we discuss lessons for routine family planning and other general reproductive health services, such as antenatal care clinics, rather than for higher-prevalence settings (e.g., STI clinics) or populations at higher risk (e.g., sex workers).

The Need to Tailor Strategies

RTI management strategies must be based on local prevalence rates of specific RTIs, health-seeking behavior, and clinical capacity. For example, the study in Zimbabwe found that few clients returned for their follow-up visit, indicating that a two-visit approach is of limited use in this context. In Hue, the low prevalence of chlamydia and gonorrhea and the unacceptable overdiagnosis of these infections using the WHO algorithm demonstrate that the algorithm is not effective for managing these RTIs in this context. Studies like the one in Hue are useful in that they assess the efficacy of current clinical practice. In Hue, switching to a syndromic algorithm that includes microscopy did not improve the diagnosis of cervical infections, but did improve diagnosis of vaginal infections.

Managing Infections Among Reproductive Health and Family Planning Clients with RTI-related Complaints

There is no consensus regarding appropriate strategies for managing chlamydia and gonorrhea in women. Given the serious complications of chlamydia and gonorrhea, even low prevalence is cause for concern. Yet in the Zimbabwe and Hue studies, as in studies conducted elsewhere, the syndromic algorithm for vaginal discharge proved ineffective in managing cervical infection. This is true even when the algorithms are correctly applied, and is due primarily to the fact that symptoms and signs do not correlate well with actual chlamydia and gonorrhea infection in women.

It may, therefore, be appropriate in some settings to drop the cervical infection arm of the WHO algorithm. An alternative might be to design and test flow charts that involve return visits and sequential use of medications for different RTI pathogens, as is the intention in Zimbabwe. This would only be appropriate in settings where a higher proportion of clients are willing to return than was the case in the Zimbabwe study. In one study in the Philippines, for example, 74 percent of patients returned for a follow-up visit (Encena, Costello, and Echaves 1998). In settings where follow-up visits have been determined to be feasible and/or common, the question remains whether this appreciably improves the performance of the algorithm and risk scores.

It is possible to diagnose and treat endogenous infections in settings with rudimentary laboratory capacity. The algorithms used in Zimbabwe did not include simple lab tests and performed poorly for vaginal infections. However, findings from Hue indicate that in settings where clinicians have the skills, equipment, and supervision needed to use microscopy and other tests, they can diagnose bacterial vaginosis and candidiasis with a high degree of accuracy. This approach represented a substantial improvement over previous infection management strategies (i.e., clinicians' judgment alone). Questions remain about the feasibility and effectiveness of incorporating such technical capacity into reproductive health programs where little or no attention has been paid to RTIs to date.

It is possible to diagnose and treat trichomoniasis in settings with rudimentary laboratory capacity. The research in Hue indicates that definitive laboratory diagnosis of trichomoniasis, an STI typically twice as prevalent as chlamydia, may be possible in some settings. While clinicians were not as proficient at diagnosing trichomoniasis as they were at diagnosing bacterial vaginosis and candidiasis, this was partly because there was more emphasis on the latter infections during training.

RTI Case Finding Among Reproductive Health/Family Planning Clients

It is not clear how cases of chlamydia and gonorrhea infection can be identified among routine reproductive health and family planning clients. Finding the large proportions of asymptomatic RTI cases among women and identifying symptomatic infections among women who do not seek care for this reason (but who may regularly attend family planning and antenatal care clinics) remain urgent challenges. Identifying and treating women with chlamydia and gonorrhea is of particular concern given their severe sequelae. The poor results of the algorithms and risk scores in identifying cases of chlamydia and gonorrhea among general reproductive health clients indicate that the tools should not be used for this purpose. An alternative method of finding and managing women with chlamydia and gonorrhea that merits testing is improving partner notification and presumptive treatment of the female partners of men with symptomatic STI syndromes, such as urethral discharge. As noted above, the urethral discharge algorithm performs well for managing infections in men. Increasing women's awareness of symptoms and the need for treatment may also be an important step in bringing more women with vaginal infections to service sites where they could be screened with relatively simple microscopy. Unfortunately, many health service delivery points do not have this capacity.

Key Technological Gaps

There is an urgent need for simple, accurate, low-cost field diagnostic tools that can be used in peripheral sites. While the Hue clinicians' capacity to diagnose bacterial vaginosis, candidiasis, and trichomoniasis correctly with simple tests is encouraging, many health posts and clinics do not have the equipment or staff capacity to make use of even these simple tools. For chlamydia and gonorrhea, the laboratory tests are too complicated and expensive for most low-resource settings. Efforts are underway at organizations such as the Program for Appropriate Technology in Health and WHO to develop simple, accurate, low-cost field diagnostic tools. While this is neither a new nor an easily implemented recommendation, we join the many others who have identified this as an urgent area for continued research.

Partner Notification

Partner notification is an essential aspect of RTI management. How best to implement partner notification—be it when a provider suspects a woman has an STI; knows she has an STI; or knows her male partner has an STI, implying that all his partners should be notified—is not well understood. Given the variable and not-so-promising results of syndromic management of vaginal discharge, and the potential social implications for a woman who informs her partner or partners that she has (or may have) an STI, this approach requires careful and considered experimentation.

Counseling

Regardless of the relative prevalence of STIs, basic information about risk is valuable to women as they seek to protect themselves from disease and choose an appropriate contraceptive method. Interactive sexuality counseling is the ideal approach. The study in Zimbabwe found that clients attending family planning clinics were comfortable discussing matters related to their and their partners' sexual behavior. However, more than 50 percent of service providers were not comfortable discussing sexual behavior issues with their clients. Other studies have had similar results. For example, trained providers in Indonesia often would not inform a woman that she had an STI because they found the topic difficult to discuss (Iskander et al. 1997). On the other hand, experiments that employed more intensive training have succeeded in enabling providers to incorporate sexuality issues into client counseling (Becker and Leitman 1997). The question of how best to train and support providers in changing the nature and content of counseling by including discussion of sensitive topics requires further research.[12] Research should also be conducted on the role of counseling to promote dual-method use.

Providers' comfort with discussing such sensitive topics as sexual behavior, how a woman might protect herself, and RTI test results is not only important to ensure that women obtain the information they need, it may also play a role in RTI diagnosis and treatment in the future. Despite its shortcomings, risk assessment may play a role when rapid, low-cost, accurate field diagnostics become available, by helping to determine which clients should receive such diagnostics, and, if so, which tests (Dallabetta, Gerbase, and Holmes 1998).

Prevention

Regardless of the shortcomings of existing tools to diagnose RTIs, there is much that can be done in terms of prevention. Even without effective low-cost diagnostic tools or access to microscopy, family planning and reproductive health services can still address RTIs directly by incorporating prevention of STIs, endogenous infections, and iatrogenic infections into their services. Prevention of STIs includes promoting condoms, promoting safe-sex practices, and counseling to increase knowledge, change perceptions of personal risk, influence behavior, and inform contraceptive method choice. When microbicides—products used vaginally to prevent infection—become available, they will provide an important means of STI/HIV prevention that women can control.[13] Prevention of endogenous infections includes discouraging douching and traditional practices such as inserting substances into the vagina, and informing women about menstrual hygiene. Prevention of iatrogenic infections requires improving infection prevention practices.

• • •

In conclusion, as outlined above, there are no easy answers to the dilemmas of RTI diagnosis and treatment in low-resource settings. However, some operational possibilities are available to family planning and reproductive health services, even in the absence of low-cost, rapid, accurate diagnostic tests. It is clear that steps should be taken to address the large burden of endogenous RTIs. Given the effectiveness of microscopy in diagnosing bacterial vaginosis, candidiasis, and trichomoniasis in settings where the equipment and expertise are available, this approach should be more widely implemented in such settings. The syndromic approach is very effective when used to manage male urethral discharge and genital ulcers. As such, it should be used more widely to manage STIs in men, which could also provide an opportunity to reach their sexual partners with appropriate treatment. Finally, prevention—including the provision of barrier methods and counseling regarding disease transmission and risk—is a proactive and necessary step that all reproductive health and family planning services can and should take.

Acknowledgments

We would like to thank the Zimbabwe National Family Planning Council's director, staff, and clients for their participation in the Zimbabwe study. We would also like to thank the U.S. Agency for International Development mission in Zimbabwe for its support of the study team. The Zimbabwe project was supported by the Population Council's Africa Operations Research and Technical Assistance Project II, which was funded by USAID. We are grateful to the Rockefeller Foundation for its support of the Hue study. Finally, we thank Janneke van de Wijgert, Deborah Burgess, and Mary Catlin for their insight and helpful comments on this chapter.

Notes

1   Existing options for prevention are not always feasible. For example, use of condoms depends on the consent of a male partner; even if women are monogamous, their husbands/partners may not be; and reducing the number of sexual partners may not be possible for women whose livelihoods depend on exchanging sex for money. When it becomes available, a microbicide (a product used vaginally to prevent infection) will be an important addition to the range of STI/HIV prevention methods because it will provide women with a method they can control.

2   See Chapter 15 for details on the dangers of IUD insertion among women with chlamydia and gonorrhea infections.

3   While it has been hypothesized that some traditional practices, as well as douching, can increase the chance of STI transmission by drying or irritating the vagina and making it more susceptible to tearing during sex, "no research has demonstrated that traditional intravaginal practices directly

influence the transmission of disease" (Brown and Brown 2000, p. 183). A large study funded by the National Institute of Child Health and Human Development is currently exploring the link between intravaginal practices and HIV transmission (van de Wijgert 2000).

4   Also known as enzyme immunoassays (EIA).

5   PCR and LCR are also used to diagnose gonorrhea.

6   Djajakusumah et al. (1998) found that among symptomatic men, the algorithm had a sensitivity of 100 percent (i.e., it was able to identify all cases of infection) and a positive predictive value of between 75 and 97 percent (i.e., between 3 and 25 percent of the clients identified by the algorithm as infected were, in fact, not infected) when compared with definitive laboratory diagnosis.

7   Moderate prevalence was defined as less than 20 percent.

8   In high-prevalence populations (greater than or equal to 20 percent chlamydia/gonorrhea, as one would find among sex workers and in some STI clinic populations) the risk scores identified 75 percent of infected women, and 56 percent of those women identified as infected were not, in fact, infected.

9   This distribution was influenced by the criteria for entry into this particular study and may not represent the general pattern of clinic traffic at ZNFPC clinics.

10   Because syndromic management cannot provide definitive diagnosis, the Zimbabwe RTI management algorithms require clients to return to the clinic for assessment after the initial dose of medication (see algorithm depicted in Figure 1). Thus, women who are treated for a suspected vaginal infection but who in fact have a cervical infection would eventually receive the correct treatment when they return with persistent symptoms despite having taken the medications prescribed. The performance of this "two-visit" approach hinges on a high rate of return for follow-up visits.

11   This shortcoming is at least partially a result of the emphasis placed on identifying bacterial vaginosis and candidiasis (at the expense of trichomoniasis) during the microscopy training, which had been done because it was thought that clue cells (that indicate bacterial vaginosis) and yeast (that indicate candidiasis) would require more microscopy skills than identifying *Trichomonas vaginalis*, a flagellated protozoa.

12   See Chapter 9 regarding an effort in Egypt to help family planning providers address sexuality issues during counseling.

13   See Population Council and International Family Health (2001) for details on the status of current microbicide research and challenges.

References

Becker, Julie and Elizabeth Leitman. 1997. "Introducing sexuality within family planning: The experience of three HIV/STD prevention projects from Latin America and the Caribbean," *Quality/Calidad/Qualité*, no. 8. New York: Population Council.

Bosch, F.X., M.M. Manos, N. Munoz, M. Sherman, A.M. Jansen, J. Peto, M.H. Schiffman, V. Moreno, R. Kurman, and K.V. Shah. 1995. "Prevalence of human papillomavirus in cervical cancer: A worldwide perspective," *Journal of the National Cancer Institute* 87(11): 796–802.

Bourgeois, Anke, Daniel Henzel, Germaine Dibanga, Gabriel Malonga-Mouelet, Martine Peeters, Jean-Pierre Coulaud, Lieve Fransen, and Eric Delaporte. 1998. "Prospective evaluation of a flow chart using a risk assessment for the diagnosis of STDs in primary healthcare centres in Libreville, Gabon," *Sexually Transmitted Infections* 74(suppl 1): S128–S131.

Brown, Judith and Richard Brown. 2000. "Traditional intravaginal practices and the heterosexual transmission of disease: A review," *Sexually Transmitted Diseases* 27(4): 183–187.

Cates, Willard, Jr. 1998. "Reproductive tract infections," in Robert A. Hatcher, James Trussell, Felicia Stewart, Willard Cates, Jr., Gary K. Stewart, Felicia Guest, and Deborah Kowal (eds.), *Contraceptive Technology*, 17th ed. New York: Ardent Media, pp. 179–210.

Coates, Thomas J., Olga A. Grinstead, Steven E. Gregorich, et al. 2000. "Efficacy of voluntary counseling and testing in individuals and couples in Kenya, Tanzania and Trinidad: A randomized clinical trial." *Lancet* 356(9224): 103–112.

Costello Daly, Celine, Anne-Marie Wangel, Irving F. Hoffman, Joseph K. Canner, Godfrey S. Lule, Valentino M. Lema, N. George Liomba, and Gina A. Dallabetta. 1998. "Validation of the WHO diagnostic algorithm and development of an alternative scoring system for the management of women presenting with vaginal discharge in Malawi," *Sexually Transmitted Infections* 74(suppl 1): S50–S58.

Dallabetta, Gina A., Antonio C. Gerbase, and King K. Holmes. 1998. "Problems, solutions, and challenges in syndromic management of sexually transmitted diseases," *Sexually Transmitted Infections* 74(suppl 1): S1–S11.

Djajakusumah, T., S. Sudigdoadi, K. Keersmaekers, and A. Meheus. 1998. "Evaluation of syndromic patient management algorithm for urethral discharge," *Sexually Transmitted Infections* 74(suppl 1): S29–S33.

Encena, Jesus, Marilou Costello, and Chona Echaves. 1998. "Syndromic approach for managing reproductive tract infections in the Philippines," in *Improving Reproductive Health: International Shared Experience: Proceedings of a Two-Day International Workshop, 4–5 December 1997, Bogor, Indonesia*. Jakarta: Population Council, pp. 69–80.

Gerbase, A.C., J.T. Rowley, D.H.L. Heymann, S.F.B. Berkeley, and P. Piot. 1998. "Global prevalence and incidence estimates of selected curable STDs," *Sexually Transmitted Infections* 74(suppl 1): S12–S16.

Iskander, Meiwita, Catherine Vickers, Subadra Indrawati Molyneaux, and Siti Nurul Qoomariyah. 1997. "Improved reproductive health and STD services for women presenting to family planning services in north Jakarta," final report on activities, Population Council, Jakarta, and the Indonesian Ministry of Health HIV/AIDS Prevention Project. New York: Population Council Asia and Near East Operations Research and Technical Assistance Project.

Kapiga, S.H., B. Vuylsteke, E.F. Lyamuya, G. Dallabetta, and M. Laga. 1998. "Evaluation of sexually transmitted diseases diagnostic algorithms among family planning clients in Dar es Salaam, Tanzania," *Sexually Transmitted Infections* 74(suppl 1): S132–S138.

Larsen, Sandra, Elizabeth Hunter, and Betty McGrew. 1991. "Syphilis," in Bertina Wentworth, Franklyn Judson, and Mary Gilchrist (eds.), *Laboratory Methods for the Diagnosis of Sexually Transmitted Diseases*. Washington, DC: American Public Health Association, pp. 1–52.

Lien, Phan Thi, Christopher J. Elias, Jamie Uhrig, Nguyen Thi Loi, Bui Thi Chi, and Nguyen Huu Phuc. 1998. "The prevalence of reproductive tract infections at the MCH/FP Center in Hue, Vietnam: A cross-sectional descriptive study," conference report. Hanoi: Population Council.

Maggwa, Baker Ndugga and Ian Askew. 1997. *Integrating STI/HIV Management Strategies into Existing MCH/FP Programs: Lessons from Case Studies in East and Southern Africa*. New York and Nairobi: Population Council.

Maggwa, Ndugga, Ian Askew, Carolyn Marangwanda, Sithokozille Simba, Hazel Dube, Rick Homan, Barbara Janowitz, Ahmed Latif, and Peter Mason. 1999. "Demand for and cost-effectiveness of integrating RTI/HIV services with clinic-based family planning services in Zimbabwe." New York and Nairobi: Population Council.

Martin, Harold L., Jr., Patrick M. Nyange, Barbara A. Richardson, Ludo Lavreys, Kishorchandra Mandaliya, Denis J. Jackson, J.O. Ndinya-Achola, and Joan Kreiss. 1998. "Hormonal contraception, sexually transmitted diseases, and risk of heterosexual transmission of human immunodeficiency virus type 1," *Journal of Infectious Diseases* 178(4): 1053–1059.

Mayaud, Philippe, Gina ka-Gina, Jan Cornelissen, James Todd, Godfrey Kaatano, Beryl West, Elizabeth Uledi, Medard Rwakatare, Lilian Kopwe, Domitilia Manoko, Marie Laga, Heiner Grosskurth,

Richard Hayes, and David Mabey. 1998a. "Validation of a WHO algorithm with risk assessment for the clinical management of vaginal discharge in Mwanza, Tanzania," *Sexually Transmitted Infections* 74(suppl 1): S77–S84.

Mayaud, Philippe, Elizabeth Uledi, Jan Cornelissen, Gina ka-Gina, James Todd, Medard Rwakatare, Beryl West, Lilian Kopwe, Domitilia Manoko, Heiner Grosskurth, Richard Hayes, and David Mabey. 1998b. "Risk scores to detect cervical infections in urban antenatal clinic attenders in Mwanza, Tanzania," *Sexually Transmitted Infections* 74(suppl 1): S139–S146.

O'Farrell, Nigel. 1999. "Increasing prevalence of genital herpes in developing countries: Implications for heterosexual HIV transmission and STI control programmes," *Sexually Transmitted Infections* 75(6): 377–384.

Peipert, Jeffrey F., Andrea Boyd Montagno, Amy Sedlacek Cooper, and C. James Sung. 1997. "Bacterial vaginosis as a risk factor for upper genital tract infection," *American Journal of Obstetrics and Gynecology* 177(5): 1184–1187.

Plummer, F.A., M. Laga, R.C. Brunham, P. Piot, A.R. Ronald, V. Bhullar, J.Y. Mati, J.O. Ndinya-Achola, M. Cheang, and H. Nsanze. 1987. "Postpartum upper genital tract infection in Nairobi, Kenya: Epidemiology, etiology and risk factors," *Journal of Infectious Diseases* 156(1): 92–98.

Population Council and International Family Health. 2001. *The Case for Microbicides: A Global Priority,* 2nd ed. New York and London: Population Council and International Family Health.

Ryan, Caroline A., Ahmed Zidouh, Lisa E. Manhart, Rhizlane Selka, Minsheng Xia, Michele Moloney-Kitts, Jaouad Mahjour, Melissa Krone, Barry N. Courtois, Gina Dallabetta, and King K. Holmes. 1998. "Reproductive tract infections in primary health-care, family planning, and dermatovenereology clinics: Evaluation of syndromic management in Morocco," *Sexually Transmitted Infections* 74(suppl 1): S95–S105.

Sánchez, Sixto E., Laura A. Koutsky, Jorge Sánchez, Americo Fernández, Jose Casquero, Joan Kreiss, Mary Catlin, Minsheng Xia, and King K. Holmes. 1998. "Rapid and inexpensive approaches to managing abnormal vaginal discharge or lower abdominal pain: An evaluation in women attending gynaecology and family planning clinics in Peru," *Sexually Transmitted Infections* 74(suppl 1): S85–S94.

Schneider, H., D.J. Coetzee, H.G. Fehler, A. Bellingan, Y. Dangor, F. Radebe, and R.C. Ballard. 1998. "Screening for sexually transmitted diseases in rural South African women," *Sexually Transmitted Infections* 74(suppl 1): S147–S152.

Sloan, Nancy L., Beverly Winikoff, Nicole Haberland, Christiana Coggins, and Christopher Elias. 2000. "Screening and syndromic approaches to identify gonorrhea and chlamydial infection among women," *Studies in Family Planning* 31(1): 55–68.

Solo, Julie, Ndugga Maggwa, James K. Wabaru, Bedan K. Kariuki, and Gregory Maitha. 1999. *Improving the Management of STIs Among MCH/FP Clinics at the Nakuru Municipal Council Clinics.* New York and Nairobi: Population Council.

Spiegel, Carol. 1991. "Vaginitis," in Bertina Wentworth, Franklyn Judson, and Mary Gilchrist (eds.), *Laboratory Methods for the Diagnosis of Sexually Transmitted Diseases.* Washington, DC: American Public Health Association, pp. 181–201.

Taha, Taha E., Donald R. Hoover, Gina A. Dallabetta, Newton I. Kumwenda, Laban A.R. Mtimavalye, Li-Ping Yang, George N. Liomba, Robin L. Broadhead, John D. Chiphangwi, and Paolo G. Miotti. 1998. "Bacterial vaginosis and disturbances of vaginal flora: Association with increased acquisition of HIV," *AIDS* 12(13): 1699–1706.

UNAIDS. 1997. "HIV testing methods," *UNAIDS Technical Update.* Geneva: UNAIDS.

UNAIDS/WHO. 2000. "AIDS epidemic update: December 2000." Geneva: UNAIDS/WHO.

van de Wijgert, Janneke. 2000. Personal communication.

van de Wijgert, J.H.H.M., P.R. Mason, L. Gwanzura, M.T. Mbizvo, Z.M. Chirenje, V. Iliff, S. Shiboski, and N.S. Padian. 2000. "Intravaginal practices, vaginal flora disturbances, and acquisition of sexually transmitted diseases in Zimbabwean women," *Journal of Infectious Diseases* 181(2): 587–594.

van Dyck, Eddy, Frieda Behets, François Crabbe, and Seth Berkley. 1996. "The STD laboratory," in Gina A. Dallabetta, Marie Laga, and Peter Lamptey (eds.), *Control of Sexually Transmitted Diseases: A Handbook for the Design and Management of Programs.* Arlington, VA: AIDSCAP Project, Family Health International, pp. 225–252.

WHO/UNAIDS. 1997. "Revised recommendations for the selection and use of HIV antibody tests," *Weekly Epidemiological Record* 12: 81–87.

Contact information

B. Ndugga Maggwa
Regional Director, Population and
  Reproductive Health Program,
  East and Southern Africa
Family Health International/Kenya
The Chancery, 2nd Floor, Valley Road
P.O. Box 38835
Nairobi, Kenya
telephone: 254-2-314-066
fax: 254-2-228-507
e-mail: bmaggwa@fhi.or.ke

Nicole Haberland
Program Associate
Gender, Family, and Development Program
Population Council
1 Dag Hammarskjold Plaza
New York, NY 10017 USA
telephone: 212-339-0676
fax: 212-755-6052
e-mail: nhaberland@popcouncil.org

Christopher Elias
President
Program for Appropriate Technology in Health
1455 NW Leary Way
Seattle, WA 98107 USA
telephone: 206-285-3500
fax: 206-285-6619
e-mail: celias@path.org

PART V
WORKING WITH COMMUNITIES AND WOMEN TO IMPROVE REPRODUCTIVE HEALTH AND RIGHTS

paragraph 7.9, Programme of Action

Governments should promote much greater community participation in reproductive health-care services by decentralizing the management of public health programmes and by forming partnerships in cooperation with local non-governmental organizations and private health-care providers.

How can communities be engaged in efforts to improve reproductive and sexual health?

---

principle 4, Programme of Action

Advancing gender equality and equity and the empowerment of women, and the elimination of all kinds of violence against women, and ensuring women's ability to control their own fertility, are cornerstones of population- and development-related programmes.

How can we work with communities to address the links between women's power and their reproductive health?

---

paragraph 4.9, Programme of Action

Countries should take full measures to eliminate all forms of exploitation, abuse, harassment and violence against women, adolescents and children.

paragraph 7.40, Programme of Action

Governments and communities should urgently take steps to stop the practice of female genital mutilation and protect women and girls from all such similar unnecessary and dangerous practices. Steps to eliminate the practice should include strong community outreach programmes involving village and religious leaders, education and counselling about its impact on girls' and women's health. . . .

How can we mobilize communities to end violence against women and girls?

17

How a Family Planning Association Turned Its Approach to Sexual Health on Its Head: Collaborating with Communities in Belize

Lucella Campbell and Mervin Lambey

The Caribbean region comprises the island nations of the Caribbean as well as several countries in Central and South America, all of which are linguistically and culturally distinct from Latin America. Across the region, serious sexual health problems have garnered little attention, with sobering effects:

- The prevalence of HIV/AIDS in the Caribbean is second only to that in sub-Saharan Africa.[1] Moreover, the proportion of HIV-positive adults who are women is substantially higher than in most other regions (35 percent, compared to 20–25 percent in Europe, Latin America, and North America and 55 percent in sub-Saharan Africa) (UNAIDS/WHO 2000). The main modes of HIV transmission in the Caribbean are sexual—through heterosexual contact or men who have sex with men. Nonetheless, most Caribbean countries lack a consistent AIDS education program or systematic, school-based sex education.
- The failure to promote Pap smears and long delays in getting results have translated into stubbornly high rates of cervical cancer. There are 35.8 cervical cancer cases per 100,000 women in the Caribbean, 4.5 times more than in North America. Cervical cancer mortality rates are over five times higher: 16.8 per 100,000 women in the Caribbean compared to 3.2 in North America. (PAHO 2001).
- Use of services to test for and treat sexually transmitted infections (STIs) is infrequent, because of stigma and the fact that services are unresponsive to clients' needs (e.g., unsympathetic staff, inadequate confidentiality, long waiting times, and delays in getting laboratory results). As a result, people tend to go to herbalists or to self-medicate with antibiotics, contributing to growing levels of antibiotic resistance.[2]

- Economic and cultural phenomena, including migration patterns and entrenched gender-based power imbalances, compromise family life and the well-being of women and children. Female-headed households, domestic violence,[3] and incest are on the rise, and increasing numbers of children in individual families are fathered by multiple absentee men.
- Girls who become pregnant are denied education because of an unwritten rule that forces them out of school; many never return to the educational system.

In this chapter we focus on changes over the past decade in the services provided by the Belize Family Life Association (BFLA), which has five clinics across the country. Like similar institutions worldwide, BFLA was originally established according to a traditional clinical family planning model. Staff were trained in the rudiments of reproductive anatomy/physiology and contraceptive methods, and this information was generally repeated by rote to clients to help them choose a method. Little if any attention was given to the client's sexual life or the context in which he or she experienced it. Spending time with clients on these issues did not fit the organizational mandate: It would neither increase the number of contraceptive "acceptors" nor contribute to couple-years of protection, the main criteria for assessing BFLA's performance.

This approach carried over to the association's outreach efforts. BFLA had little experience engaging the community directly. It was isolated not only from the community it served, but also from other nongovernmental organizations (NGOs) serving the community. Typically, outreach staff made sporadic visits to the community, where they would present lectures on the benefits of family planning and on the various contraceptive methods available. On occasion, the lectures would include information on reproductive anatomy/physiology or HIV. There might be time for a few questions, but the flow of information was generally one way. BFLA staff members also appeared occasionally on radio shows. Typically, these appearances consisted of interviews with doctors or other staff members, or five-minute taped lectures, again with an almost exclusive focus on contraception.

With nowhere to turn for help with their sexual and reproductive health problems, many women raised them with staff of BFLA, hoping for a sympathetic ear or for professional guidance. They talked about poor communication with partners; partner infidelity and fears of contracting HIV; incidents of incest, sexual and emotional abuse, and domestic violence; and problems they had managing difficult teenagers. BFLA's staff, however, had limited ability to help people address the social dimensions of sexual and reproductive health issues and little to offer besides contraception. In the absence of institutional support for counseling on these issues, providers' responses to the needs of their clients varied. Some subtly sidestepped the issues, while others offered clients whatever information they had at hand.

RECOGNIZING THE NEED FOR CHANGE

In the mid-1990s, in response to needs expressed at the country level, the International Planned Parenthood Federation/Western Hemisphere Region (IPPF/WHR) and BFLA launched a community-based sexual health project that reflected their acknowledgment of the importance of meeting a broader range of sexual and reproductive health needs and the limitations of the conventional approaches common to the work of many IPPF/WHR affiliates. The goals of the project were ambitious: to improve sexual health and to transform the association's approach to community education. This expanded vision would require a significant shift in the values, mission, and modus operandi of BFLA.

A TRADITIONAL FAMILY PLANNING ASSOCIATION ENGAGES A COMMUNITY

Belize, bordered by Mexico, Guatemala, and the Caribbean, is the only English-speaking country in Central America. Approximately 46 percent of its ethnically diverse population is "poor" or "very poor" (PAHO 1999). Nationwide, 22 percent of households are headed by women; in Belize District this figure reaches 33 percent (PAHO 1999). Primary school is free and compulsory up to age 14, but over one-third of children (36 percent) do not complete primary school (PAHO 1999).

Two of the three leading causes of morbidity among women are related to reproductive health: complications of pregnancy and abortion (PAHO 1999). Unmet need for contraception, at 51 percent, is significantly higher than the average for the region (Central Statistical Office et al. 1992). Adult HIV/AIDS prevalence is high, at 2 percent at the end of 1999 (UNAIDS/PAHO/WHO 2000).

BFLA has played an important role in providing contraception nationwide. However, a sexual health approach, which requires a broader array of services and a more dynamic engagement with clients, presented a challenge to its traditional philosophy and program. Board members required sensitization to ensure their understanding and support. The laboratory required equipment to conduct testing for STIs and to offer Pap smears. Existing staff required retraining to help them adapt the counseling process to clients' sexual and other reproductive health concerns, and new staff needed to be recruited. Perhaps most importantly, the relationship with the community, built on one-directional didactic monologues about contraception, needed to be replaced by frank, two-way communication on sexuality and reproductive health. This dialogue, in turn, would help reconfigure BFLA's clinic-based services in a manner that was truly client-centered.

LAYING THE GROUNDWORK FOR COMMUNITY DISCUSSIONS

An effective community-based program would require new relationships with the community, new educators, new content, and new measures of success. The use of community volunteers was crucial, because it would augment BFLA's limited human resources, offer communities "onsite" help, and, most importantly, facilitate community ownership of the project.

BFLA project leaders began by identifying individuals in the community who could provide leadership and support, largely by contacting established village leaders and informally canvassing community members about who had influence.

This was the first time BFLA staff had engaged the established community leadership—village council members, health care delivery staff, and, to a lesser extent, religious and business leaders—in shaping a local intervention. They described the new project, received feedback, sought support, and asked about the community's concerns. They also identified links between these concerns and sexual health issues and asked how BFLA staff could best mobilize community involvement. The community leaders offered to bring together the first group of community members when BFLA was ready to initiate the discussions that were to be the cornerstone of the association's new approach.

The next step involved recruiting community volunteers from among the individuals recommended by village leaders. Thirty individuals were selected to facilitate group discussions in ten communities. These trained facilitators would be charged with holding meetings with community members once or twice monthly and providing feedback to BFLA. Although a few of those selected were teachers and nurses, most were housewives; in one community, many also served as volunteer government health workers and thus began with established community relationships and credibility. The facilitators were not paid, although their expenses were covered and the project staff provided them with bicycles.[4]

An experienced trainer developed and led a five-day workshop for facilitators.[5] He was supported by the IPPF/WHR program advisor and, in the later stages of the project, was joined by a gender specialist.[6] In the course of the workshop, the facilitators-in-training were taught to help people articulate their sexual health concerns. They were discouraged from giving information and offering their opinions. Instead, they were encouraged to raise questions or to elicit questions and comments from other people in the group and to allow people's understanding to evolve through self-reflection.

Most of the facilitators-in-training had not thought about many of the issues that arose, let alone discussed them in a group setting. For the first time they had to face—and express—their feelings about subjects such as homosexuality, adolescent contraceptive use, and masturbation. Not only did they have an opportunity to express their perspectives and learn from others, some also continued the discussion outside of the sessions. One woman reported examining her "private parts" for the first time, having learned that this was not "sinful." She later said: "This moralizing thing is all in our heads."

Exercises were designed to help facilitators confront their own feelings on sexual issues, recognize their own ability to address matters of concern, and ultimately recognize the power of communities and individuals to effect change. Exercises included defining sexuality and reproductive health; examining the factors that prevent people from seeking treatment when they believe they have an STI; and enacting role-plays about common sexual and reproductive health dilemmas. Through this process the facilitators-in-training came to realize that sexuality and sexual health were an active part of their everyday experience. By the end of the workshop, the newly trained facilitators were able to develop exercises for other participants. For example, a small group developed an exercise to explore "frigidity" and asked the larger group for a definition. Suggested definitions included "cold" and having "no feeling toward sex." Participants then suggested possible causes, including infidelity, abuse, and fear. This was followed by a role-play in which a man comes home and immediately asks his wife for sex. The role-play was stopped at this point, so that the facilitators-in-training could suggest reasons for the wife's reluctance. They suggested that she might have another sex partner, not be satisfied, or be tired. They were then asked to offer solutions. Suggested solutions included encouraging the couple to improve their communication with each other, having the man respect the woman's desire, and so forth.

Facilitators came to the workshops uncertain of their capacity to handle sexuality topics and left confident in their skills. As one participant said, "It was wonderful to see how we all could think."

Tools for a Changing and Demanding Role

Facilitators were provided with a community outreach manual for guiding group discussions, which was designed so that it could be adapted for use in different contexts.[7] It has since been supplemented in Belize by five simple guides. The content of the manual is described below:

- *Making it happen.* This section explains the facilitator's role to help community members identify their sexual and reproductive health problems and concerns; help people develop strategies to overcome underlying problems at the community level; provide information on specific concerns; link people with the family planning association and other referral points; explore barriers to use of sexual and reproductive health services; and provide feedback to BFLA on strategies to improve services and outreach.

It also outlines the process of community outreach, including recruiting participants (suggestions include talking with community organizations, such as sports teams, market vendors, and church groups, or, more informally, simply gathering a group of friends), identifying needs, and planning and conducting community discussions. Tips for each of these steps and suggestions on sources for further help are provided.

- *Facilitation and activity guide.* This section highlights key sexual and reproductive health concepts and suggests topics for community discussions, including gender, male–female communication, parent–child communication, family planning and sexual/reproductive health, STIs/HIV, and how to make sex safer (see Boxes 1 and 2).
- *Sexual and reproductive health reference materials.* These include brief fact sheets about family planning, STIs and HIV/AIDS, making sex safer, cervical cancer screening, teen pregnancy, unsafe abortion, and safe motherhood.
- *Referral information.* These locally developed supplements to the manual identify facilities that will accept referrals for infertility management, STI treatment, domestic violence, adolescent services, and other concerns.
- *Facilitation tools.* This section includes tips on facilitating lively group discussion, examples of ways to introduce participants to one another and make them feel comfortable, and tips on how to handle common problems (e.g., when no one talks, or when a few people dominate the discussion).

GETTING STARTED

Community leaders helped announce the upcoming discussions, organized the sessions, and introduced the volunteer facilitators and staff of BFLA, thus legitimizing the effort. Often, they arranged to make a public space available for the meetings. Once the discussions had begun, facilitators relied on church announcements, community radio bulletins, and word of mouth to generate further interest. Public notices were placed where groups congregated, such as soccer fields, health clinics, village shops, or post offices. The notices invited people to "Come join a discussion and help improve our community life" and stated the topic of the next week's discussion, such

---

Box 1. Communication between partners: Fishbowl exercise (30–45 minutes)

Purpose: To practice using good partner communication and analyze the problems that arise between sexual partners.

Getting ready

Prepare four or more situations for people to role-play. In each situation, there should be an issue or problem to discuss. Here are some examples:

- Woman whose partner is threatening to leave her. She wants him to use a condom when they have sex.
- Woman whose partner has had children with other women. She depends on him for money for her family.
- Girl with an older boyfriend. He wants her to have sex and she is not sure she wants to. She really loves him.
- Man who wants his partner to use family planning. She is not sure she wants to.
- [Write in your own]

What to do

Ask for volunteers to play the role of the man and the woman and to practice communicating with each other as they act out these scenarios. The rest of the group watches and helps to analyze what works and what could be done better. It may be helpful to make lists reflecting the group's definition of what constitutes good communication (e.g., two-way communication, listening, empathy) and what constitutes bad communication. If possible, everyone should have a turn role-playing and observing.

Facilitation tip

Before commenting, give those who did the role-play the first opportunity to say what they think went well, and what they wish they had done better. Then the observers' comments will feel more helpful and less critical.

Source: Lovich 1996.

---

as "Addressing domestic violence" or "How do you feel about AIDS?" Notices also indicated the time and location of the meeting. Topics for future discussions were chosen in consultation with participants. The size of the groups tended to grow as women, who predominated at the first meetings, started to bring their partners. Groups ranging from eight to more than 20 participants gathered in locations as diverse as community centers, the BFLA clinic, house bottoms (the open space below people's homes, which are built on stilts), and occasionally the sitting area in bars.

HOW THE DISCUSSIONS FUNCTION

The facilitators began the first discussion by asking about problems in the community. Participants were concerned about jobs, drainage and garbage disposal, violence, drugs, and housing. The facilitators then helped community members make links, where appropriate, between these issues and sexual and reproductive health; they focused the discussion by explaining that while they might not be able to help with jobs,

---

Box 2. STIs: A simple matter? Role-play (45–60 minutes)

Purpose: (1) To identify some of the problems that men and women face in dealing with partners when they suspect that they themselves have an STI; and (2) to identify strategies men and women can use to communicate with each other and to get the help they need.

What to do

Divide the participants into two groups. Ask each to prepare a role-play.

Group 1: What does a woman say or do with respect to her partner when she suspects she has acquired an STI?

Group 2: What does a man say or do with respect to his partner when he suspects he has acquired an STI?

Each group then performs the role-plays.

Discussion

1. What is different about the way that the man and the woman have reacted? Why do you think this is so?

2. What could help the woman? What could help the man?

Source: Lovich 1996.

---

they might be able to help address sexual and reproductive health problems. Then they asked what people thought was meant by "sexual and reproductive health." In the course of the discussion, issues were raised such as the difficulty of raising children, adolescent problems, domestic violence, suicide, incest, family planning, communicating with one's partner, and gender roles. These exchanges helped the facilitators identify the sexual and reproductive health issues of primary concern to the community around which future discussions could be shaped.

Initially there was considerable resistance to the chosen topics because people were not accustomed to talking about their personal lives. To maintain the interest of group members, facilitators followed up with resistant or particularly shy individuals between sessions to elicit concerns they might not yet be comfortable enough to articulate in a group setting. Gradually, participants began to see themselves in the stories of others and their reticence diminished. As one of the facilitators explained, "It's as if we opened a dam and the water burst."

For example, in discussions about gender, the facilitators asked provocative questions, such as "What do you think men talk about when they talk about women?" and "What does a woman expect from a man?" Often, women said that their partners did not listen to them or that their opinions were not considered. They also discussed their anxieties about finding ways to avoid having men walk out on them. The subject of gender conflict also surfaced. A commonly expressed source of conflict had to do with men's expectation of sex on demand at the end of their working day, which was based on their assumption that women had been idle all day. In addition, men spoke of feeling overwhelmed by women's expectations of them and of almost always feeling misunderstood. The discussions also unearthed considerable distress about partner violence against women. The discussions about gender often grew heated, challenging the facilitators to hold the group together and help the men and women to see that it was normal to have differences and productive to examine other points of view. Some men walked out of the meetings early on, but in time both men and women expressed satisfaction with the opportunity to gain insight into other perspectives and to work toward common ground.

Listening to polarized perspectives expressed openly and explored in detail forced participants to rethink their long-held assumptions. Women, in particular, overcame their reluctance to raise sensitive subjects with spouses. Women who attended without their husbands expressed an eagerness to have their husbands participate. As one woman explained, "I think it would really help my husband to hear what some of these people have to say. Maybe he might start to listen to me more."

These new community discussions bore no resemblance to BFLA's previous mode of dealing with the community, which had been focused on family planning and was technology-centered and provider-dominated. The emphasis of the discussions, even when contraception was the subject, was on the underlying personal and social barriers inhibiting effective use. Facilitators asked participants about their attitudes toward contraception and their resistance to particular methods. They sought to learn about—and to help the participants become more aware of—the belief systems, life circumstances, and relationship characteristics that may prevent individuals from using contraceptive methods even when they want to.

Discussion of AIDS, which had previously centered on transmission and prevention, now explored participants' feelings, fears, and experiences in relation to the illness. With HIV prevalence rates rising, facilitators helped community members explore what they could do to help reduce their risk of acquiring HIV and to support people living with HIV/AIDS. Women brought their partners to hear about risk behaviors, observe a condom demonstration, practice communicating in a constructive, respectful two-way exchange, and explore the practical and emotional needs of individuals living with HIV/AIDS.

When the community groups talked about STIs more generally, the facilitator helped them understand why many people avoid being tested. Many reported going directly to a pharmacy for medication without a proper diagnosis. They also described lack of privacy and long delays at public clinics.

EARLY ACCOMPLISHMENTS:
SELF-ASSURANCE, COMMUNICATION, AND COHESION

One of the most immediate tangible results of the project was community members'
increased self-assurance in speaking about sexual and reproductive health matters.
Women who were silent at their first meetings, except for the odd giggle when "vagina" or "clitoris" was mentioned, soon began to admit to feeling more comfortable
with their bodies, even to the point of inspecting their genitalia, an activity they would
never have engaged in previously. This self-assurance extended to greater communication with partners about sexual and reproductive health issues. As one community
worker remarked:

> Some husbands have now started coming to meetings and listening. They listen, too,
> when you make house visits; before it was always behind a curtain, lately they are
> beginning to talk. . . . This lady has eight children, and when she did not want to have
> sex her husband started fighting her . . . she came to me, and I told her to tell him what
> you feel about it and he listened. Women have also begun to talk about things [and to]
> tell their husbands.

One woman in the community said, "My husband and I now talk about everything in our house, and he agreed that he only wants two children so that he could
attend to them well."

The level of intimacy and candor generated by the meetings fostered cohesion
among community members. The meetings also resulted in an increased sense of ur-
gency about community development matters that led to action in areas beyond sexual
and reproductive health concerns, such as political participation. A housewife and
mother of three commented, "I don't mind taking time from my work to come to
these meetings, because something good is happening here." At the encouragement of
their communities, six BFLA facilitators ran for and succeeded in gaining seats on
local village councils. While these individuals had long served as community health
workers, they had not previously held formal leadership positions.

TWO STEPS FORWARD, ONE STEP BACK

BFLA continues to face challenges. Several staff retreats and training sessions had to be
held before BFLA staff—who were overseeing the program and the community facilitators—began to internalize the shift in philosophy and programs, and new staff and
technical capacity had to be added to institutionalize the shift effectively. For example,
the original workplan had called for both qualitative evaluation and comprehensive
documentation of the project, but BFLA had neither the personnel nor the expertise

to conduct these activities. Additional staff were hired to enhance the agency's evalua-tion capacity and other areas of work in which BFLA had little previous experience.

Other problems unfolded as the project was implemented. It was difficult to recruit male facilitators, and newly trained facilitators of both genders were hesitant to relinquish their comfortable, well-defined roles as teachers imparting factual informa-tion for the relatively unstructured roles of facilitating discussions focused on participants' feelings and experiences. The transformation ultimately required careful selection of facilitators, retraining, and the confidence that came from experience. Follow-up training was provided during facilitators' meetings with their designated staff supervisor and during larger meetings with all facilitators that took place about once a year.

Despite the continuing emphasis on training, retraining, and supportive super-vision, facilitators were sometimes unable to respond to sensitive situations that arose in the community discussions. One facilitator spoke about trying to help a victim of incest. She needed guidance not only to help this individual, but also to deal with the complex ethical and legal issues surrounding reporting such matters. In discussions with BFLA staff it was agreed that responsibility for reporting the situation lay with the individual and not the facilitator, but that the facilitator should encourage the individual to do so. Many of the facilitators—particularly those who were also govern-ment outreach workers—struggled with the new participatory approach. The govern-ment program had fostered a language of "us" and "them." These facilitators therefore perceived themselves as acting on behalf of BFLA rather than as members of and spokespeople for their communities. This attitude was explored in follow-up work-shops, and efforts to help the facilitators adapt to their new role are ongoing. More generally, the experience of facilitators tends to follow a pattern. At first they are afraid that they are not sufficiently "professional" in their interactions with the community. As time goes on, they develop confidence and become innovative in their efforts to generate discussion. Slowly but surely, they are identified as trusted leaders. People look to them for help.

Perhaps the greatest challenge faced by BFLA was helping service-delivery staff confront the limits of a formerly clinic-centered program and the information and service package at its core. The clinic-based program had to be modified to match the approach adopted by the community outreach program. This was accomplished by allowing clinic staff to participate in the facilitators' training, exposing them to the facilitators' community work, and providing them with specialized training in client-oriented sexual and reproductive health counseling.[8] In this way, clinic staff were ulti-mately able to internalize the organization's philosophical shift and ensure that it was reflected inside the clinic, as well as within the community. Over time it became clear that some of the factors impeding the achievement of sexual health were related to contextual variables that only community members can change—including religion, culture, norms, status, perceptions, and accepted practice. On the other hand, many aspects of the information and services provided by BFLA would need to be improved considerably to maximize their effects on sexual and reproductive health. The steps taken by BFLA to improve and expand its clinic services in response to community needs are discussed below.

TRANSLATING DISCUSSION INTO ACTION

Generating discussion about sexual and reproductive health was just one of the program's objectives. The next challenge was to take action on the issues raised. Once a month, the 30 facilitators met with their designated BFLA supervisors to advise them of community concerns, which tended to fall into two broad categories: problems that BFLA could address through its clinic services and programs, and problems that were beyond the scope of the clinic and could only be remedied through community action.

Perhaps the strongest validation of the new approach is that communities have begun to take responsibility for supporting the discussions and taking action in the areas of concern they have identified. Village health committees have been established in almost half of the nearly 70 communities in which the discussions have been conducted. Facilitators nominate village health committee members and provide them with appropriate guidance. The nominees join facilitators at BFLA orientation meetings that cover strategic planning, developing and using workplans, and monitoring and supervision. The facilitators themselves sit on the village health committees and are often elected president.

In response to the concerns raised during the discussions and one-on-one conversations with community members, the facilitator develops a workplan that outlines the subjects to be discussed in the coming month. The facilitator's role is to guide the discussion, provide relevant data, elicit suggestions for addressing concerns, help with setting priorities, decide on strategies to address concerns, and help community members develop concrete plans to implement the ideas. Over the course of the project, the content of the community action plans has evolved. Early plans focused on adolescent issues, with an emphasis on providing young people with information on puberty, relationships with peers and parents, drugs, and so forth. Many facilitators believed that this initial focus was indicative of discomfort among adults about dealing directly with their own sexual and reproductive health concerns. Later plans reflected recommendations for addressing a broader range of issues directly related to the sexual health of the adult community (e.g., domestic violence, relations with partners, infidelity, and STIs). Because the community identifies its top priorities, some of these recommendations have extended beyond sexual and reproductive health concerns to such areas as nutrition, diabetes, and hypertension.

Once the community action plans are developed, BFLA focuses on collaborating with community representatives to implement recommendations related to sexual and reproductive health. Some innovative recommendations for community action include having neighbors take turns caring for dying AIDS patients to relieve family members under stress; using some community discussions to counsel participants on the needs of AIDS patients; and holding special sessions for men on the issue of domestic violence.

Community action is also manifested in other ways. In the town of Belmopan, for example, when the government hospital could no longer accommodate the BFLA clinic on its premises, community members approached the United Nations Human Rights Commission for funds and secured a grant to build a prefabricated clinic. They also helped build the clinic.

INSIDE THE CLINIC WALLS

Building on its better relations with communities, BFLA has also responded to service-related concerns that arise during community discussions and those that are reported by community facilitators during monthly meetings. Facilitators help BFLA prioritize concerns based on the extent of community need, the association's capacity and resources to meet competing demands, the potential benefit to a community of one intervention over another, and other criteria.

In recognition of community concerns about violence against women in the home and the inadequacy of referral services, BFLA hired a part-time psychiatric nurse-counselor at one clinic. She is available six hours per week for free consultations on violence and other issues requiring individual counseling, as well as for occasional community sessions. In addition, the association opened a Saturday clinic to respond to the needs of working men and women. In introducing this new service the facilitator's opening comment was, "The family planning association is *one a we*," meaning, "The family planning association is one of us."

In response to community concerns about confidentiality and delays in obtaining STI results, BFLA adjusted its protocols to increase confidentiality and reduce the waiting time for test results. Only the doctor and laboratory technician have access to test results, which are now handed to the client by the receptionist in a sealed envelope. Staff are trained to counsel people before and after they receive their test results. Clients who are treated for infections are required to return two weeks later to ensure that the infection has cleared. Staff also encourage clients to refer their partners, but because partners often do not show up, clients are given information to take home and advice on handling the situation.

In addition to identifying ways to help community members care for AIDS patients, BFLA responded to community concerns by conducting a small-scale survey of 16 individuals living with AIDS, with the objective of improving the care they receive based on their expressed needs. The survey found that AIDS patients wanted counseling for themselves, their families, caregivers (nurses), and neighbors to increase sensitivity to their situation and reduce their sense of shame; they also indicated that there was a tendency among some AIDS patients to spread infection, and that this problem needed to be addressed. These and other findings were shared with the community and with relevant NGOs and public-sector groups. As a result, the government has formed a task force to address the issue of people living with AIDS.

Community members also expressed concern about young people. Parents had used the sessions on adolescent development to air their confusions about managing "these young people of today." The level of concern in this area was so intense that BFLA developed a focused effort to work directly with disadvantaged teens (see Box 3).

More generally, the community project has infused BFLA staff with its innovative spirit. The information, education, and communication department has reoriented its approach to advertising and invites all staff to contribute ideas for outreach; even the employees of the accounts division contribute ideas. New advertisements show people speaking about the importance of sexual health and community participation, rather than the sterile image of a nurse delivering a monologue to a client across a desk. Community facilitators and outreach group members participate in developing radio shows, the appeal of which is reflected in an increasing volume of calls from listeners.

The quality of the provider–client exchange has also improved. The project assigned a visiting nurse to observe these exchanges, document their content and style, and make recommendations. The nurse found that when a woman comes for a contraceptive method, for example, a BFLA staff nurse listens closely to what the woman is saying and elicits elaboration and questions. The nurse might ask, "When you were talking you said ————. Do you want to talk more about this?" Pap smears, STI testing, and discussions about condoms are now a routine part of the visit, and nurses discuss these service options with all clients.

Since BFLA's new approach was initiated, the association has seen a substantial rise in the number of individuals who come to its clinics. In 1994, before the project began, the association's clinics saw 16,181 clients. This number increased almost 6

Box 3. A special effort to reach disadvantaged teens

Parents tend to describe adolescent culture in disparaging and despairing terms. Statements such as "[teenagers] would hold someone up as easily as they would get a job" are not uncommon. The community discussions on bringing up adolescents helped BFLA understand the links between having few places to go, limited economic prospects, and being at risk of poor reproductive and sexual health. Many of the most disadvantaged young people were gang members, who were unemployed, unskilled, and not in school. A BFLA youth program responded by providing space for teenagers to rechannel their energies, often into developing economic, social, and cultural skills.

BFLA hired two youth officers to lead its youth project, which focused on four youth groups. Two of these groups address sexual and reproductive health issues directly and assist teens in developing job skills.[a] Each group is described briefly below.[b]

- *Belize Youth with an Aim for Prosperity* trains participants, mostly males ages 16–21, in entrepreneurial job skills such as barbering and catering, and provides training in business accounting and practices.

- *The RAD Squad* (Ready for Action and Development) functions as a "big family," offering a vehicle for young people ages 16–24 to form friendships and function effectively as a group. Its primary activities include volleyball and basketball games and discussions of sexuality. In addition to their weekly get-togethers, squad members talk to other friends about sexual health issues and pass out BFLA pamphlets. They have also collaborated on the development of a newspaper, which they named *The Youth with the Wickedness Slam*.

- *The Under-twenty Club* is a group of adolescents being trained to work as reproductive health peer counselors at BFLA and in their schools. More recently, older members have begun focusing on citizenship issues by increasing their own and other young people's knowledge of their basic rights and the laws that govern them, and developing leadership skills. The club also produced a series of call-in radio programs hosted by a young psychologist. The radio programs dealt with sexual health issues from a youth perspective, using an approach that kept the issues "real" rather than shrouded in professional jargon. One program episode hosted a sex worker and a judge to discuss prostitution— a radical and creative departure from BFLA's earlier radio format.

- *ASTRAL* is a dance and drumming group that received training in sexual and reproductive health and is now using its performances to educate audiences on such issues as adolescent pregnancy, teen parenthood, relationships with parents, intimate relationships, and AIDS. ASTRAL members are primarily unemployed, out-of-school adolescents. Their performances, conducted either free or for a small fee, take place in schools, at community centers, and at "block-os"—community street-corner fundraising events featuring food and music.

(continued)

---

percent during the project's first year, and another 10 percent the next. Overall, the number of clients increased 30 percent over a five-year period. Most of this increase is attributable to visits for reproductive health services other than family planning, a direct result of BFLA's broader philosophy and the community's heightened awareness of its own needs. Many of these visits were spurred by involvement in BFLA's community discussions. Client records indicate that 90 percent of new client visits from the community of Corazol, for example, to the neighboring Orangewalk clinic are prompted by contact with a community facilitator or by participation in community discussions. In the communities of Orangewalk and Dangriga, the corresponding

(continued from previous page)

In its efforts to engage adolescents, BFLA has developed a common core of sexual and reproductive health information it wants to transmit, and a repertoire of interactive methods such as role-plays, art projects, and games to keep young participants engaged. At meetings of each of these groups, an adolescent participant picks the topics for the session; a role-play might deal with ways to support a friend who has been kicked out of her family for getting pregnant, for example.

The teen programs, all of which are mixed (boys and girls), have faced serious challenges. There are gender tensions, such as boys' use of derogatory terms to refer to girls; social pressures to feel included and fierce social competition among the girls; unease with the subject of sexuality and reticence to take on a peer counseling role; problems with sexual violence, depression, and drugs; and tensions between in- and out-of-school youth. BFLA has responded to these challenges in the following ways:

- Organizing an intensive three-day workshop to promote team building among the in- and out-of-school youth.
- Organizing occasional female-only groups.
- Arranging for some group members to participate in regional and international training opportunities to enhance their group leadership skills.
- Organizing "booster" sessions to allow for further exploration of priority issues.
- Deflecting attention from disparities in literacy levels by having group members report on their activities verbally, rather than requiring written reports.

This project operates from a youth center, which is managed by a director of youth services and an assistant, both of whom were recruited especially for the project. The center, which also provides sexual health counseling and services, is located in one of the most depressed areas of Belize City. This site was selected following discussions with several of the communities to be served. In recognition of its success, BFLA has now received additional funding to support its work with out-of-school youth, as well as support for the construction of a youth center in BFLA headquarters.[c] This center will replace the current site.

[a] The job skills training component was undertaken in partnership with the National Development Foundation of Belize with funds from the Peace Corps. This element of the youth project has since been discontinued because of lack of funding.
[b] These groups now fall under the umbrella of the Youth Advocacy Movement, a growing movement of young people throughout the Caribbean who work with family planning associations to shape and implement adolescent sexual and reproductive health programs.
[c] Funding for these initiatives is being provided by the Summit Foundation.

figure is 50 percent, and in Belize City, where community activity is minimal, only 5–10 percent of new visits are prompted by these activities.

Because clients pay for services, the increased client load has been accompanied by an increase in clinic income, permitting continued expansion. At the Orangewalk clinic, for example, the income generated from client services increased from US$20,145 in 1994 to US$69,044 in 1998.

Perhaps the most tangible demonstration of the success and extent of the alliance between BFLA and the community was the fact that the community outreach component was sustained during a period of reduced funding. While less staff follow-up was possible during this time, the activities did not stop. The volunteer nature of the work appears to have sustained the commitment of the facilitators. An approach tied largely to paid staff would not have survived funding gaps. A second round of funding from the European Union was received, allowing BFLA to continue its work in communities.

BFLA's community involvement approach has allowed the association to carry the message of sexual and reproductive health to communities across Belize, combining its own resources with the human resources and enthusiasm of the communities themselves. In the process community members have been empowered to become active participants in improving their own sexual health.

Acknowledgments

We acknowledge the dedication of the management, staff, and board of the Belize Family Life Association. We also acknowledge the contributions of the community facilitators, village health committees, peer counselors, participating community members, and the various agencies that provide support to BFLA, including those who provided and received BFLA referrals. Finally, we are grateful for the support of the European Union and other donors.

Notes

1   As of December 2000, 390,000 people in the Caribbean were living with HIV/AIDS; the adult prevalence rate is 2.3 percent, compared to 0.5 percent in Latin America (UNAIDS/WHO 2000).

2   As in many developing countries, it is not unusual for pharmacists to dispense drugs over-the-counter, without a prescription, when clients present with particular symptoms. Ampicillin is one of the most readily dispensed drugs.

3   Studies in some Caribbean countries indicate that 30 percent of adult women have been physically and/or sexually assaulted by an intimate partner (Heise, Ellsberg, and Gottemoeller 1999).

4   The bicycles were provided with support from the Japanese government. More recently, BFLA has begun experimenting with having the facilitators distribute condoms and pills, for which they earn a percentage of sales revenue.

5   The workshop was led by Tony Klouda, a trainer with extensive experience developing and leading training activities dealing with sensitive subjects.

6   The specialist, Patricia Mohammed, is a lecturer and director of the Gender Studies Unit at the University of the West Indies, Jamaica.

7   The manual was written by Ronnie Lovich, a nurse and counselor involved with the project. See Lovich (1996) for more information.

8   The specialized counseling training was provided by Ronnie Lovich.

References

Central Statistical Office, Ministry of Finance, Belize Family Life Association, Ministry of Health, Division of Reproductive Health, and Centers for Disease Control. 1992. *1991 Belize Family Health Survey.* Atlanta, GA: U.S. Department of Health and Human Services, Centers for Disease Control.

Heise, Lori, Mary Ellsberg, and Megan Gottemoeller. 1999. "Ending violence against women," *Population Reports,* Series L, no. 11.

Lovich, Ronnie. 1996. *Community Outreach Workers' Manual.* European Commission Project: Belize, Guyana, St. Lucia FPAs. New York: IPPF/WHR.
Pan American Health Organization (PAHO). 1999. "Country health profile: Belize," www.paho.org/English/SHA/prflBEL.htm, accessed 4 January 2002.
———. 2001. "Cervical cancer: A brief snapshot of the situation in Latin America and the Caribbean, 2001," www.paho.org/English/HCP/HCN/CCOverview.htm, accessed 4 January 2002.
UNAIDS/PAHO/WHO. 2000. "Epidemiological fact sheet on HIV/AIDS and sexually transmitted diseases: Belize," update. Geneva: UNAIDS/WHO.
UNAIDS/WHO. 2000. "AIDS epidemic update: December 2000." Geneva: UNAIDS.

Contact information

Lucella Campbell
Senior Program Advisor
International Planned Parenthood Federation/
  Western Hemisphere Region
120 Wall Street, 9th Floor
New York, NY 10005
telephone: 212-214-0259
fax: 212-248-4221
e-mail: lcampbell@ippfwhr.org

Mervin Lambey
c/o The Old General Hospital
Belize City, Belize
telephone: 501-2-44399
e-mail: mlambey@hotmail.com

18

"Let's Be Citizens, Not Patients!": Women's Groups in Peru Assert Their Right to High-Quality Reproductive Health Care

Bonnie Shepard

Problems with the quality of reproductive health care can be found throughout the world. In Peru, however, the nature and scope of these problems has been particularly well documented by both feminist organizations and established population and family planning institutions. Peru is one of the poorest countries in Latin America, with 37 percent of its 26.1 million citizens living below the poverty line, a figure that rises to 61 percent in rural areas (National Statistics Institute 1999, 2000). Maternal mortality is high, estimated at 185 maternal deaths for every 100,000 live births, one of the highest rates in Latin America (National Statistics Institute 2000). The differences in health conditions and indicators between large cities and outlying provinces are particularly marked. Furthermore, many service providers cannot easily communicate with the 27 percent of the population whose first language is Quechua, rather than Spanish (United Nations 1995).

In the early 1990s, a consortium of Peruvian feminist nongovernmental organizations (NGOs)[1]—Consorcio Mujer—conceived a project to enable local women to advocate for and collaborate in the improvement of reproductive health services in their own municipalities.[2] Its strategy was to involve local women and service providers in assessing the quality of care and engaging directly with health authorities in follow-up discussion about how to better meet users' needs. Unlike projects that invoke the term "community involvement" to mean perfunctory consultation, this project required community women to take responsibility as self-empowered citizens.

Linking users' needs to citizenship and sexual and reproductive rights was a logical and coherent step for the feminist consortium. As Latin American countries underwent democratization in the 1980s and 1990s, the concept of citizenship emerged within the

Latin American women's movement—especially in the regional meetings to prepare for the 1995 United Nations World Conference on Women in Beijing—as the theoretical and political foundation of discussions about women's status and empowerment. In order for women to exercise full citizenship, both the society at large and individual women would need to recognize female rights and autonomy in all spheres of life (e.g., occupational, political, economic, cultural, religious, and sexual) and be able to exercise such rights. A truly democratic society would thereby imply a shift from female dependence and submission toward equality and power sharing in governance and in the myriad decisions that affect women's lives (Hola and Portugal 1997).

In applying this concept of citizenship to the health sector, Consorcio Mujer aimed for a shift from a paternalistic model of interaction between providers and users toward an emphasis on community participation and users' rights. To appeal to goals that were already paramount in the health sector's agenda, Consorcio Mujer framed its project as one that would improve quality of care, a central concern in several national health projects funded by major agencies such as the Inter-American Development Bank, the World Bank, the United Nations Population Fund (UNFPA), and the U.S. Agency for International Development (USAID). To unite the concepts of quality and citizenship, the consortium placed users' rights and women's participation at the center of the concept of quality, while building on the quality-of-care framework developed by Bruce, which encompasses choice, information, provider–client interaction, technical competence, continuity of care, and access to a range of related services (Bruce 1990).

This approach stands in contrast to the paternalistic model, which is based on the belief that services for the poor are a matter of charity, not of the human right to health care. A corollary is that the provider knows what is best for the user. To Consorcio Mujer, community participation meant that users should participate in setting goals for health care provision and in helping providers achieve these goals. Sensitive to past abuses, the consortium emphasized users' rights related to voluntary participation in health care services, informed consent, nondiscrimination, and access to high-quality health care, regardless of ethnic group or socioeconomic class. Box 1 provides a comparison of the citizenship and paternalistic models of health care.

In 1992, when Consorcio Mujer conceived this project, there was little interaction between public health authorities and the women's movement, but the time was right to initiate dialogue. The health sector was being decentralized, resulting in the transfer of greater decisionmaking power to local officials. In addition, health-sector reforms mandated community involvement in setting priorities and in transforming local health centers into self-sufficient entities with community oversight boards.[3] With this in mind, each of the six Consorcio Mujer NGOs participating in this project

> **Box 1. Comparison of two models of health care provision**
>
> | Citizenship model | Paternalistic model |
> | --- | --- |
> | Users have rights of access to health services, to freedom of choice, and to be treated with dignity. | Health services benefit users, and are provided to low-income people as a favor. |
> | Community participation means that users are involved in setting goals. | Community participation means that community organizations help achieve providers' goals. |
> | Equal relationships: Providers listen to users' concerns nonjudgmentally, and their responses take users' concerns into account. | Vertical relationships: Providers know what is best for users. |

selected a community in which it had a tradition of work with both providers and local women's organizations: three were in the capital city of Lima; one each was in the Amazonian jungle, the Andean highlands, and on the rural coast.

DEFINING CLIENTS' PERSPECTIVES ON QUALITY OF CARE

In 1994 Consorcio Mujer began gathering information on how clients view quality of care. A number of studies had documented these issues in the past, but had concentrated on family planning; only two had incorporated clients' perspectives. Therefore the consortium focused its initial evaluation on women's own perceptions of health care, and on the full range of women's health services. The evaluation examined capacity for and the quality of basic gynecologic, contraceptive, and obstetric services, including the diagnosis and treatment of reproductive tract infections. In the six municipalities, the appointed NGO used standardized instruments to survey providers and at least 30 users and to conduct direct observations of provider–client interactions, with the clients' permission, in small health posts, larger health centers, and maternity hospitals. Some questions were specific, but many were open-ended, for example, "Was there any point during the medical visit when you felt ashamed?"[4]

The findings documented a range of problems:

Disrespectful treatment. Women reported being subjected to insults, angry shouting, and belittling. Nearly half (48 percent) suggested the need for improvement in providers' interpersonal skills. When asked which aspects of health care were most important for building trust, 57 percent highlighted "good treatment." In all, 17–30 percent of respondents in each municipality felt shame as a result of being rebuked or belittled by a provider.

Providers' failure to greet users and introduce themselves. The proportion of providers who greeted the client ranged from 15 percent to 60 percent.

Waiting time. Waiting time was more than one hour for 48 percent of women.

Inadequate information. Women complained of perfunctory and incomplete counseling. For example, they reported that providers did not explain diagnostic procedures and follow-up treatment. Many felt the explanations offered were not fully understandable. Only 17 percent of providers gave any explanations before or during vaginal exams, for example. In Cusco and Piura, only 8–9 percent of providers explained Pap smears, and 9–23 percent provided information on breast self-exams. According to Consorcio Mujer staff, "The information given to users is scant. . . . When users have vaginal infections, generally the professional says, 'It's inflamed'" (Consorcio Mujer 1998, p. 42).

Interruptions, lack of privacy, and presence of third parties. Women described frequent interruptions by other personnel while they were undergoing exams. Twenty-eight percent had no privacy during their exam because of the presence of third parties; 8–19 percent felt shame because of this. Overall, 60 percent of women reported feeling shame at exposing their genitals. (While one might expect that such modesty would lead to preference for a female provider, only 10 percent of respondents rated having a female provider as being of high importance.)

The findings were compiled into a report and discussed with local women's organizations, frontline providers, and municipal health authorities. These discussions often took place under the auspices of multi-sectoral committees that had been organized by the government in the mid-1990s to provide regular opportunities for communication between private and public actors involved in promoting health in a region or district.[5] The discussions were designed to reach agreement about courses of action to remedy the problems identified. There were difficulties, however, in attaining an adequate response from local authorities. Although the local women's groups and the frontline providers were dedicated to the process, they were not in a position to effect changes throughout large municipalities. The providers and users who had participated in the evaluation were from several health centers in the region, hence the findings could not be applied directly to improve services at any one center. Furthermore, because the decentralization of the health sector was still in its initial stages, central-level guidelines were still defining many municipal workplans.

The experience in Piura exemplifies the challenges of gaining consensus across a number of administrative levels. In Piura, the only rural area included in the consortium's project, a day-long assembly was convened to review the outcomes of the quality-of-care evaluation. Representatives of NGOs and the Rural Women's Network,[6] all of the midwives in the area, and municipal authorities attended, including representatives from Centro IDEAS, the member of the consortium that had conducted the evaluation. Midwives presented findings from the provider interviews, and women from the community presented a summary of users' input. In addition to deficiencies in service quality, women had highlighted the need to address health problems not traditionally dealt with by clinical services, including domestic violence. Comments from both midwives and women from the community noted the need for more holistic services. However, when the midwives presented their workplan for the year, it was as if these reports had never been made. The central authorities had already mandated two campaigns promoting and providing free Pap smears and two promoting and providing free sterilization. An NGO representative stood up and asked, "Wait a minute. What does this have to do with everything we just heard?" But there was little that could be done; funding was tied to directives from Lima.

While the municipal discussions led to frustration, the interaction between women and providers was generally viewed as valuable. For example, users complained that while the Pap smears provided through the centrally mandated campaign in Piura were free, when women returned for their results they were often told to pay a fee. Not surprisingly, some women in this cash-poor region went home without their results. These complaints helped providers grasp the frustration and distrust such campaigns generated in the community.

In addition to facilitating discussion, Consorcio Mujer used two other tactics to promote users' rights as the linchpin of quality of care. First, it designed a public media campaign with the slogan "Let's Be Citizens, Not Patients!" and distributed literature as part of the country's Safe Motherhood Day campaign. The consortium redoubled its efforts to influence quality-of-care evaluations at the central levels of the ministry and offered the ministry use of its research instruments and outcome indicators. These negotiations, initially promising, were truncated as controversy over the government's sterilization campaigns led to a growing rift between the ministry and some of the NGOs.[7]

A REVISED STRATEGY FOR COMMUNITY PARTICIPATION

Following the first set of experiments in provider–client dialogue, Consorcio Mujer decided it needed a new strategy, one that would have more specific geographic focus and build provider–client interaction around specific health center operations. The strategy would focus on collecting site-specific data on participating health centers and on training both clients and providers. The participating NGOs met with municipal health officials to select one health center in each project area. With an eye toward replicating the project beyond these pilot sites, the NGOs chose health centers that had been designated "network coordinators" as part of the national decentralization scheme.[8]

A NEW LOOK AT QUALITY OF CARE AT THE SIX SITES

While the results of the 1994 user surveys were useful for diagnosing general problems in a geographic region, the sampling strategy did not provide any one center with reliable information. In 1997 Consorcio Mujer conducted new user surveys on quality of care at each of the six pilot sites. The most common complaints cited paralleled the findings of the 1994 evaluation: disrespectful treatment, long waiting times, lack of privacy, and inadequate information. A number of new complaints surfaced in the 1997 surveys, however, including:

Pressure to be sterilized or accept intrauterine devices. This type of pressure was reported in the three sites outside of Lima. In the early 1990s, the Peruvian family planning program's overwhelming emphasis on provider-dependent and long-acting methods focused mainly on provision of IUDs; overt and systematic pressure on providers to persuade users to be sterilized had not yet emerged at the time of the 1994 evaluation.[9] This significant change was apparent in the 1997 surveys, however. As a community health promoter in Carabayllo, Lima, reported in 1998, "Last year they made the mama tie her tubes, whether she wanted to or not, like a kid who has to obey the father's rule."

Lack of culturally appropriate services. Failure to respect Quechua childbirth practices was of concern in all six sites.[10] The incompatibility between Western hospital-based childbirth practices and Andean customs has long been common knowledge in Peru and is one of the main obstacles to increasing rates of hospital-based births.

Inappropriate fee-collection practices. Users at five sites reported problems with providers charging for services that are officially free of charge. Women at all six sites reported mistreatment of indigent women who requested fee waivers. The collection of fees is a relatively new practice in the public sector, and the money collected is often retained by health centers to purchase supplies and equipment and to supplement the low salaries of permanent employees.[11] A users' committee member in Cusco explained, "If we have money, they treat us well. . . . [Rural women] don't like to come to the city to give birth, because they have no money; the doctor ignores them and the nurses yell at them and insult them."

Users were also asked to characterize good-quality treatment, and many willingly talked about positive experiences in the health system, again emphasizing the importance of personal interaction:

> *She treats me kindly. I have a lot of trust and confidence in her and she is a good doctor. Several friends and I see her and we like her a lot.*

> *She calls me by my name, and doesn't say anything negative about my having sexual relations and not being married; in other places they scold you.*

> *She talks to me like a sister so that I'm not afraid during my labor; she helps me get off the bed and gives me advice.*

KEY TO THE NEW STRATEGY: THE TRAINING WORKSHOPS

Consorcio Mujer developed separate but overlapping workshops for providers and users on quality of care, users' rights, and sexual and reproductive rights. The providers' workshops were attended by the direct service providers, auxiliary nursing staff, and, in some settings, the health center director. For the users' workshop, the consortium invited leaders of community-based organizations (such as food committees and mothers' clubs) who also worked as health promoters. These women were selected because they would have enough health and leadership experience to replicate the workshop in the community. Most of these women were poor and had only primary-level education.

Each workshop consisted of four half-day sessions. Participants' goals were to:

- Define the concepts of sexual and reproductive rights and users' rights;[12]
- Critically analyze the attitudes and assumptions underlying the paternalistic model of health care;
- Reflect on their own experiences as users of health services, paying particular attention to problems that had been identified in the surveys;
- Suggest new models of provider–client interaction; and
- Generate concrete proposals for improving quality at their health center.

The consortium emphasized different issues in the providers' and users' workshops. Providers dealt first with their own experiences as users and with users' rights, and then concentrated on issues related to quality. These included the tension between quality and productivity, and quality-improvement strategies. Users dealt with self-esteem, rights, citizenship, and gender issues before they turned to the topic of quality of care.

Consorcio Mujer trainers used various communication strategies to promote reflection about quality-of-care issues and to stimulate positive role-playing. For example, participants analyzed an actual provider–client transaction that had been observed in one site (see Box 2).

In the final stage of the training, participants in both workshops developed specific proposals for improving services and formed implementation teams. The hope was that the two teams (called quality committees among the providers, and users' defense committees among the women) would engage in ongoing dialogue.

RESPONSE TO THE WORKSHOPS

What Providers Learned

Providers demonstrated openness to learning, recognized the need for quality improvement, and were aware of remaining obstacles, including a need for further training to deal with gender and sexuality issues. A provider in Piura said: "We learned that

---

Box 2. Speaking to deaf ears: An exercise to analyze a provider–client interaction

The user, a 24-year-old high-school graduate, is a vendor. She has come to the clinic because of a delayed menstrual period and has received a positive pregnancy test result. The provider is a midwife with 20 years' experience.

Provider: Sit down, my love. [She asks the number of children and the date of the user's last period] Little mother, did you do a [pregnancy test]?

User: Yes, doctor. [She gives her the lab report]

Provider: Who prescribed this?

User: I did. I came to the center and took the test, but I don't want to have more children now. I have many problems.

Provider: What's going on with this, little girl? Why don't you want to be pregnant?

User: [Laughs nervously] Things are not well at home, we are still building the house, and I have no money.

Provider: Do you have sons or daughters?

User: Two daughters.

Provider: So many little women? Now let's try for the little man. We're going to have this little child, the last one, little mother, because then we'll take care of you with pills or little tubes in your arm. Look, like these. [Shows the pictures of oral contraceptives and Norplant®] We won't do anything foolish, we'll respect this little boy child, and we'll love him very much as well.

User: I was taking Lo-Femenal, so why did I get pregnant?

Provider: You didn't take them correctly, my daughter.

User: *No.* I took them correctly.

Provider: But surely you forgot one.

User: No, I didn't.

Provider: I'm going to give you some pills so that you don't get nauseous. Next time you come, I'll do your analyses.

User: But, doctor, I'm not nauseous.

Provider: It doesn't matter, take them anyway, they'll be good for you. [She doesn't indicate how many times a day, or for how long]

Source: Consorcio Mujer 1998. This interchange was documented during the 1994 evaluation.

---

the users wanted us to ask them about sexuality. So now, we ask in a friendly way. But we still have some prejudices, and have asked Centro IDEAS for more training." Staff from the health center in the rural coast region commented:

> *They gave information on users' rights to us and to the users, thus initiating communication between us. Before we had problems. We saw things one way, and they saw them in another.*

> *The exercise where we put ourselves in the shoes of the users—[in which I was] remembering a time when I was treated terribly—influenced me. No one paid attention to me, and I got very demoralized.*

> *The course was very interesting. It allowed us to view ourselves objectively and see how we treat users. It was very useful to see their perceptions.*

A comment from a clinic director in Lima exemplifies the change in attitude that the consortium's workshops aimed for: "Before, the providers were the authority, and the patients asked us to help them as a favor. Now we say, 'We are employed thanks to the patients.'"

In all six sites, the workshop also revealed providers' frustration at feeling pulled between a concern for users' rights and institutional pressures to sterilize women. As one doctor exclaimed, "What about my rights? Who is going to look out for me when I apply quality principles and am fired for not meeting my quotas?"

The providers were committed to participating in the workshop. In many sites, the sessions lasted for several hours beyond the scheduled time, sometimes until 10:30 p.m. In one site, an unsympathetic administrator scheduled an obligatory meeting to conflict with the workshop; the staff reacted by rescheduling the session for the evening, after work hours.

What Users Learned

The response among users was equally favorable, particularly with regard to the focus on rights. The previous training provided by NGOs to these grassroots women's organizations had focused on improving their effectiveness as community leaders, and did not link personal issues in women's lives such as lack of self-esteem to their ability to organize for their rights as citizens. Latin American feminist organizations—in their programs to promote citizenship among grassroots women's organizations—have learned the importance of participatory training methods for women in groups to support each participant's ability to "reconstruct oneself as a bearer of rights." The user trainees in Consorcio Mujer's project underwent this process to enable them to demand respectful and safe services. Participants voiced pride in their increased ability to ask questions, complain about mistreatment, resist coercion, and engage in discussion with providers on quality issues.

> *We didn't know about self-esteem. We learned to love and value our bodies and ourselves. Before, we let ourselves be mistreated, but no longer.*

> *The concept of users' rights was new; it fit us like a ring on a finger. . . . We had complained before but without legal grounds.*

> *Now we understand that human rights include the right to health. This caused us to think deeply. Why do we let them mistreat us? Why aren't we capable of reacting or asking for what we want?*

The emphasis on self-esteem was important. We learned we can say no. We give and give, always for others. . . . Women always feel guilty.

The women's own views of what they deserved evolved over the course of the workshop. This process was summed up by a trainer in Piura:

What is new about the module is the concept of citizenship and rights. While the women already had some idea of these concepts, they were able to internalize them. The women reflected deeply. At the beginning of the training, they said that the quality of the services was just fine. Then, as we probed more into the different aspects of users' rights, the incidents of violations emerged—having to do with lack of privacy, inadequate information, mistreatment. . . .

At the beginning, I didn't think that the women were going to open up, but I was wrong. Little by little, they began to talk about everything they had left unsaid, and to express it with all their emotions. One woman wept as she described how she had been humiliated.

The providers understood about users' rights much more easily than the users. . . . [For the users] it was difficult to grasp the concept, because they only envision themselves as users and not as bearers of rights.

AFTER THE TRAINING: STRIKING A BALANCE

After the training, the two groups came back together. Throughout the project, the relationship between health care providers and community health promoters struck a balance between cooperative goodwill and tension. For example, community health promoters fiercely resented continuing to receive peremptory commands from health care providers as the predominant style of interaction: "Bring us 30 women on Tuesday for Pap smears." Difficulties also arose from provider resistance to users' new status and sense of entitlement. In one site, providers did not appreciate having users' comments included in the evaluations of individual care providers. In another site, the users' committee tried wearing special aprons to signify a semiofficial status, and joined the staff when they opened the waiting room suggestion boxes and reviewed users' comments. Although this action was negotiated by Consorcio Mujer and both sides agreed in principle, it did not work in practice. A user explained, "One woman went to the meeting to discuss the complaints, but she found that the language they used was too sophisticated. The women from the Mothers' Club didn't want to go any more, and the providers felt invaded."

In another site, according to the providers, members of the users' defense committee arrived unannounced and sat in the waiting room observing. When they were asked what they wanted, they said, "We're here to supervise you." Providers refused to negotiate directly with the users' defense committee, explaining, "This community is very combative. We were afraid to enter into a formal relationship with them, because we don't have the means to live up to their expectations."[13]

In spite of these difficulties, in five of the six sites the relationship between the two groups remained generally friendly and cooperative after the workshops. A trainer in one site observed, "We have not noticed a negative reaction from the providers to women's participation. They view the women as allies." A user at another site remarked, "We had a positive attitude . . . that we were there to help them reach the people most in need. Before, we just criticized and didn't offer to help."

SHARED SOLUTIONS

The focus of post-training meetings was on solutions. Equipped with a new perspective about the rights of users, users and providers negotiated remedies for the various problems that had been identified. Most of the following solutions were implemented at particular sites; in some cases, however, several sites arrived at similar plans.

Promoting Respectful Treatment

- Rotate staff who treat users well into positions requiring public contact. In one Lima site, for example, a friendly cleaning woman was promoted to admissions.
- Establish procedures for firing, transferring, or disciplining personnel who are consistently the focus of mistreatment complaints. A doctor in the same Lima site lost her post as clinic director as a result of community pressure.
- Provide follow-up training to address assumptions and attitudes underlying rude behavior.

Ensuring that Providers Introduce Themselves

- Require providers to wear name badges.

Reducing Waiting Time

- Create chart retrieval routines to limit waiting time for women who arrive without their health cards.
- Post someone to direct clients to their proper destination.
- Establish procedures to serve clients in the order in which they arrive.

Protecting Privacy

- Establish a private area in which a user can state the reason for her visit.
- Place signs on examination room doors indicating whether the room is "free" or "occupied."

Eliminating Pressure to Be Sterilized

- Establish a waiting period between the counseling visit and the sterilization procedure. (This practice, originally instituted in one site, has now become part of the Ministry of Health's guidelines.)
- Conduct a community survey to prove to officials that there is no unmet need for sterilization to decrease pressure to fulfill unrealistic quotas.

Counseling

- Enforce a 15-minute minimum visit time to compel providers to spend more time offering information and counseling.

Promoting Cultural Sensitivity

- Introduce selected elements of natural childbirth and allow women to give birth in the squatting position with family members present.
- Use Quechua-speaking auxiliary staff to translate for users during visits.

Ensuring Access and Appropriate Fee-collection Practices

- Enforce guidelines on free services.
- Establish a savings plan during each antenatal visit to cover childbirth expenses (obstetric care is free but supplies must be paid for by the patient).

Although only limited evaluations of quality have been carried out since these measures were instituted, providers and users in all six sites have testified that services, while not perfect, have improved. Follow-up training of providers has consolidated some gains, while staff turnover has eroded others. Providers' comments point to adjustments in both the technical aspects of clinic operations and in their own attitudes:

> We have to be realistic. We have been raised a certain way and consciously we know how we should be, but we can't live up to it. We have raised the problem that it is difficult to work on these issues with the community when we ourselves still have machismo inside us.

> We made the changes needed and applied a second survey, and we saw improvements in satisfaction with admissions, the cashier, and the first aid room. But our basic problem is that we have few personnel and many patients. The problem of waiting time can't be solved.

> Above all, the change has been within us.

Users have also found changes "within themselves." Comments from women who had participated in the project indicate an increased ability to assert their rights as users:

> Now we can complain and denounce mistreatment. We communicate with the superiors.

> I had decided to not get my tubes tied, but then one day a very angry nurse came to my house and asked, "Why would you want more children if you can't feed them?" I replied, "Miss, I'm not going to do it and no one can make me." Because if I want to, they can tie them, and if I don't, they can't force me. The nurse came for the second time, but I didn't want to meet her. . . . I had already been trained, so I told her that no one could make me, that this is my right and my body.

CONCLUSION: THE NECESSARY ELEMENTS FOR CHANGE

Consorcio Mujer developed both a framework and a process of dialogue that challenged a paternalistic health care system and advanced a system of health promotion based on citizenship and equality. Clients, both individually and in groups, had to internalize the conception of themselves as bearers of rights. Providers had to begin to respect users' rights and to view respectful service delivery as a duty rather than a charitable function. Promoting such change required participatory training methods and time.

Another element in the relative success of Consorcio Mujer's training strategy was that its rights-based framework for change was followed by discussions and workshops to develop concrete proposals for improvements in service delivery and by actions to carry out the proposals. The combination of intensive interventions for attitude change, immediately followed by an opportunity to put these new principles into action, was a powerful strategy. While this strategy guided the process, some combination of the other facilitating factors was also necessary for success. Exceptional structural supports were in place through which the consortium was able to prod the system most effectively in some sites. These included:

- The availability of well-functioning, government-sanctioned multi-sectoral committees to serve as a forum for dialogue, pool resources on joint initiatives, and coordinate work. The existence of these committees was probably the single most important factor influencing success in some of the sites;
- Donor and government support of large-scale parallel and complementary projects designed to improve the quality of care;[14]
- Generally receptive attitudes among health officials toward community oversight, because of the introduction of such oversight mechanisms as part of health-sector reform; and

- A long-standing and trusting relationship between the Consorcio Mujer NGOs and local service providers and community-based women's organizations.

Consorcio Mujer did intensive work during 1999 to document the project's experiences, resulting in three publications (Consorcio Mujer 2000a, 2000b, 2000c), an account of the experiences at each of the sites, and training manuals for providers and community health leaders on quality of care and users' rights. According to the project coordinator, the demand for these publications has been lively. Only a more rigorous long-term evaluation could begin to take account of the ripple effects in the communities and elsewhere in Peru.

This chapter highlights the role of NGOs in effecting meaningful improvements in the quality of women's health care. Community oversight of quality of care in the provision of health services can be a delicate process; it is helpful to have an external entity managing it and monitoring the dynamics. The NGOs heard the views of both sides before bringing them together to engage in discussions and negotiation. Because users and providers speak different languages and operate from different places in the system, the NGOs played the role of mediator.

Finally, this chapter provides evidence of the ability of a rights and citizenship framework to stimulate collaborative partnerships between health care providers and the people they serve. The goal of democratic participation can only be realized when the less powerful actors in a system gain more power. Reaching this goal involves simultaneously promoting changes in people's attitudes and devising organizational, political, and economic structures that stimulate power-sharing and mutual respect.

Acknowledgments

Sylvia Madalengoitia of Centro de Estudios Sociales y Publicaciones (CESIP), the project coordinator, gave invaluable assistance through her overview of Consorcio Mujer from its inception and by helping to coordinate my travel. Luz Maria Gallo and Virginia Agüero of Centro IDEAS in Piura, Magda Matteos and Rosario Salazer at Centro de Estudios y Promoción de la Mujer Amauta in Cusco, and Maribel Becerril of Centro de Estudios y Promoción Comunal del Oriente in Tarapoto provided insights and introductions to the users and providers they had worked with, as did Ida Escudero of CESIP, Rocío Gutierrez of Movimiento Manuela Ramos, and Yngeborg Villena of Centro de la Mujer Peruana Flora Tristán in the Lima neighborhoods where they worked. I owe a special thank you to the health officials, service providers, and members of users' defense committees who gave generously of their time to talk about their experiences. The writing of this chapter was made possible by generous support from the Ford Foundation and the David Rockefeller Center for Latin American Studies at Harvard University.

Notes

1   The Consorcio Mujer members involved in this project include Movimiento Manuela Ramos, Centro de la Mujer Peruana Flora Tristán, and Centro de Estudios Sociales y Publicaciones in Lima; Centro de Estudios y Promoción de la Mujer Amauta in the Andean highlands; Centro IDEAS in the rural coast zone; and Centro de Estudios y Promoción Comunal del Oriente in the Amazon region.

2   The documentation of the project presented in this chapter is based on reports and documents produced by Consorcio Mujer, on my personal knowledge of the project as a program officer for the Ford Foundation during the period 1993–98, and on semistructured interviews I conducted at the six sites with NGOs, health officials and providers, users' committees, and members of multi-sectoral committees during a two-week period in December 1998.

3   For more information on reform of the Peruvian health sector, see Ugarte and Monje 1999.

4   Such questions proved much more productive than asking a general question about a client's level of satisfaction, the answers to which tended to indicate falsely high levels of satisfaction.

5   The committees, organized in the mid-1990s with the encouragement of the Ministry of Health, included representatives from the health sector, other ministries, municipal officials, NGOs, and, occasionally, community organizations. The ministry hoped that by institutionalizing such communication, the resources of all institutions active in health promotion in one geographic area could be directed toward common goals and strategies.

6   The Rural Women's Network is an organization of peasant women in the Piura area with district-level subnetworks of more than 1,000 women.

7   The sterilization campaigns, which began in 1995, led to rights abuses throughout the country. During the campaigns, health care providers were given monthly quotas for numbers of sterilizations, which were enforced with both threats and incentives from the Ministry of Health. Given low pay and lack of job stability, few providers could afford to ignore these pressures. The campaigns ended abruptly in January 1998 when related human rights abuses were exposed in the media by Giulia Tamayo of CLADEM Peru, a women's rights network.

8   In the decentralization scheme, each network might include the maternity hospitals, health centers, and health posts in a health region. The institution designated as the coordinator of the network was in a key position to implement new programs and guidelines.

9   The levels of intimidation of users differed among the six project sites, depending on provincial fertility rates and on the willingness of regional, subregional, and health center directors to resist pressures from above. One United Nations professional described how Quechua women began to flee into the hills whenever the public health midwife came to their village, because they were afraid of being coerced into being sterilized.

10 Andean women traditionally labor in a warm and dark environment among family members. They ingest hot broths and teas, and the customary position when giving birth is to squat with the use of a birth pole. Postpartum practices include a restricted diet and burial of the placenta.

11 Some health officials would not admit that fees are used to supplement salaries, while others confirmed that doing so is a widespread, but unofficial, practice.

12 The new General Health Law, passed in July 1997, included a section on users' rights. Consorcio Mujer trainers gave participants in both workshop groups a poster with a list of users' rights as established by law. Ironically, the law was passed in the middle of the sterilization campaigns.

13 In most sites, the NGOs had a long history of work with both the health center and the local women leaders and could build on previously established trust. In this site, however, the Consorcio Mujer NGO was reaching out to a completely new geographical area, one in which the local women's organizations had had a confrontational relationship with the health system. It lacked sufficient history with these organizations to influence their stance and enable an effective dialogue. Based on the author's analysis of interviews at the six sites and interviews with the project director, it appears that the dialogues were most effective when the NGO had carefully negotiated and clarified the terms of the dialogue and prepared both groups in advance. This was easiest where there was a historical working relationship.

14   The World Bank, USAID, and UNFPA were promoting infrastructure improvements and quality-
      of-care initiatives during the project period.

References

Bruce, Judith. 1990. "Fundamental elements of the quality of care: A simple framework," *Studies in Family Planning* 21(2): 61–91.

Consorcio Mujer. 1998. *Calidad de Atención en la Salud Reproductiva: Una Mirada desde la Ciudadanía Feminina* [Quality of care in reproductive health: From the perspective of women's citizenship]. Lima: Consorcio Mujer.

———. 2000a. *Compromiso para Fortalecer la Participación Ciudadana desde los Servicios de Salud: Modulo de Capacitación a Personal de los Servicios de Salud* [The health services' commitment to strengthen citizen participation: Training manual for health service providers]. Lima: Consorcio Mujer.

———. 2000b. *Fortaleciendo las Habilidades Ciudadanas de las Mujeres en Salud: Modulo de Capacitación a Líderes de Salud* [Strengthening women's citizenship skills in health: Training manual for health leaders]. Lima: Consorcio Mujer.

———. 2000c. *Se Hace Camino al Andar: Aportes a la Construcción de la Ciudadania de las Mujeres en Salud* [Forging paths: Resources for the construction of women's citizenship in health]. Lima: Consorcio Mujer.

Hola, Eugenia and Ana María Portugal (eds.). 1997. *La Ciudadanía a Debate* [Debates on citizenship], Ediciones de las Mujeres no. 25. Santiago, Chile: ISIS Internacional and CEM.

National Statistics Institute. 1999. *National Household Survey (ENAHO) of the National Statistics Institute (INEI) 4th quarter, 1995 and 1997*. Lima: National Statistics Institute.

———. 2000. *Encuesta Demográfica y de Salud Familiar 2000* [Demographic and family health survey 2000]. Lima: National Statistics Institute.

Ugarte, Oscar and José Antonio Monje. 1999. "Equidad y reforma en el sector salud" [Equity and reform in the health sector], unpublished paper. Lima: Universidad del Pacífico.

United Nations. 1995. "Core document forming part of the reports of states parties: Peru," submitted to the UN treaty bodies. HRI/CORE/1/Add.43/Rev1. http://www.hri.ca/fortherecord1999/documentation/coredocs/hri-core-1-add43-rev1.htm.

Contact information

For Spanish and Portuguese speakers
Sylvia Madalengoitia
Centro de Estudios Sociales
   y Publicaciones (CESIP)
Coronel Zegarra 722, Jesús María
Lima 11, Peru
telephone: 51-1-471-3410
e-mail: mina@cesip.org.pe

For English speakers
Ana Guezmes
Centro de la Mujer Peruana Flora Tristán
Parque Hernán Velarde no. 42
Lima 1, Peru
telephone: 51-1-433-0488/0694/2765/
   1457/9060
fax: 51-1-433-9500
e-mail: ana@flora.org.pe

19

Action Research to Enhance Reproductive Choice in a Brazilian Municipality: The Santa Barbara Project

Margarita Díaz, Ruth Simmons, Juan Díaz, Francisco Cabral,
Debora Bossemeyer, Maria Yolanda Makuch, and Laura Ghiron

For many decades the family planning field has focused efforts to expand contraceptive choice on the introduction of new fertility-regulation methods. Great hopes were placed on the contributions of technology. This chapter presents findings from a project that has used a different approach, arguing that the addition of new technology alone accomplishes little. The approach is founded on the idea that technology can fulfill its potential only when introduced into settings that have the capacity to provide services of good quality. Because public-sector services often lack this capacity, efforts to broaden contraceptive choice may require upgrading deficient service systems and fostering client-centered care rather than simply expanding the types of methods available.

The project discussed here is part of an effort by the World Health Organization (WHO) to implement an approach to contraceptive introduction that emphasizes quality of care, a client-centered orientation, and a reproductive health philosophy (Simmons et al. 1997; Spicehandler and Simmons 1994). This approach shifts attention from an exclusive emphasis on a specific technology to a broader, holistic view of factors relevant to technology introduction. These include attention to the social context that affects method choice; the currently available method mix; the organizational capacity of programs to ensure quality for existing, as well as new, methods and services; and the strong role that participatory approaches can play in guaranteeing that interventions are client-centered and appropriate to the context. Within this framework the central issues are understanding the needs of a community and the match between these needs, the capacity of services, and the technologies available. The approach emphasizes three stages of work: assessment, research, and expansion of research findings for policy and program development. It is currently being implemented in nine countries, including Brazil.[1]

The Brazil case—with a particular focus on action research conducted in the municipality of Santa Barbara d'Oeste—is the focus of this chapter.

The chapter shows that in order to make reproductive choice a reality in Santa Barbara d'Oeste it was necessary to reorient the municipal health system to increase access to and the availability of care and to provide better-quality reproductive health services. The project engaged not only the providers and their immediate supervisors, but also the municipal authorities, community members, and researchers, in an intense participatory process. From its inception, the project looked beyond family planning to reproductive health. Adding contraceptive methods not previously available in this service setting was an important component of the process, but by no means the most essential one. Perhaps the most important lesson from the project is that substantial change was possible within the municipal health system, and that this change was brought about with technical assistance from the research team but with limited infusion of other external resources.

THE SETTING

Brazil's constitution has guaranteed women the right to family planning since 1988. In 1984 the government committed itself to a national reproductive health policy through the creation of a national program of integrated health care for women, known by the acronym PAISM. Although PAISM is not fully implemented even to this day, the breadth of its vision has served as a standard by which the policies of other countries can be gauged. In guaranteeing the right to family planning, the government approved the provision of a range of contraceptive methods, including the pill, the intrauterine device (IUD), barrier methods (including condoms and the diaphragm), and periodic abstinence. Injectables were added to the list of methods approved by the Ministry of Health in 1996, and male and female sterilization in August 1997.

Program practice stands in stark contrast to policy in Brazil. A 1993 nationwide assessment of contraceptive service delivery, conducted as the first stage of the WHO-sponsored strategic approach to contraceptive introduction, indicated that public-sector availability of and access to contraceptive services of adequate quality were extremely constrained (Formiga et al. 1994). Few public-sector facilities provided the full range of approved methods, and many provided none at all. Provider bias against such methods as the IUD was widespread, and access to tubal ligation, for which there is high demand in Brazil, was limited.[2] Vasectomy was provided in only a small number of public-sector facilities.

Reproductive choice and improvements in reproductive health were further hampered by problems in the structure and quality of care-giving. Technical competence and counseling services were weak. Further, physicians working in the municipal sector were paid extremely low salaries and were, therefore, eager to minimize their time at clinics, effectively reducing women's access to already limited services. Stories of women waiting in line from 4:00 a.m. solely to obtain an appointment for a reproductive health consultation in the distant future were not uncommon. In some service settings, women were required to schedule a series of appointments—for an educational session, a Pap smear, receipt of the Pap smear result, and consultation with a specialist—before they finally obtained an IUD.

Overall, the needs assessment showed that access to methods that were already approved and theoretically available in the public sector was, in reality, extremely limited. Therefore, adding new contraceptive technologies was not a priority for Brazil. Instead, there was a need to improve the provision of approved methods in the context of a service system characterized by higher quality and greater responsiveness to client and community needs. Active work with the managerial system would be necessary to make these improvements possible. The assessment concluded that widespread introduction of methods not then authorized should await Ministry of Health approval of their use and be undertaken only when public-sector service capabilities had been improved (Formiga et al. 1994). Several areas of study were recommended, among them: (1) research to assess ways of enhancing the capacity of services to provide approved contraceptive methods with adequate quality and client orientation; (2) service-delivery research on whether and how contraceptive options for women and men could be broadened; and (3) introductory research to assess the service-delivery implications of adding injectables to public-sector services.[3]

STEP ONE: USING A PARTICIPATORY PROCESS

In the second half of 1994, the municipality of Santa Barbara d'Oeste and the Center for Research on Maternal and Child Health (CEMICAMP—a nongovernmental organization affiliated with the University of Campinas) began a collaborative, action research project (hereafter referred to as the Santa Barbara project) to explore the research questions outlined above. The project constituted the second stage of implementing the strategic approach to contraceptive introduction. It was conducted with funding from WHO and technical assistance from the Population Council office in Brazil and the University of Michigan. Key members of the research and technical assistance team had participated in the aforementioned 1993 nationwide assessment. The aim of the project was to establish a participatory process involving members of the Santa Barbara d'Oeste community, local health authorities and providers, and researchers in identifying needed improvements in reproductive choice, access, quality of care, and client orientation that were feasible given the resource limitations of the municipal health system.[4]

Santa Barbara d'Oeste, a municipality in central São Paulo State, was selected by the research team as the locale for this project because its family planning services were severely deficient; it is located near the implementing research agency, CEMICAMP; its health secretary and the mayor had a strong commitment to improving services; and the health secretary had requested support from CEMICAMP. Santa Barbara d'Oeste is an almost exclusively urban community with a population of 170,000, the majority of whom live within walking distance of a health facility. The municipality has one private-sector hospital. Public-sector health services are concentrated in 11 health centers/posts. Roughly three-quarters of the clinical care appointments in these facilities are with female clients.

The participatory nature of the Santa Barbara project constituted a marked departure from standard administrative procedure. In theory, decisionmaking about municipal health services occurs through a municipal health council with representation from workers' unions, women's groups, and other community organizations. As in many other Brazilian municipalities, a municipal health council did not exist in Santa Barbara d'Oeste because the process of "municipalization" was not complete.[5] Neither were there regular meetings between health authorities and providers to guide the provision of services, solve problems, and address emerging needs. To implement project activities, an executive committee was established, comprising members of the health secretariat of Santa Barbara d'Oeste, government officials, service providers, collaborators from CEMICAMP, representatives from a local women's organization, and adolescents.[6] This participatory structure ensured a feedback mechanism for various stakeholders, including community members. The purpose was to ensure relevant input from the community and providers on the interpretation of diagnostic results, the identification of needed interventions, and the implementation and evaluation of their effectiveness. The executive committee approved all the major interventions undertaken by the project.

The involvement of community representatives on the executive committee was facilitated by the municipal coordinator of PAISM, who informed various community groups—particularly those interested in public health—of the new project. He also supported the formation of a local women's organization, SOS Mulher, to participate in the project. Women who had been active in other local organizations provided leadership to SOS Mulher. The fact that most members were of higher social and economic status than typical users of public-sector services may in part explain why their participation in the project eventually waned. The active participation of SOS Mulher members during the crucial, early stages of the project ensured that women's reproductive health concerns were ably represented on the committee and reflected in the interventions. There were, however, issues of access and community reach to which these women were not attuned.

Key members of the research team maintained close contact with the health authorities in Santa Barbara d'Oeste and played a leading role in shaping the agenda of executive committee meetings, conducting and presenting results from the diagnostic assessment, and making proposals for interventions. Interaction between the research team, health service providers, and health authorities was facilitated through regular field visits by the research team to Santa Barbara d'Oeste and through training activities for providers and community representatives as described below.

STEP TWO: A DETAILED DIAGNOSIS

The Santa Barbara project is grounded in the intellectual tradition of "organization development" (French and Bell 1995), which entails collaborative diagnosis of organizational problems, identification of interventions and ways of facilitating implementation, and evaluation of effectiveness. To initiate improvements in the municipal health system's capacity to provide more and better reproductive health services, the research team conducted a baseline diagnostic study of four aspects of the Santa Barbara d'Oeste service system: (1) availability and accessibility of services; (2) quality of services; (3) physical and human resources; and (4) the management system. To ensure a diversity of perspectives, the research included community-based focus-group discussions with men and women (both users and nonusers of public services), interviews with women who had received care from a gynecologist and with users of other clinic services, interviews with providers at the 11 municipal health facilities and with clinic and municipal administrators, patient-flow analysis,[7] and observation of clinic functioning and the care provided by gynecologists.

Availability and Accessibility of Services

The research carried out in Santa Barbara d'Oeste found a persistent pattern of limited availability of and constrained access to women's health services, especially family planning. Of the 1,826 average monthly consultations provided by gynecologists at the 11 municipal facilities in 1995, less than one-tenth were for family planning. Over half were for Pap smears. The remainder were for antenatal care (11 percent) and general gynecologic services (30 percent). In addition:

- Although gynecologists were expected to see 16 women during a four-hour clinic session, they typically attended fewer women and saw them hurriedly. This allowed them to stay at the clinic for a shorter period of time. Some staff members felt frustrated because they witnessed women's distress as they struggled to gain access to care. However, these staff members did not have the confidence or authority to make changes, and their motivation to initiate change was low.

- Pregnant women were given priority in obtaining appointments, leaving even fewer slots for those in need of family planning and other reproductive health services.
- Medical personnel were used inefficiently. Gynecologists spent more than half of their time doing Pap smears, giving patients Pap smear results, or dispensing routine contraceptives, tasks that could be delegated to appropriately trained auxiliary personnel.
- A complex system of appointment scheduling curtailed demand, obliging women to arrive at the health post in the middle of the night and to stand in line for hours to obtain "walk-in" care or to make an appointment.

Focus-group discussions with community women were dominated by the theme of difficulties in gaining access to services. The majority spoke of enduring long waits only to be informed that there were no slots left and to return another day, or worse, to be scolded for not coming early enough.

> This is wrong. You go there and they only have one doctor. Only one for a lot of people. . . . If you complain what do they do? They say, "You wake up earlier and you come here earlier." It happened to me one day. I left home early, and when I arrived, because there were two more women in front of me in line, they didn't give me the appointment.

> Me too, me too. And when we complain the attendant always says, "You insist too much. What a lot of insistence." If you don't insist, you don't get anything.

Many women indicated that they have no alternative sources of care and therefore often neglect or take risks with their own health, even taking medications prescribed for friends or family members who have what they perceive to be similar conditions:

> We didn't take care in the right way; because to go to the health post is so far, we don't have the money to go; women do not have time to go.

> Here is one woman who feels a pain and goes to the other's house and then they pass the medicine. Then here in this way people help each other [by] giving [each other] medicine.

> Either they go to the doctor or take someone else's medicine.

Women's sense of powerlessness and the low priority accorded many of their needs were reflected in sarcastic replies to the question of where women seek family planning services:

She even has the possibility of having two children before she gets the consultation. (Everybody laughs)

If she has the means, she can go to a private doctor; but if she doesn't, then she goes to the health post.

There were no reproductive health services directed at men and nonpregnant, unmarried adolescents. Municipal health facilities would not provide condoms to men, and vasectomy was available only in the private sector, and at very high cost. Both men and women participating in focus groups repeatedly indicated that the municipal facilities should pay attention to reproductive health services for men as well as women.

Quality of Care

The baseline research assessed quality of care in terms of the six-element framework outlined by Bruce (1990): choice; information giving; interpersonal relations; an appropriate constellation of services; technical competence; and continuity of care. The observational assessment showed that improvements were particularly needed in the technical dimensions of care, in the information and choices provided to users, and in the interpersonal dimensions of care-giving. Patient-flow analysis revealed that waiting times were long and record keeping was inadequate to permit continuity of care.

During the few opportunities available to observe consultations with women who came specifically for contraception, observers noted that the level of technical quality was good. However, gynecologists seeing women with other types of reproductive health needs revealed poor knowledge of contraception and neglected discussion of family planning even when such a service was clearly indicated. Gynecologic exams were sometimes incomplete or of poor quality: Half of the physicians omitted a breast exam, and when one was performed it was not always thorough. Providers only intermittently washed their hands or used gloves for patient examinations. Referrals were not always given when necessary, and, frequently, pertinent information was not recorded on the patient's chart.

The quality of interpersonal relations between physicians and patients was mixed. During the observed interactions, physicians were cordial. They established a friendly relationship with women, although in an authoritarian style that provided little opportunity for the women to ask questions. Privacy was not maintained; for example, staff entered examination rooms and left the doors open while patients were being examined. Consultations tended to be rapid, lasting an average of five to six minutes. Waiting time for a consultation ranged from two and a half to four hours.

Some women complained that the physicians gave them too little information or treated them poorly:

> *I always go there to the [health post]. I go there but I don't like the doctors there very*
> *much. They don't pay attention to us. We talk and talk and they don't say anything*
> *about the exam. They only say it's good and give a prescription.*
>
> *They also make mistakes. There are some who don't say the right thing. . . .*

Gynecologists providing antenatal care attended only to the medical aspects of pregnancy and neglected psychological and information needs. In one case, a 15-year-old
girl who was pregnant for the first time was given no information about her pregnancy
and was not asked whether she needed a referral to a psychologist or social worker.

Nurses received mixed evaluations. Some were perceived as gentle and accom-
modating, while others were described as unhelpful, rude, and unwilling or unable to
assist women with their problems. When women came to the health post because they
felt ill, they were sometimes told they did not have a problem, or that they could
receive care only in the case of major illness. Examples were given of women with
serious health conditions who could not obtain access to services. However, even when
women were specifically asked about the quality of care, the conversation returned
spontaneously to the difficulties in obtaining care. When access is a major barrier, the
question of quality becomes subordinate.

The Management System and Supplies

The management system gave no attention to the pressing problems of service availability or quality of care. Technical oversight and supportive supervision of municipal
facilities were lacking. Staff motivation was poor and turnover was high.

While a management information system (MIS) was in place, it did not differentiate among the various elements of reproductive health care, thus making the tracking
of contraceptive service provision and other key elements of care impossible. Data
from the system were not adequate to allow effective supervision, appropriate reimbursement from the government,[8] or assessment of supply needs, particularly for contraceptives. The pattern of irregular and insufficient supplies of contraceptives was
partially a result of these deficiencies in the MIS. Focus groups with men from the
Santa Barbara d'Oeste community demonstrated that local residents resented the fact
that they could not count on receiving contraceptive supplies at the health post:

> *How do they expect us to do family planning to control births when they don't have*
> *methods? I have never seen methods or condoms given at the health posts. . . . There are*
> *women who don't have the money to buy these medicines. And it is the poorest ones*
> *who have more children, because they don't have the [resources] to prevent [having*
> *them].*

STEP THREE: ENHANCING ACCESS *WITH* QUALITY

What was striking throughout the focus-group discussions was the way in which participants repeatedly returned to the question of access when issues of quality were raised. People would say: "Once you get an appointment, the treatment is good." This is not to imply that everyone was satisfied with the quality of care received, but receiving care was the predominant concern. Expert observation of services during the diagnostic assessment identified the need for quality improvements, and the diagnosis of the management system identified severe deficiencies in the areas of supervision, technical support, management information, and supplies. It was thus apparent that enhancing both access to and the quality of care, including expanding contraceptive choice, would be essential and that these objectives could only be accomplished if the municipal health service system were strengthened and reoriented.

Even before the results of the diagnostic assessment were available, the executive committee had identified areas in need of attention. Some interventions, such as training, were initiated immediately. Findings from the diagnostic assessment were later presented to the executive committee by the research team and were extensively discussed. Community members on the executive committee played a key role in this discussion by confirming the findings and adding anecdotal evidence from their experiences and those of their friends and families. They also used the forum as an opportunity to raise other areas of concern, such as the lack of drugs in the health care system. Some providers reacted defensively to the findings. Careful facilitation by the research team kept the meeting constructive by engaging all stakeholders. Hearing the voices of community members was particularly influential for providers and health authorities.

Five areas of intervention to improve access to and quality of services were subsequently identified by the executive committee: (1) training; (2) developing an improved management information system; (3) improving the availability of contraceptive supplies; (4) recruiting additional personnel; and (5) developing client-focused systems of appointment-making and service delivery.

Training Municipal Health Care Providers

In 1995 CEMICAMP conducted a five-day general training session for physicians, nurses, auxiliary nurses, a social worker, and community representatives.[9] This session was followed by additional training on specific topics for particular municipal health staff from all 11 facilities. Through role-plays, discussions of case studies, group activities, games, and hands-on training, the program covered four broad areas: (1) the philosophy of reproductive health with a focus on women's needs; (2) the characteristics of a high-quality family planning service-delivery system, including job descriptions, definition of functions, scheduling, and patient flow; (3) counseling and communications skills; and (4) all contraceptive methods, including, but not limited to, those approved by the Ministry of Health.

The training for gynecologists was supplemented by one week of individualized practical training in contraceptive screening, IUD insertion and follow-up, and management of complications and side effects, conducted at the CEMICAMP family planning clinic. Subsequent monitoring and supervision by trainers reinforced the acquisition and implementation of skills. Because some municipal gynecologists were unable to attend the first general training, additional lectures were given to gynecologists in 1996 to update their technical knowledge of contraception and general gynecology.

Auxiliary nurses (typically high-school graduates trained for six months to one year), attendants (typically primary-school graduates trained for approximately one month), and the receptionist received an additional three days of classroom training, supplemented by a one-day practicum for auxiliary nurses on Pap smear collection and breast exams. A one-day workshop for all health center/post staff on sexuality, gender issues, sexually transmitted infections (STIs), and HIV/AIDS completed the training intervention. The sexuality component of the training helped participants expand their understanding of sexuality to include both the physiology of sexual organs and reproductive functions and the social, religious, and cultural dimensions of sexuality. Through a question-and-answer session, participants' understanding of the link between sexuality and sexual and reproductive rights was enhanced. Providers also gained a clearer appreciation of the close relationship between gender issues and the health of women and men.

The family planning training methodology[10] used a series of exercises to help health care providers shift from the belief that they must decide what is best for the client toward accepting women as capable of making their own choices. The intention was to help providers understand that they should assist women in making free and informed choices. Providers were encouraged to offer clients information about the range of contraceptive options available, check their medical history, and facilitate reflection on various aspects of their lives, so that they could consider their method options in that context. For example, if the pill was discussed, women would be encouraged to think not only about how they would feel about the daily regimen, but also about their sexual lives and whether they needed dual protection. During role-plays, trainers challenged providers' conventional advice to women. For example, a trainer playing the role of a 30-year-old woman with five children who was using the pill encouraged providers to see that her contraceptive choice was reasonable and to refrain from making the standard suggestion that she obtain a tubal ligation.

Creating More Appointment Space for Clients

A key bottleneck in the service system was the limited time available for appointments with gynecologists, who, in Brazil's public-sector services, are responsible for women's health care, including family planning. To create more appointment time, some tasks were shifted from gynecologists to nursing and auxiliary staff, and gynecologists were hired for health posts that had none. The job functions of the nursing and auxiliary staff were expanded to include collecting Pap smears and providing normal results; doing breast examinations on a routine basis; and providing family planning education and refills for pill and condom users. The training had laid the groundwork for this shift in responsibilities. Because auxiliary and nursing staff could provide these services, women seeking them no longer needed an appointment. They could walk in on any day during clinic hours and be served. In addition, the appointment-scheduling process was changed to ensure that each gynecologist saw 16 women per clinic session and to allow women to schedule appointments any day of the week and within a reasonable period of time.

Initially, researchers worried that there might not be sufficient resources within the municipal health system to recruit additional health personnel. And because public-sector salaries are extremely low, it was feared that it would be difficult to identify motivated individuals to fill these positions. In large part as a result of the health secretary's support, both the resources for recruitment and the medical personnel were found, making it possible for five gynecologists to join the municipal health staff. With the project's emerging success increasingly visible, even more positions were made available and were filled.

Supplies and the Management Information System

The diagnostic research had shown that certain administrative procedures and the existing management information system were not supporting the provision of high-quality, client-oriented care. One problem—the irregular and insufficient supply of contraceptives—was initially resolved by requesting supplies from the Ministry of Health and by making local purchases with municipal funds. This solution worked only in the short term, however, and supply problems recurred. Subsequently, a new MIS system was established to improve the tracking of family planning services.

STEP FOUR: CREATING A MODEL FOR
CLIENT-ORIENTED REPRODUCTIVE HEALTH CARE

While the aforementioned interventions conducted at the 11 facilities increased service access and quality, they could not substantially change service availability. The quantity of contraceptive services increased during the first months of the project but subsequently reached a plateau. Family planning services were not given the priority they deserved, and the reproductive health needs of men and adolescents could not be met by the existing service-delivery system. A more basic structural innovation was needed. Upon the advice of the research team, the executive committee decided to create a model reproductive health referral center within the more centrally located of the two existing secondary-level service-delivery points. Additional staff, including one gynecologist, two psychologists, and one nurse, were recruited and trained to provide contraceptive and other reproductive health services at the center.

The new center, which opened in 1995, would exemplify high-quality care and client-oriented services with an emphasis on family planning, and it would be a referral center for the rest of the municipality. Two factors facilitated the recruitment of physicians who were willing to see a full slate of clients and to give priority to providing family planning services within the context of a broader reproductive health philosophy. First, the health secretary gave important political and financial support, and additional funds for this effort were identified from existing budgets. Second, the reproductive health services provided at the new center—which demanded a higher level of provider competence than the norm—began to be viewed as a medical specialty by physicians and other providers, thereby enhancing the prestige of participating clinicians. The center was designed to provide adults and adolescents with contraceptive education, counseling, and services; Pap smears; gynecologic consultations (for women with abnormal Pap smear results); breast examinations; some gynecologic emergency care; antenatal care (for adolescents); and, for family planning clients, services for STIs.

A broadened range of contraceptive options is consistently available at the referral center, including Depo-Provera®, IUDs, pills, diaphragms, condoms, and vasectomy. Men, women, and adolescents residing in Santa Barbara d'Oeste are eligible to receive care in the facility. Vasectomy provision began in 1996, after the research team trained a gynecologist to perform the procedure and trained relevant staff to provide counseling. The service includes individual and couple education, psychological screening, clinic services, and follow-up. The newly organized clinic provided men, who previously had no access to reproductive health services in the municipal program, with access to vasectomy, condoms, and education about contraception and STIs.

The lack of reproductive health services for adolescents in the municipality had been seen as a major problem from the earliest days of the project. While the executive committee recognized that relevant training for health care providers was essential, they also knew that without information dissemination about the newly created center, adolescents were unlikely to come for reproductive health services other than antenatal care. The adolescent portion of the project therefore had three components: implementing services specifically designed for adolescents; training adolescents as health agents; and creating a support group for pregnant adolescents.

Space for adolescents was created within the reproductive health referral center, and special times were devoted to providing them with services. Forty adolescent health agents were selected from among 200 adolescents who attended a participatory workshop on problems related to adolescent sexual and reproductive health that had been organized in the city's schools. The function of these health agents was to help communicate the availability of adolescent-specific services. Those selected were trained to provide sexual and reproductive health information to their peers in schools, in the community, and in the referral center. They were also trained to distribute condoms to adolescents who did not wish to go to the referral center. In addition to building the adolescents' technical knowledge of reproductive health and communication skills, the training focused on sexual and reproductive rights, gender and sexuality, and intrafamily relations. The training used participatory techniques and was conducted in 14 three-hour sessions, held once a week.[11]

A support group for pregnant adolescents was organized to provide assistance during pregnancy and to prepare them for delivery and motherhood. The support group also attended to the social and emotional aspects of pregnancy and other aspects of reproductive health, including contraception and prevention of reproductive tract infections (RTIs). A female psychologist employed at the referral center was in charge of the sessions. Referral center staff were trained to attend to the needs of pregnant adolescents, and all pregnant adolescents coming for antenatal care throughout the municipal health system were informed about the support available at the referral center.

Although the model clinic considerably expanded reproductive health service options, it is nonetheless limited in its capacity to serve all needs. For example, the center provides STI services only for family planning patients and antenatal care only for adolescents (the other municipal facilities must meet the demand for adult antenatal care).

RESULTS: MORE AND BETTER SERVICES
FOR MANY MORE CLIENTS

A formal evaluation of the Santa Barbara project took place in late 1996 and 1997, using the same instruments and approaches that were used for the baseline diagnostic research, along with data generated by the new MIS.[12] Evaluation results confirmed that the changes instituted between late 1994 and 1996/7 in Santa Barbara d'Oeste were effective.

Access to reproductive health care improved significantly. Gynecologists were seeing more women: the average number of gynecologic consultations per month increased 48 percent, from 1,826 in 1995 to 2,693 in 1997 (see Figure 1). The referral center made a major contribution to increasing overall access, with the client load at the center increasing 83 percent between 1995 and 1997. The number of clients seen at the other ten facilities also increased, albeit less dramatically (by 37 percent on average). In 1997, gynecologists at the referral center alone saw an average of 791 women per month, accounting for 29 percent of all gynecologic visits in the system.

As important as the number of gynecology consultations is their content. Shifting the responsibility for handling Pap smears or pill refills from physicians to nurses greatly improved access, both to routine services and to physician appointments. This increased access did not result in a loss of quality. According to the research team's observations, the nurses and auxiliary nurses who had been trained to perform breast exams and Pap smears performed these tasks well. As a result, by 1997 the gynecologists were spending far more time on antenatal and family planning consultations. Family planning consultations with gynecologists rose from 8 percent of all consultations in 1995 to 25 percent in 1997 (see Figure 2). As a result, the number of new users of all contraceptive methods increased considerably between 1995 and 1997 (see Figure 3). Municipal family planning services, which had been almost nonexistent at the beginning of the Santa Barbara project, were easily accessible by 1997.

The goal of providing contraceptive choices to clinic users was met, thereby addressing one of the key elements of quality of care. Several key interventions produced this result. Assistance with procurement of supplies ensured that methods approved by the Ministry of Health were more regularly available. Training had encouraged providers to discuss a wider range of options with potential users. Revised appointment scheduling and the creation of the referral center had brought access to care with a philosophy of reproductive choice within reach.

Contraceptive choice was also enhanced by responding to community interest in increasing men's access to family planning (Penteado et al. 2001). Before the project, vasectomy was available only in limited sites in the private sector, and at very high cost. By March 1999, 535 vasectomies had been performed free of charge at the refer-

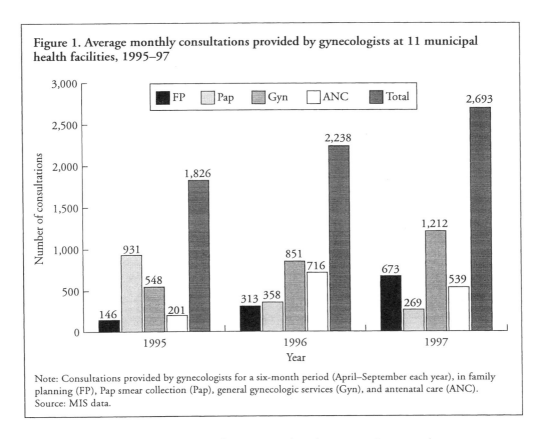

Figure 1. Average monthly consultations provided by gynecologists at 11 municipal health facilities, 1995–97

Note: Consultations provided by gynecologists for a six-month period (April–September each year), in family planning (FP), Pap smear collection (Pap), general gynecologic services (Gyn), and antenatal care (ANC). Source: MIS data.

ral center. Condom distribution also increased at the center. Because the new management information system does not collect data on men, the number of men who received condoms from the center is unknown; however, the number of women who were registered as new users of condoms over the six-month evaluation periods (April–September) increased from 5 in 1995 to 44 in 1997. With the introduction of these services in the referral center, men's ability to participate effectively in fertility regulation increased substantially.

Exit interviews with clients confirmed the importance of increasing access, with female clients most frequently citing improvements in appointment scheduling, waiting time, and the availability of gynecologists. Men who underwent vasectomy reported being extremely satisfied; some noted that they could never have obtained the surgery had it not been free of charge.

Finally, mechanisms designed to involve the community and make health services more responsive to community needs are being sustained. This has not been an easy process. It required continued attention from the research team in the project's early years, and particularly after municipal elections resulted in a new mayor and new health authorities, who initially were opposed to continuing the Santa Barbara project.

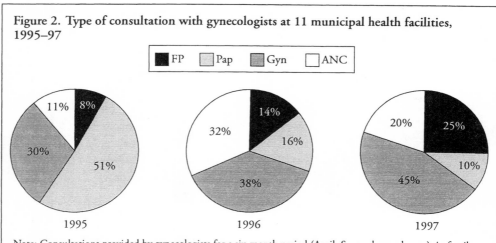

Figure 2. Type of consultation with gynecologists at 11 municipal health facilities, 1995–97

Note: Consultations provided by gynecologists for a six-month period (April–September each year), in family planning (FP), Pap smear collection (Pap), general gynecologic services (Gyn), and antenatal care (ANC). Source: MIS data.

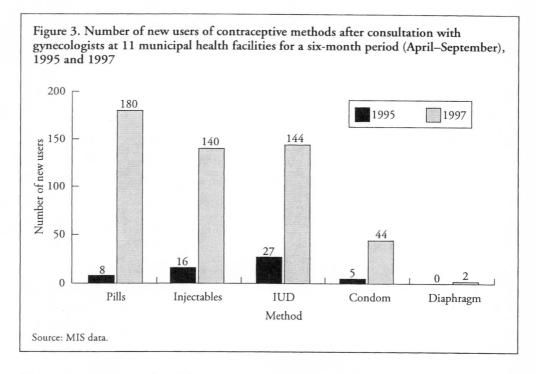

Figure 3. Number of new users of contraceptive methods after consultation with gynecologists at 11 municipal health facilities for a six-month period (April–September), 1995 and 1997

Source: MIS data.

The new mayor considered the vasectomy program a political risk and saw no reason for continuing a project that had been initiated by the previous health secretary. However, when community representatives from the executive committee strongly defended the value of the new system and services, the mayor changed his mind and has since become a major supporter of the project.

The participatory process has become institutionalized and functions well, although the research team no longer attends executive committee meetings on a regular basis. The executive committee continues to meet, although not as routinely as in previous years. The voices and concerns of different sectors of the population, including adolescents and community women, continue to be directly represented on the committee.

When participation in SOS Mulher declined, representatives from community-based women's groups linked to two churches and working on public health issues were recruited to participate on the executive committee during a large community meeting held to report on the project's progress. Because they were more representative of users of municipal health services, the new members could more readily identify service gaps. For example, they pointed out that sections of the city quite distant from the referral center continued to have limited access to health care. In 1997, at the community's request, the project provided 14 women with 15 weekly training sessions on all aspects of reproductive health to enable them to become health promoters who could provide support to women in their local communities. One of the women who participated subsequently became an active community health leader and was given additional training. She strongly advocated for the establishment of a second referral center in an isolated section of Santa Barbara d'Oeste. The mayor granted this request and a second referral center was established in 1999. Other trainees have acted as community health promoters, referring patients to the center when the need arose. During a national campaign in 1999 promoting Pap smears these promoters went from house to house asking women when they had had their last Pap smear and emphasizing the importance of the test. With the exception of the reproductive health training described above, these initiatives were undertaken without support from the research team.

REMAINING CHALLENGES

Although the health service innovations introduced by the Santa Barbara project have been maintained and health authorities have added further innovations, vigilance will be required to sustain them over time. For example, physicians at health posts (although not at the referral center) have begun exerting pressure to return to previous scheduling patterns, which served their interests rather than patients' needs and rights. For a time, because of lack of supervision, they succeeded. In response, a supervisor was recruited and provided with technical training from CEMICAMP; appointments have since been more closely monitored and abbreviated physician schedules have become less common.

Consistent supervision and technical competence remain concerns. For example, some providers were reluctant to provide updated information about the increased duration of IUD effectiveness; they feared their patients might believe they were providing incorrect advice rather than updated technical information. High public-sector turnover also presents problems. When two key gynecologists left the referral center, their replacements demonstrated strong interpersonal skills but weak technical competence. The current plan is to use the referral center to provide on-the-job training to newly recruited staff at both the center itself and at other municipal health facilities.

WHO is no longer providing support to the Santa Barbara project. However, the research team continues to provide limited technical assistance to Santa Barbara d'Oeste in the context of the recently initiated Reprolatina project, funded by the Bill and Melinda Gates Foundation. The objective of this initiative is to expand innovations previously tested in Santa Barbara d'Oeste and three additional municipalities to other regions of Brazil and Latin America. Participation in the network of municipal partners established by the Reprolatina project is likely to stimulate Santa Barbara d'Oeste to sustain and enhance the earlier innovations.

CONCLUSION

The Santa Barbara project demonstrates several points: (1) changing a public-sector system so that it is oriented toward client-centered reproductive health care is possible; (2) community involvement in this process is feasible and beneficial; and (3) women's contraceptive choice should first be enhanced by improving overall access and quality. Because of the interventions put in place to respond to problems identified by the diagnostic assessment, many women and men who previously were not able to obtain reproductive health and family planning services from the municipal health sector are now able to do so. Services—especially family planning services—are more readily available and of better quality. Vasectomy, which was not previously available, is now being offered in the context of improved service delivery. The same is true of injectables, which, while not officially approved at the time the project began, were nonetheless provided. Methods that previously were inconsistently or not at all available, such as the diaphragm, oral contraceptives, and IUDs, are routinely offered. Adolescents and men now receive reproductive health services. The explicit aims of the project—to improve the availability of and access to contraceptive and related reproductive health services, and to expand contraceptive choice through increased access to existing methods and the addition of new methods—have been realized.

One of the key lessons learned is that change within the public sector is possible. However, this shift would not have been possible without expert training and ongoing technical assistance. The project's success depended upon a participatory "organization development" process involving multiple stakeholders. The new specialized women's reproductive health center was instituted using existing public-sector resources. Once the value of the intervention (both the systemwide service improvements and the establishment of the specialized center) became apparent, it was relatively easy to gain commitment from municipal authorities to redirect existing resources toward the goal of improved reproductive health care. The decision to establish the referral center was an important practical as well as political choice. First, because increasing access to a range of family planning methods was at the core of its mission, the center legitimized the concept of family planning services as a key element of municipal health care. Second, the prestige attached to the center allowed it to attract providers who were motivated to provide family planning services in the context of high-quality reproductive health care. Finally, the center serves as a steady resource to the other municipal facilities engaged in reproductive health care—it is a laboratory in which new services can be developed and providers trained and apprenticed.

Perhaps the most important lesson learned is that without a participatory process, the reproductive health innovations described here would long since have been abandoned. Because these interventions serve the needs of the community, and because local people have been associated with their implementation throughout and were therefore ready to defend their continued existence, the innovations of the Santa Barbara project are now viewed as an established part of the municipal health bureaucracy and as community property. Initiatives are now undertaken directly in response to community pressure without inputs from the research team—the engine that drove the process of organization development at the beginning of the project. Community members—especially women and adolescents—have come to see that they can play a key role in shaping the scope and quality of health services to meet their community's needs. Reaching this stage took much longer than the project's initial two-year funding period.

The Santa Barbara health team, like any other organization, needs external inputs to sustain innovations in client-centered approaches. Because state and federal health authorities do not provide such inputs, support from the external research team continues to play an essential role. The newly initiated Reprolatina project seeks to ensure that the innovations in Santa Barbara d'Oeste are sustained and that they can help serve as models and catalysts for replication in Brazil and elsewhere.

Acknowledgments

The Santa Barbara project was supported by funds from what was then the World Health Organization's Strategic Unit for the Introduction and Transfer of Technologies for Fertility Regulation, UNDP/UNFPA/ WHO/World Bank Special Programme of Research, Development, and Research Training in Human

Reproduction, Geneva. We are indebted to Anibal Faúndes, President of CEMICAMP, for his ongoing support to the project. We gratefully acknowledge the support of Carlos Gonzalez, the PAISM coordinator, and Carlos Cavalcante, Secretary of Health of Santa Barbara d'Oeste when the project was initiated. Eliana Hebling provided valuable research support. We also wish to thank the municipal health care providers and the community of Santa Barbara d'Oeste who graciously gave their time and energy to this project.

Notes

This chapter was modified and reprinted with permission of the Population Council from Díaz, Margarita, Ruth Simmons, Juan Díaz, Carlos Gonzalez, Maria Yolanda Makuch, and Debora Bossemeyer. 1999. "Expanding contraceptive choice: Findings from Brazil," *Studies in Family Planning* 30(1): 1–16.

1   The approach is implemented by various national teams with technical and financial support from WHO in collaboration with the International Council on Management of Population Programmes (ICOMP), the University of Michigan, the Population Council, and Reprolatina, a nonprofit organization in southern Brazil. In-country financial support is also provided by the United Nations Population Fund, GTZ, and the U.S. Agency for International Development.

2   Even before female sterilization was legalized, this method accounted for over one-third of contraceptive use in Brazil.

3   Service-delivery research on injectables was recommended because, although some injectables were already provided in the public-sector health system at the time of the assessment, discussions were in progress to formally include these methods in the Ministry of Health norms.

4   The participatory approach used in this project is discussed in detail in Díaz and Simmons 1999.

5   The decentralization of decisionmaking authority to the municipal level is referred to as municipalization.

6   Adolescents were invited to join the executive committee later in the project, after the addition of an adolescent component.

7   Patient-flow analysis is a technique for tracking the exact amount of time patients spend in specific activities in the health facility from the moment they arrive to the time they leave.

8   Public health facilities in Brazil are reimbursed by the federal government for services provided.

9   SOS Mulher members had identified the need for better health education for women in the community; participation in the training enabled these women to provide health education at municipal facilities.

10   The methodology was developed by Margarita Díaz.

11   The training was coordinated by Margarita Díaz and Francisco Cabral.

12   For a detailed discussion of the evaluation results see Díaz et al. 1999.

References

Bruce, Judith. 1990. "Fundamental elements of the quality of care: A simple framework," *Studies in Family Planning* 21(2): 61–91.

Díaz, Margarita and Ruth Simmons. 1999. "When is research participatory? Reflections on a reproductive health project in Brazil," *Journal of Women's Health* 8(2): 175–184.

Díaz, Margarita, Ruth Simmons, Juan Díaz, Carlos Gonzalez, Maria Yolanda Makuch, and Debora Bossemeyer. 1999. "Expanding contraceptive choice: Findings from Brazil," *Studies in Family Planning* 30(1): 1–16.

Formiga, José Noble, S.G. Diniz, Ruth Simmons, E. Cravey, P. Hall, S. Sorrentino, Margarita Díaz, L. Bahamondes, Juan Díaz, and Maria Yolanda Makuch. 1994. "An assessment of the need for contraceptive introduction in Brazil," document no. WHO/HRP/ITT/94.2. Geneva: World Health Organization.

French, Wendell and Cecil Bell. 1995. *Organization Development,* fifth ed. Englewood Cliffs, NJ: Prentice Hall.

Penteado, Luis Guilherme, Francisco Cabral, Margarita Díaz, Juan Díaz, Laura Ghiron, and Ruth Simmons. 2001. "Organizing a public-sector vasectomy program in Brazil," *Studies in Family Planning* 32(4): 315–328.

Simmons, Ruth, Peter Hall, Juan Díaz, Margarita Díaz, Peter Fajans, and Jay Satia. 1997. "The strategic approach to contraceptive introduction," *Studies in Family Planning* 28(2): 79–94.

Spicehandler, Joanne and Ruth Simmons. 1994. "Contraceptive introduction reconsidered: A review and conceptual framework," document no. WHO/HRP/ITT/94.1. Geneva: World Health Organization.

Contact information

Margarita Díaz
Reprolatina
R. Maria Teresa Dias da Silva, 740
Campinas, SP Brazil
CEP 13084-190
telephone: 55-19-3289-1735
e-mail: mdiaz@reprolatina.org.br

ReproSalud: Feminism
Meets USAID in Peru

Debbie Rogow and Susan Wood

For close to two decades, Peru has carried out a vigorous population policy aimed at promoting contraceptive use in general and, for the last decade, long-acting and permanent methods in particular. These efforts—heavily supported by the U.S. Agency for International Development (USAID) and other donors—have fallen far short of their goals. As is true throughout Latin America, overall contraceptive prevalence rates have risen in Peru. But family planning services remain inaccessible and/or unwelcoming to millions of women, especially in rural areas, where 20 percent of women have an unmet need for contraception (Moyano et al. 1997). Factors contributing to this unmet need include low quality of care, poor treatment by providers, distrust of the government program (including a much-criticized sterilization campaign), women's lack of decisionmaking power, and inadequate access to information.

The government's narrow focus on contraceptive delivery has been coupled with neglect of other aspects of reproductive health and choice, with particularly dire consequences for women and girls living in rural areas. Maternal mortality remains stubbornly high at 265 deaths per 100,000 live births nationally, with the rate in rural areas estimated to be twice that in urban zones (Moyano et al. 1997). Several factors contribute to this situation, one of which is unsafe abortion. Abortion is illegal in nearly all circumstances and, consequently, is often performed under unsafe conditions. Despite this fact, every year one in three Peruvian women and girls who are pregnant seek abortion (WHO 1998). Obstetric services are also inadequate: Few women obtain antenatal care, and one-half of all births occur at home. Again, the lack of services has a greater effect on rural women, who have an average of 5.6 children, compared to a national average of 3.5 (Moyano et al. 1997).

In recognition of the failure of narrowly configured family planning services to improve the reproductive health of Peruvian women in greatest need, one of the world's leading population donors and one of Peru's strongest feminist organizations joined forces. In an unprecedented move, USAID awarded the Manuela Ramos Movement nearly $20 million for a five-year project to enable some of Peru's most disenfranchised women to take action on behalf of their own reproductive health and lives. What made this effort so daring was not just the unprecedented level of funding for an activist nongovernmental organization (NGO) by a major bilateral donor, but the very nature of the project itself.[1]

The project, called ReproSalud, was designed by Susan Brems, the former director of the Population, Health, and Nutrition Division of the USAID/Lima Mission. ReproSalud was conceived as a uniquely multifaceted project that linked women's contraceptive use and reproductive health to initiatives to improve their personal, social, and—in an approach hitherto unheard of in USAID population/family planning projects—economic power. Within six regions of the country, provinces and districts were chosen based on their high poverty, low contraceptive prevalence, and relative accessibility, including an absence of terrorism. The project had three key components:

- Education and support for women to learn more about their own reproductive health;
- Education and support for women to advocate for improved quality of care from local health care providers;
- Income-generation schemes, including a credit system and several collectively owned businesses, to improve women's economic status, which was hypothesized to be linked to their reproductive well-being.[2]

In an equally remarkable departure from traditional programs, the ReproSalud design called for local women—who often have little self-confidence, little education and mobility, and no experience with project design—to define which reproductive health problems the project would address, and to articulate and help implement the solutions. The long, slow work of gender-sensitive development would involve listening to women.

The unusual partnership and the unorthodox design of this large-scale population effort attracted significant attention to ReproSalud. However, Brems, an anthropologist, was the first to explain that this project was hardly reinventing the wheel:

> There is nothing new here in terms of reproductive health. What is new is that we are, with the mandate of Cairo [the 1994 International Conference on Population and Development], actually implementing what has been learned from the field of development. Decades of work and research in development have generated the same basic lessons: community participation and working from the ground up. These essential principles are talked about all the time, but they get short shrift in implementation. Community participation often turns into getting local folks to do the work without giving them real ownership. It's easy to have a town meeting, but building actual capacity at the local level is a different process.

> *[With Cairo], we have had to erase traditional assumptions about what im-*
> *proves people's lives. We have had to acknowledge how many of our activities are so-*
> *cially constructed (e.g., by gender and power). We needed a different framework.*

FINDING AND SUPPORTING LOCAL PARTNERS

The Manuelas[3] started by adapting their organization to accommodate a large-scale USAID cooperative agreement and then established and staffed eight ReproSalud field offices in the selected regions. Regional staff were trained and began to seek out local women's organizations to become partners in a self-help effort to improve women's reproductive health. The process of building these partnerships is at the core of the ReproSalud approach.

The partnership process involves the same basic steps in each region. ReproSalud staff visit all the villages in an area and inform the mothers' clubs and food cooperatives about the project. They explain that the project's focus is reproductive health, and use a flip chart to illustrate the full range of reproductive health issues. They invite the groups to apply to become involved in the process as a partner, or official subgrantee. The first step is for interested groups to submit a letter and a list of members, so that ReproSalud staff can determine whether the group is an authentic organized entity. From among the submissions—often up to 20 from each cluster of villages—the ReproSalud staff promoters select the five most promising groups, based largely on the group's length and breadth of experience. The group is then asked to prepare and present a sociodrama, or skit, about an urgent reproductive health problem affecting the lives of women in their community; all five groups come together for the day of sociodramas. ReproSalud staff use the skits to assess the level of social organization in the group. (For example, do they articulate a problem, think through a coherent en-actment, take time to rehearse the actors? Do they interact as a group or does one leader appear to have disproportionate control?) From this process of listening to the women enact their concerns, ReproSalud selects its subgrantee partner group or groups.

Once the partner groups are chosen, ReproSalud staff return to the village and, over several months, work closely with the women on a range of activities outlined below:

- They carry out a baseline survey in which they ask community members about their reproductive health history, knowledge and use of contraception, contraceptive attitudes, and basic information about family life, including economic decisionmaking, health practices, and attitudes toward domestic violence.
- They conduct a 12–15-hour workshop, in three-hour sessions over one to two weeks, involving members of the partner group. Called an *autodiagnóstico*, or "self-diagnosis," the workshop complements the baseline survey with qualitative information about women's self-perception and experience. As part of

---

Box 1. Giving women voice: Self-diagnosis workshops and advocacy activities

The *autodiagnósticos* are more than a research tool; they have proven to be valuable interventions. In turning to women for their own analysis, or "diagnosis," of their most pressing needs, the Manuelas succeed in empowering women from the start. A number of women from the local partner groups attend the *autodiagnóstico* workshop. Although the women have been introduced to basic concepts in reproductive health through a flip chart at an initial presentation, at the *autodiagnóstico* the Manuelas allow the women themselves to define reproductive health. The women participate in exercises that encourage them to think about themselves, their reproductive health, and their status as women. For example, one of the initial exercises, called "A Girl from this Community," traces the reproductive life cycle; if women do not mention specific events such as menarche, childbirth, or menopause, ReproSalud staff promoters prompt them. The participants also begin to share their beliefs about their sexual and reproductive anatomy and physiology by drawing images of their bodies and filling in the body parts with whatever names they know. This "body mapping" helps women become more comfortable talking about their bodies and, at the same time, informs ReproSalud staff about women's beliefs and the terminology they use. In analyzing their health problems, they participate in a "problem tree" exercise, which uses the image of a tree to help them analyze the "roots" of a given problem as well as its "fruits," or consequences. (Problem tree exercises are described in greater detail in Chapter 21.)

From the *autodiagnósticos*, participants learn about: (1) the problems they share; (2) their bodies, sexuality, and health; (3) the resources available to them to solve their problems; and (4) the opportunity to change their lives by working together. As women learn that they do not face their problems alone, many begin to feel empowered in ways they have never before experienced, as illustrated by comments from ReproSalud staff and participating women:

> *What lies behind our success is the methodology we use. This starts with the autodiagnóstico, which is the first time these women have thought about themselves.*

> *They listened to me and said they wanted to support me in what I cared about. Nobody ever said that before.*

Furthermore, in the course of the *autodiagnóstico*, the participants agree on a single priority reproductive health problem on which they will focus in their partnership with ReproSalud.

---

the process, participating women identify a priority reproductive health problem. The workshop also promotes a sense of solidarity and enthusiasm among the women (see Box 1 for a more detailed description of the *autodiagnósticos*).

- Twelve members of the group then plan a project that focuses on the identified health issue. ReproSalud provides the basic model for the project—training peer educators—but the women learn how to specify objectives, activities, a time frame, and material needs. During this design phase, organizations from neighboring communities are invited to participate as associate partners.

- The group elects two sets of leaders: project administrators (who manage the project and the money) and community-based promoters (who are peer educators and not the same as ReproSalud staff promoters, who work for the project's regional offices). ReproSalud staff compile a budget providing nominal support for project leaders as well as material provisions.

- The project administrators attend a training course (together with administrators from other subprojects in the region), where they learn basic financial
  management (e.g., budget monitoring, cash flow, and financial record keeping), in addition to basic project management skills. Community-based promoters participate in a two-week peer educator course that covers basic
  reproductive anatomy and physiology, the identified priority health issue, self-
  esteem, gender relations and human rights, communication skills, and family
  planning.
- The community-based promoters return home to organize week-long workshops to convey what they have learned to other women in the community.
  With help from ReproSalud staff, they teach their neighbors all they can about
  the topic that has been identified as the priority health issue.

As the project proceeds, the groups begin their advocacy work with local health
and municipal officials. Often this stage is difficult at first, particularly for women for
whom culture, language, education, and gender have traditionally created an impen-
etrable barrier precluding the possibility of communication with the educated, male,
Spanish-speaking officials who control services that are vital to them and their families. Women have learned to articulate their concerns about the health system to each
other, but directly addressing municipal authorities takes courage. As one local leader
described it, "The first time we went up the steps, we were all shaking." To help them
prepare, the ReproSalud staff promoters assist the women in organizing their presentations, which include information about their priority health concerns and project
activities and requests for service improvements, and accompany them when they
meet with the authorities, at least for their first meeting. A young ReproSalud staff
promoter described the women's growing confidence:

> They go right up to the [public health] authorities. At first, you can see he thinks they
> don't know anything about family planning. They tell him about their analysis of their
> problems, the causes, their needs, and their plans. And then he sees how much they do
> know! For me, this is the best moment.

UNEXPECTED TURNS IN THE ROAD:
RESPONDING TO WOMEN'S UNCONVENTIONAL WISDOM

The Manuelas had been carrying out grassroots health education with women for
almost 20 years. They knew that if local women were to define priority issues and
implement solutions, ReproSalud would need an unusual level of flexibility, especially
for such a large-scale project. A number of surprises, however, forced them to reshape
the program in response to what women told them. These surprises have had a lasting

effect on the project and on what we can learn about programmatic approaches to reproductive health. This chapter highlights two of the major shifts required of ReproSalud because of its commitment to listen to women.

Responding to Women's Concerns About Reproductive Tract Infections

The first unexpected turn came with the initial opportunity that women had to sit and speak together—in the *autodiagnósticos*. Chief among the goals of the workshops was for participants to identify their priority reproductive health problem. The conventional wisdom was that family planning would be the single greatest need. The Manuelas expected women to emphasize problems of unwanted pregnancy, unsafe abortion, maternal mortality, unmet need for contraception, and domestic violence.

Indeed, all of these problems were cited by women. "Too many children" was the priority in a number of villages, as were childbirth complications, abortion, and teenage pregnancy. In virtually every workshop across Peru, domestic violence and disrespectful, inadequate treatment by local health care providers were also pressing concerns. But the reproductive health issue named as the number-one priority in the greatest number of villages was reproductive tract infections (RTIs). Indeed, 56 of the women's groups identified this as their most pressing concern, followed by "too many children" (35 groups), and difficulties with birth (18 groups). Other problems cited as urgent reproductive health issues were vaginal inflammation, uterine prolapse, menopause, and uterine swelling.

Few people would have predicted that RTIs, known locally as *descensos* or *agua blanca* (roughly translated as "vaginal discharge" or "white water"), would be chosen throughout the country as the most compelling reproductive health concern for women. (See Box 2 for a discussion of Peruvian women's perceptions of RTIs.) Despite indications from the few studies conducted in Peru that RTIs, including sexually transmitted infections, are extremely common (at least in urban areas), the topic was virtually ignored by most health authorities and USAID.[4] As Susan Brems remarked:

> Look how important RTIs are to the Peruvian women. It's their number-one concern
> in this project. Yet RTIs have not been deemed important in many public health and
> population circles.

Many health professionals regard RTIs as an intractable problem. The equipment and supplies for widespread testing and treatment are beyond the resources available to many reproductive health programs. Efforts to train providers in syndromic management are of limited value, given that such pathogens as chlamydia and gonorrhea are largely asymptomatic in women.[5] Even among symptomatic women, the syndromic algorithm for vaginal discharge has been found to be inadequate for managing these pathogens because of the poor correlation of symptoms and signs with

---

Box 2. Women view RTIs as a single disease, with many problems at its root

Even more surprising than the fact that RTIs were most often named as the number-one priority was the apparent reason that they are considered so important. The *autodiagnósticos* revealed that women view RTIs as part of one illness that is chronic, difficult to cure, and leads to uterine cancer. They believe that discharge changes color as the disease progresses, from white or clear at the start, to pink, and then to red with the onset of cancer and approaching death. Furthermore, they see this disease as closely related to the other priority problems they identified. Indeed, an analysis of the "roots" of RTIs in the problem trees drawn by women showed that women include as causes of this disease many other reproductive health concerns (e.g., problems with modern contraception, too many children, complications during pregnancy and childbirth, abortion, and so forth).

This holistic view of reproductive health prompted ReproSalud to encourage women to design their projects in ways that addressed their concerns. For example, if women emphasized too many children as a principal cause of RTIs, more information about family planning was included. If they attributed the disease to poor diet after delivery, then nutrition was added to the educational sessions. And cancer was given greater attention than originally expected, as a result of the belief that RTIs lead to cancer.

---

infection.[6] In places like rural Peru, these limitations are compounded by the fact that women tend not to seek help from the public health system because of distrust in modern medicine, resentment of disrespectful treatment by providers, lack of money to pay for medicine, and lack of time to walk miles to wait all day in a health center.

By simply asking women for their input, however, the Manuelas learned that women did not like living with chronic RTIs. One of their first steps was to contract with leading international RTI researchers at the University of Washington who were already working on this issue in Peru to design a prevalence study of selected infections. ReproSalud solicited the participation of women from their partner groups in 25 communities (most of which were rural, but some of which were provincial cities or urban slum areas). The research team took wet smears from 780 women ages 18–67 and conducted a number of laboratory tests.[7] While a full analysis is still pending, the initial findings revealed a 40 percent prevalence of bacterial vaginosis and a 16 percent prevalence of trichomoniasis.[8] The results confirmed that the women were right: RTIs are a serious public health problem in Peru.

ReproSalud staff conveyed what they were learning from the *autodiagnósticos* and the prevalence research to local health authorities. The reactions were positive, as typified by the following comment from the medical director of Chavin Hospital:

> *Manuela Ramos and ReproSalud did a study last year on reproductive tract infections.*
> *We learned how much there is; it gave us a new understanding. Their work has been*
> *very productive, throwing a light on something we had not seen.*

The core of ReproSalud's response was to develop an interactive curriculum for training its staff and for preparing community-based promoters to begin teaching their neighbors about how to identify, treat, and prevent common infections.[9] The one-week workshop begins with the generic ReproSalud training model: an overview of female and male anatomy and physiology; attention to issues of self-esteem, sexuality, and communicating with one's partners; and women's rights, including the right to refuse unwanted sex, to be safe from physical abuse, and to control one's fertility. This last aspect includes information on contraceptive methods.

The workshop then addresses RTIs. Participants learn that some infections are transmitted sexually while others may result from poor hygiene. They learn that infections can be symptomatic or asymptomatic. They discuss the steps and costs of diagnosis and treatment, as well as the long-term sequelae of untreated infections. They learn the need for treatment of infected individuals and about condom use to prevent infection and reinfection. Most importantly perhaps, they reaffirm their right to promote their own health and enact role-plays demonstrating how to explain the risk to husbands and partners. Participants also learn which hygiene practices (e.g., regular external washing) are helpful and which (e.g., internal douching) may be harmful.

The women who have participated in these workshops are proud not only of their newfound knowledge but of the realization that they can do something to promote their own well-being, as illustrated by the comments of several women from the Andean town of Acopalca:

> We didn't know what caused agua blanca or how to treat it. Now I know it may come from hygiene and it may be transmitted sexually, it depends on the disease.

> Before, I didn't know what agua blanca was, where it came from, and what to do to treat it. Now I know that if I itch or have little granules in my discharge, I need to go to the health center right away. I also know I need to get a Pap; I get it twice a year. I had never done it before.

> The doctor told me the discharge is from anxiety. I told him I went to a training and I know it's not from that! He remained silent.

Health professionals have also noted a change, as documented by the comments of several providers:

> Women never used to come for discharge problems. Now they come, especially from the communities where ReproSalud is working on this problem. . . . Unfortunately, I lack many of the medications I need to treat these infections; I only have some of them.

> Last week a woman came in to talk about agua blanca. She proceeded to describe her problem to me. She asked for her treatment. This surprised me! With the other women,

we have to ask, to draw them out. They don't want to tell us. The women who have been trained by ReproSalud talk openly about their bodies. They are not inhibited.

They [women trained by ReproSalud] are definitely more open, not so distrusting. It is easier to establish rapport. They come and tell me, "I have agua blanca." The women from the other communities are still shy. They lower their heads, they don't answer my questions.

Efforts to diagnose RTIs must confront the limits and affordability of medical technologies, unequal provider–client relationships, and gender dynamics in sexual behavior. While it will take a number of years to determine ReproSalud's full effect on RTI prevalence, the problem of RTIs is being recognized as a more complex, but ultimately less intractable, issue. More women are willing to seek diagnosis and treatment, and a number have reported that they are better able to discuss treatment and prevention with their partners. Further, while technical capacity remains a challenge in resource-poor settings, some providers are responding to women's input with efforts to upgrade the quality of services.

The Call to Work with Men

The Manuela Ramos Movement had learned in the course of two decades how much women valued having a separate place where they could listen to and support each other. While ReproSalud reaffirmed and supported this desire, participating women had also revealed another powerful need—the positive engagement of their male partners. The women decided to include men in the project, because "The men can change if they learn what we are learning." Women were going home enthusiastic about the experiences and knowledge they had acquired, and their husbands took note. Some were initially resentful that their wives had access to information—and, in the case of community-based promoters, cash—that they lacked.

At first my husband questioned my participation and disagreed about my going. But I invited him and he talked with the people from ReproSalud. Now he agrees.

He says, "You have more education than I do. Now you're going to earn more money than I do. You are wearing the pants in the family."

But more often, the men were enthusiastic and curious and simply wanted to participate along with their wives. As a 55-year-old male participant explained, "I went to the training to learn."

ReproSalud staff initially debated whether and how including men might shift resources away from women's control. To explore how best to involve men while ensuring that women's activities remained autonomous, the Manuelas hired a Mexican consultant with programmatic experience in gender relations. His recommendation was to begin to train staff to handle gender issues more comfortably and then later train local male community-based promoters. These men, often the husbands of female community-based promoters, would then conduct workshops for other men in the community.

The male workshops are highly participatory and unlike any other learning experience the men have had. Men draw images of their bodies, engage in recollections of personal childhood experiences, create collages, and enact role-plays. They learn about male physiology and about sexuality. The content of the workshops is similar to that of workshops for women, but emphasizes issues of masculinity, violence, and communication. The trainers emphasize a "family harmony" approach that incorporates: (1) voicing one's own childhood experiences with violence and reflecting on the attitudes these experiences fostered; (2) learning to talk about problems rather than losing one's temper; (3) abstaining from violence against women and children; (4) learning that sexuality can be a source of pleasure for both partners when there is no violence and no risk of disease or unwanted pregnancy; and (5) understanding the toll that each pregnancy and birth takes on a woman's body. Through a range of exercises, participants explore the pressures they feel to conform to traditional gender roles, and they learn about the relationship between these traditional roles and health problems such as stress, heart disease, risk of sexually transmitted infections, and alcohol-related disease. The exercises have led to discussions about alcoholism and violence, forced sex, communication with women, and women's basic human rights.[10]

Parallel workshops for young people were also conducted in some communities (again, in response to women's requests), and a number of young men were reached through them. These workshops contributed to the work with men by dealing with gender socialization issues for young women and young men. For example, young men learned to understand how girls feel about being sexually harassed; several girls have since spoken of boys who have stopped harassing girls.

In interviews up to one year after these workshops, men were eager to discuss what they had learned and how much they had valued the experience. Participants and their wives reflected about the workshops' effects on their relationships:

Before, I drank a lot and hit my wife. Then I felt bad and wondered why I did it. Now I drink less and I do not hit her. I talk to my oldest daughter and encourage her to study.

Now I converse with my wife, in better conditions. . . . If she doesn't want relations, I can't demand it, sometimes the women don't want it. Since the talks, my wife and I take care. I prefer natural ways, according to her period, and from time to time, the condom. Before, we knew nothing. We didn't take care at all.

I can talk to him more openly now. For example, I used to be embarrassed if he touched me a lot. I can tell him now where it feels good, in the vagina, the clitoris. He asks me and I can tell him.

Before, when our husbands hit us, we sat quietly and cried. Now we are not afraid. We can file a complaint; some women are doing that. Before, no. We were just cooking and crying. My husband was very difficult before. Now he went to the men's training. And he is more affectionate.

A treasurer for the project had this to say:

Thirty men were trained. About 100 more men are in the community. The husbands who have been trained understand better. Before, they brutally forced sex. They hit, especially when they were drunk. Now, no more. I am so proud.

Changes in men's attitudes toward their partners weave their way into a myriad of behaviors that are difficult to measure. Nonetheless, several outcomes were identified in a one-year qualitative evaluation undertaken in Andean villages, including those where the above-cited participants reside. Interviews suggested a dramatic drop in alcohol consumption and physical abuse by male workshop participants. In one setting where data on alcohol sales volume were available, the village merchant reported a 50 percent drop in consumption since the workshops had been held the previous year. Local municipal authorities reported a drop in incidents of domestic violence in ReproSalud communities.

REPROSALUD: OVERALL PROGRESS

Initially, ReproSalud had not anticipated focusing on reproductive tract infections or working directly with men. But the project took the advice of local women and today both of these issues are cornerstones of its work. Both areas were part of the larger process of building the capacity of communities to address needs identified and expressed by women. After five years, close to 250 organizations had been selected as partners and received grants and technical support. Approximately 2,220 additional community groups are working indirectly as associates of the primary subgrantee organizations. Most have completed their first project and have begun follow-up activities, often including advocacy among local authorities for improved health services. The number of individuals who have participated directly in ReproSalud educational activities now exceeds 89,500 women and 46,700 men. Project evaluations have found that those participants have passed on what they have learned to another 650,000 friends and family members. It is anticipated that by its tenth year, the project will have reached well over one million people.

Ongoing monitoring and evaluation of the ReproSalud project has always been a priority. Before and after each community workshop, project staff have conducted assessments of knowledge, attitudes, and practices among a sample of participants. Data generated from these assessments showed increases in the number of contraceptive methods participants could name and greater knowledge of how these methods work. There were also striking increases in participants' understanding of the fertile phase of the menstrual cycle (ranging from 29 to 50 percent), recent experience discussing family planning with partners (60–98 percent), and stated intention to begin using a contraceptive method within the next year (40–68 percent).

In 1999 the Manuelas began to evaluate the effects of ReproSalud. The evaluation, which took the form of case studies, assessed changes in women's empowerment and in knowledge, attitudes, and practices related to contraception. Researchers were sent to three areas (two in Andean regions, one in the Amazon) where work was most advanced. Interviews were conducted with male and female community-based promoters or administrators who had participated in the workshops. Separate interviews were conducted with health and municipal officials.

The preliminary findings suggest wide-ranging and remarkable achievements. Women reported significant increases in self-esteem and comfort with their bodies; greater knowledge about reproductive health; enhanced decisionmaking regarding sex, family matters, and cash flow; increased influence in community affairs; and greater rapport with their partners. For the Manuelas, the achievements of ReproSalud are closely linked. They have seen that improving women's comfort with their bodies led to improvements in reproductive behaviors, including increases in contraceptive use among women in need; that helping men grapple with their own concerns related to self-esteem resulted in reductions in violence; and that providing women with knowledge, solidarity, and confidence enabled them to advocate effectively for improved services. A 24-year-old Andean mother who lives two hours by foot from the nearest town put it more eloquently:

> Before, my husband hit me. Sometimes, when he thought he was right, when he drank. I was afraid before to go to the health center. And I was afraid of the [contraceptive] methods.
>
> Since I became a [community-based] promoter, I am not the same person. I learned about how to live together with my husband, to talk together, to do things together.
>
> My husband also went to the training for men. Now he doesn't hit me anymore. He doesn't drink and he doesn't hit me. And my husband asks my opinion, for example, we ask each other's opinion about whether to sell an animal, whether he will leave for work. We don't see women crying in the street anymore from being hit.

I am not afraid of the family planning methods anymore. Now we discuss that we want to use family planning. We decided on the injection. I am on my second injection now. I didn't get a Pap because I didn't have the money. But I want to, because the Pap tells if the uterus is healthy.

We women respect ourselves and each other more now. The other women appreciate us, for what we have taught them. And the men respect us more, too. I feel I am happier because of what I am doing.

While no one denies the value of these changes, donor interests still often center on increases in use of health care services, and particularly on family planning use. As part of the 1999 evaluation, the Manuelas conducted a quantitative analysis of service use in selected areas. In the Chavin region, family planning visits increased among women in ReproSalud communities. One hospital recorded a 400 percent increase in family planning visits by residents of the local ReproSalud community, as compared with a 51 percent increase from residents of nearby control villages and a decline in the number of visits made by residents of the urban center where the hospital is located (see Table 1).

The patient log at a hospital in Huari indicated a 105 percent increase in family planning visits from the ReproSalud community, compared with a 39 percent increase among residents of control villages and a 26 percent increase among local urban residents (Table 1). Moreover, many interviewees reported using the rhythm method correctly, whereas they had previously used it incorrectly or used no method. Anecdotal evidence also suggests that potentially harmful behaviors, (e.g., douching, heavy lifting during pregnancy) are less common. Parallel evaluations in other regions indicate similar results, although on a less dramatic scale. Overall, the evaluation showed that the changes were greatest in those villages where ReproSalud has been working for nine or more months; they also tended to be greatest among those individuals closely involved with the project as community-based promoters or subproject coordinators.

Complications related to birth was the priority problem identified in Huaripampa Bajo, and the health center in nearby San Marcos is encouraging women to come for antenatal care and delivery. Data from available health center obstetric logs documented a gradual rise in clinic deliveries among women in this village.

Both patients and health providers have reported improvements in the quality of services:

Before, they didn't take good care of us at the hospital . . . they said we were bothering them. We told the director that we had rights, that they needed to take care of us. Now they attend to us well, they take care of us quickly.

Table 1. Family planning visits per month before (1997) and after (1998) ReproSalud workshop

	Before	After	% change
Chavin			
ReproSalud communities[a]	3	15	+400
Control villages[b]	39	59	+51
Urban center	23	14	−39
Total	65	88	+35
Huari			
ReproSalud communities[a]	22	45	+105
Control villages[b]	62	86	+39
Urban center	138	174	+26
Total	222	305	+37
Canchabamba			
No control or urban sites[c]	5	10	+100

[a] The ReproSalud communities served by Chavin are Chuyo and part of Huarimayo; in both communities, the identified problem was "too many children." The ReproSalud community served by Huari is Acopalca, where the identified problem was *agua blanca*.
[b] The figures for control villages include total visits from women in all other rural communities served by the health center.
[c] Canchabamba health post serves only the Canchabamba community, with referrals sent to San Luis Health Center.

I go to the health center in Chavin. You wait and wait. Now we demand to be seen more rapidly.

The women were complaining that they were not treated respectfully and that they had to wait too long. . . . We are improving patient flow. Now they get a card and start moving through; before we had a longer process with their records. So the waiting time is less. We have also done some training with all levels of staff about how to treat patients. We check for improvements through a suggestion box. The forms have drawings for the illiterate women.

Chavin is a region where ReproSalud has been successful in working with providers to upgrade services incrementally. Providers were urged to provide more respectful treatment, and patient- and record-flow modifications were made in order to reduce waiting times. This success underscores an essential point: If women do not see the desired improvements in the quality of care, they are unlikely to translate the increased interest in improving their reproductive health and avoiding unwanted fertility into greater use of services. Notwithstanding its remarkable achievements, ReproSalud does not have the authority or influence to improve the accessibility and quality of services on a large scale. Meeting donor interests in increased family planning and use of reproductive health services, therefore, lies beyond the project's control and ultimately depends upon parallel efforts by the Ministry of Health and local health care providers.

THE VULNERABILITY OF AN UNORTHODOX ALLIANCE

The partnership between a traditional population donor and a feminist NGO has been, in the case of ReproSalud, mostly synergistic. The experiment has relied upon flexibility and patience on both sides. First, the complex procedures required by USAID strained the Manuelas' administrative capacity. Realizing the Manuelas would need to strengthen their institutional capacity if the project was to succeed, USAID relied on a technical officer to provide extensive technical assistance and managerial support throughout the project's first years. The officer explains some of what it takes to cultivate such alliances:

> There must be a commitment on the part of the entire donor agency to support and develop feminist organizations to become institutionally capable of administering large projects. In working with the Manuelas, this was much easier, because if Susana [Galdos, ReproSalud's director] saw we had a concern, she always just looked at us and said, "Be frank." Breaking down the old polarity between population donors and feminist groups will take time—inviting groups to come to meetings, getting to know leaders personally, learning from them, developing small collaborative activities, and ultimately, providing the institutional support to foster their success. Donors must take the initiative to establish greater trust.

While the administrative obstacles have been taxing for both parties, the political challenges have been even greater, especially for the Manuelas. Early on, they endured criticism from other feminist groups for cooperating with a donor whose goals explicitly included fertility reduction. Later, they faced criticism because ReproSalud was mistakenly associated with the government's attempt to impose sterilization quotas on providers.[11]

In 1999 the Manuelas faced perhaps their greatest challenge. Ironically, the biggest threat to the stability of ReproSalud came from the new policies of the donor. The U.S. government—in response to domestic anti-choice politicians—reinstated the "gag rule," a policy of refusing to finance any project that provides abortions, advocates for abortion reform, or even allows its staff to attend international meetings that call for the decriminalization of abortion. The Manuelas had to choose between the availability of USAID resources to continue the project and their rights to freedom of expression and assembly. Although they were not then engaged in activities to decriminalize abortion in Peru, the Manuelas had worked for many years to change abortion laws in the country.

The Manuelas realized that although their own philosophy and values had not changed in 20 years, USAID/Peru, its valued partner for the past five years, was vulnerable to shifts in U.S. policy. After considering their options, the Manuelas decided that they could not abandon their obligation to the hundreds of thousands of beneficiaries ReproSalud was reaching, so they reluctantly signed the "gag rule" amendment. Nevertheless, they wrote a letter of protest to U.S. President Bill Clinton, decrying the antidemocratic assault on Peruvians' right to free speech; parts of this letter were read by U.S. Secretary of State Madeleine Albright at a formal event at the White House. In addition, the Manuelas have begun seeking alternative sources of funding.

As ReproSalud enters its sixth year, the Manuelas have taken a hard look at their own potential contribution in various regions of Peru. The intensive approach used by project staff is probably most cost-effective in settings where women are least empowered and/or have lowest contraceptive use rates—generally speaking, in places where traditional family planning efforts have failed. In areas where ReproSalud sensed its goals had been largely met, the project formalized agreements for the local health services to incorporate the community-based promoters into their programs and has decreased its presence, focusing its resources instead on communities where the need is greatest.

LESSONS FOR THE FUTURE

This chapter has focused on one of the most fundamental lessons that ReproSalud's experience offers—the importance of listening to women and building their capacity to make decisions about their own lives.[12] As the project's associate director says, "We approached this work with the right philosophy: the direct participation of women in improving their own lives." This approach enabled ReproSalud to appreciate and undertake two lines of work they had not anticipated: addressing RTIs and working with men. Even at this early stage of the project, each of these areas of work has already generated valuable lessons:

- RTIs require greater attention than they currently receive. They were the single most important reproductive health problem identified by thousands of women involved with ReproSalud. Clearly, there is a need for more data on prevalence, as well as for greater investments in identifying, developing, and instituting practical clinical responses.
- Men value the opportunity to talk openly with one another in a supportive environment. Furthermore, inroads into the seemingly intractable problem of domestic violence can be made. The men's workshops, sustained community exposure to anti-violence messages, and provision of anti-violence education within a context of reproductive health and family harmony all seem to have contributed to reductions in domestic abuse.[13]

It will take time to gather and analyze the broader lessons of the ReproSalud experiment. (Indeed, in part because of the project's success, and in recognition of the fact that programs that promote democracy and gender equity require sustained investments of time, USAID has extended the project for another five years.) In the meantime, the international reproductive health community is taking note of what has so far been learned:

- Women living in poor, rural communities are, in contrast to popularly held views, quite interested in and willing to discuss sexuality and gender. The task is to listen and to share power, rather than to impose solutions.

- Given confidence in the value of a project and a sense of their own ability to lead, women will often involve their husbands. ReproSalud leaders emphasize that the central involvement of men would never have taken place had the staff not been committed, above all, to listening to women and giving them control over the project.

- While feminist NGOs such as the Manuela Ramos Movement can help create the conditions for women to take action to improve their reproductive health—including increased use of services—the government must assume its responsibility to ensure that services are of acceptable quality. Both the "demand" side and the "supply" side must be driven by women's expressed needs.

- Enabling women to overcome the structural obstacles that impede the achievement of their reproductive health and their social and economic well-being requires a long-term investment in building the capacity of community organizations and increasing economic options. The kind of change brought about by this kind of development work is profound and far-reaching, but it happens one woman at a time; there is no technological magic bullet.

- Traditional population donors and feminist NGOs can collaborate effectively toward mutual goals.

If there had been no Manuela Ramos Movement, there would be no ReproSalud today; an organization with a clear gender perspective at its heart has been key to ReproSalud's success. There are experienced feminist organizations in much of the world; yet, to date, no donor other than USAID has provided support for a large-scale, essentially feminist project.[14] To achieve the kind of results that ReproSalud is beginning to demonstrate, donors need to consider building sustained major partnerships with mature women's organizations.

Acknowledgments

We express our gratitude to Barbara Feringa (formerly a Population Leadership Fellow working with USAID/Lima) for reviewing the chapter and for providing essential factual corrections and useful insight. We also thank Benno de Keijzer for his material related to ReproSalud's work with men. We appreciate the assistance of the ReproSalud staff in Lima and the regional team in Chavin for extensive efforts on our behalf. Finally, we wish to acknowledge the International Women's Health Coalition, which provided substantial support toward the preparation of this chapter.

Notes

1   ReproSalud accounts for close to 25 percent of the population budget of the USAID/Peru Mission.

2   A discussion of ReproSalud's income-generation component is beyond the scope of this chapter; we focus here on its educational activities, which have been its principal focus.

3   The name Manuela Ramos is considered so ordinary and common in Peru as to signify "everywoman," somewhat like Fulana in Brazil or Jane Doe in the United States. The founders of the Manuela Ramos Movement wanted to express that their organization works for all women. Members of the organization are often called "Manuelas."

4   Available data—drawn mostly from urban populations—suggest high prevalence of RTIs in Peru. For example, a study among clients of family planning clinics in Lima found a prevalence of bacterial vaginosis of 30 percent among women with the symptom of vaginal discharge and 25 percent among asymptomatic women (Sánchez et al. 1998). In a second study, carried out in a sample of women in Lima, researchers found that 33 percent had at least one of three pathogens under study: herpes simplex virus type 2, *Chlamydia trachomatis*, and *Treponema pallidum* (which causes syphilis) (Sánchez et al. 1996).

5   Syndromic algorithms—step-by-step visual flow charts—were developed to assist clinicians in deciding, based on a presenting client's symptoms and clinical signs, what RTI syndrome she or he might have and what medications could be used to treat the majority of organisms responsible for that syndrome.

6   See Chapter 16 for further discussion of the limitations of current tools for managing RTIs.

7   These included vaginal pH determination, potassium hydroxide whiff test, Gram's stain, and polymerase chain reaction.

8   The higher rate of bacterial vaginosis found by the ReproSalud study may result from their use of a more careful research protocol (see note 4 for a discussion of the lower rate found by other studies). For example, it is common among Peruvian women to treat vaginal discharge with various douche preparations that can temporarily remove the pathogen; in this study, all women were instructed not to douche or to use vaginal contraceptive foaming tablets for two days before the exam. Quality control for laboratory procedures is also an issue in resource-poor settings; the ReproSalud study may have benefited from greater resources for such controls. The description of ReproSalud's research was provided by Susana Chavez, ReproSalud's clinical research coordinator at the time.

9   ReproSalud designed different curriculums around the specific reproductive health priorities that emerged in various communities; hence, there were separate training workshops on RTIs, "too many children," unsafe birth, and adolescent pregnancy. The community-based promoters attended the workshop that focused on the particular problem identified in their community.

10 In some villages, the men had already been exposed to anti-alcoholism and anti-violence messages from evangelical missionaries; these messages, while not placed in a gender context, laid some groundwork for ReproSalud trainers seeking to address these issues.

11 See Chapter 18 for more details on the sterilization campaign and its ultimate demise.

12 For further reading on ReproSalud see Coe 2001, Galdos and Feringa 1999, and Rogow 2000. ReproSalud produces a bulletin in Spanish about program activities called *De Retamas y Orquideas* [Of broomflowers and orchids].

13   Using the framework of family harmony to approach the topic of domestic violence is a strategy
      employed by other projects discussed in this book. See, for example, Chapter 22.

14   It is not necessary that an organization characterize itself as "feminist" per se. The essential point
      is that women's empowerment and a gender perspective be at the core of an organization's work.

References

Coe, Anna-Britt. 2001. "Health, rights and realities: An analysis of the ReproSalud Project in Peru."
    Takoma Park, MD: Center for Health and Gender Equity.

Galdos, Susana and Barbara Feringa. 1999. "Creating partnerships at the grass-roots level: The ReproSalud
    Project," in *Confounding the Critics: Cairo Five Years On*, conference report. Cocoyoc, Mexico:
    Health, Empowerment, Rights, and Accountability, pp. 26–32.

Moyano, Jorge Reyes, Luis H. Ochoa, Vilma Sandoval F., Hans Raggers, and Shea Rutstein. 1997.
    Encuesta Demográfica y de Salud Familiar [Demographic study of family health]. Calverton, MD:
    DHS/Macro International, Inc.

Rogow, Debbie. 2000. *Alone You Are Nobody, Together We Float: The Manuela Ramos Movement, Quality/
    Calidad/Qualité* no. 10. New York: Population Council. (Also available in Spanish.)

Sánchez, Jorge, Eduardo Gotuzzo, Joel Escamilla, Carlos Carrillo, Irving A. Phillips, Cesar Barrios,
    Walter E. Stamm, Thoda L. Ashley, Joan K. Kreiss, and King K. Holmes. 1996. "Gender differ-
    ences in sexual practices and sexually transmitted infections among adults in Lima, Peru," *Ameri-
    can Journal of Public Health* 86(8, part 1): 1098–1107.

Sánchez, Sixto E., Laura A. Koutsky, Jorge Sánchez, Americo Fernández, Jose Casquero, Joan Kreiss,
    Mary Catlin, Minsheng Xia, and King K. Holmes. 1998. "Rapid and inexpensive approaches to
    managing abnormal vaginal discharge or lower abdominal pain: An evaluation in women attend-
    ing gynaecology and family planning clinics in Peru," *Sexually Transmitted Infections* 74(suppl 1):
    S85–S94.

World Health Organization. 1998. *Unsafe Abortion: Global and Regional Estimates of Incidence of and
    Mortality Due to Unsafe Abortion with a Listing of Available Country Data*, 3rd ed. Document no.
    WHO/RHT/MSM/97.16. Geneva: World Health Organization.

Contact information

Susana Moscoso
Associate Director, ReproSalud
Movimiento Manuela Ramos
Av. Juan P. Fernandini 1550
Lima 21, Peru
telephone: 51-1-423-8840
e-mail: smoscoso@manuela.org.pe

"If Many Push Together, It Can Be Done": Reproductive Health and Women's Savings and Credit in Nepal

Tom Arens, Denise Caudill, Saraswati Gautam,
Nicole Haberland, and Gopal Nakarmi

Nepal, nestled between India and the Tibetan region of China, is among the poorest countries in the world. Annual GNP per capita is approximately US$200, with over half of the population living on less than US$1 per day (UNICEF 1998). While daily life presents challenges to most Nepalis, pervasive gender inequities make many difficulties even more daunting for females. This bias begins early in life. Child mortality is 24 percent higher among females than males (Pradhan et al. 1997). Adult literacy rates of 41 percent for men and 14 percent for women reflect a historical bias toward boys in education (UNICEF 1998). Even today, in many rural areas less than 40 percent of primary school students are girls (Central Bureau of Statistics 1995).

For most girls, adolescence also brings marriage; half of women ages 20–24 were married by the age of 17, with 6 percent of currently married women in a polygynous union.[1] Early childbearing follows: 51 percent of 19-year-olds are already mothers or pregnant with their first child. As adults, most women in Nepal work more hours per day than men. During the harvest season many women begin work at 4:00 a.m. and do not stop until 10:00 p.m. In contrast to most other countries, women in Nepal do not live as long as men.

Given these conditions, it is not surprising that most women experience serious reproductive health problems. Total fertility is high, at an average of 4.6 children per woman. Yet, in 56 percent of all births mothers receive no antenatal care. During childbirth, only 9 percent of women are assisted by a doctor or trained nurse-midwife, 23 percent are assisted by traditional birth attendants, 56 percent by friends and relatives, and 11 percent have no assistance. The maternal mortality ratio in Nepal has been estimated at 539 deaths per 100,000 live births.

Almost a third of married women of reproductive age say they do not want to become pregnant but do not use contraception. Among the 29 percent who use a modern method, 46 percent rely on female sterilization, 21 percent on male sterilization, and 17 percent on injectables.

There are scant data on sexually transmitted infections (STIs) and reproductive tract infections (RTIs) in Nepal. HIV prevalence remains low, at 0.24 percent of adults ages 15–49 in 1997 (UNAIDS and WHO 1998). Concern about HIV is increasing, however, given an expansion in commercial sex work, migrant worker flow to and from India, and increases in injection drug use.

This chapter describes how a community development and family planning program in Nepal reoriented itself to a broader reproductive health approach. In so doing it sought to expand the range of clinical services available to poor rural women, including addressing more complex and controversial issues such as the availability of high-quality, early abortion services, and to address some of the social and economic issues that perpetuate women's poor reproductive health.

THE BOUDHA-BAHUNIPATI FAMILY WELFARE PROJECT: A CONVENTIONAL BUT COMPREHENSIVE APPROACH

Kavre and Sindhupalchowk Districts, situated in the Middle Hills east of Kathmandu, are the sites of the work described in this chapter. Here, as in most other rural districts, health and development indicators are generally worse than the national average. Poverty is pervasive and few roads are navigable by car. Government health services, if they operate at all, are of poor quality.

The Boudha-Bahunipati Family Welfare Project (hereafter BBP) was founded in 1973 as an experimental program of the Family Planning Association of Nepal and World Neighbors and now operates through eight indigenous nongovernmental organizations (NGOs) formed at each original program site.[2] Prior to the inception of the project described in this chapter, BBP provided family planning and basic curative services through its primary health clinics and community outreach programs and operated development projects such as agroforestry, fodder and livestock production, and development of sources of safe drinking water. Clinic-based services included antenatal care, labor and delivery, and provision of contraceptives (including injectables, pills, and condoms). Clinics that have been in existence for five or more years are at least 50 percent self-supporting. Family planning education sessions and some services were also provided in the community. For example, nurses and clinic assistants offered contraceptives on a regular schedule at "depo points" (named for Depo-Provera®)

in more remote communities. BBP clinicians also responded to calls for assistance with difficult home births.

Clients occasionally requested help dealing with other reproductive health problems. If a woman had an RTI, staff either provided medication (based on clinical assessment) or referred the client to other government or NGO clinics with better technical capacity. Clients were counseled that their partners must also follow a treatment regimen, but staff doubted whether clients relayed this information to their partners.

Women also approached staff for assistance in aborting unwanted pregnancies. Because abortion is illegal in Nepal, staff explained that they had no means to terminate the unwanted pregnancy, and suggested that the woman have the baby and return afterward for contraception. Women with complications of spontaneous or induced abortion typically did not present to the BBP clinics; they went instead to a well-equipped hospital about one hour by private vehicle from one of the main BBP sites. BBP staff were frustrated and concerned that they were unable to provide direct assistance to women needing abortions or postabortion care.

Selected development efforts were offered along with the basic maternal and child health and primary health care program. These included fodder production, agroforestry, improvements to livestock and livestock health, provision of safe drinking water, and literacy training. While BBP assisted in initiating these activities and provided ongoing guidance, it also helped to organize community-based user groups around such community needs. These user groups included all household members—both men and women. User group members contributed to a fund to cover activities such as drinking water system maintenance. When the funds collected exceeded expenses, the groups extended loans to community members at agreed-on interest rates. These development activities were gender neutral as originally conceived.

TWO DECADES LATER: THE REDESIGN

The traditional BBP approach compartmentalized activities (i.e., health and development services were fielded separately) and did not always include specific interventions to support women's interests. Nonetheless, it yielded important results over the years. Majhigaon, a project village in which BBP had been working for more than 15 years, was compared with nonparticipating villages in a 1989 evaluation. In Majhigaon, the proportion of households with access to adequate supplies of food year-round increased from 13 percent in 1983, to 49 percent in 1986, to 73 percent in 1989. Communities in which BBP programs were active had increased access to safe drinking water and were more likely to have planted trees and grass for fodder on terrace lands and reforested formerly eroded hillsides.

There had also been positive effects on health. The Majhigaon survey found that 38 percent of married women of reproductive age used family planning versus 29 percent in a comparison village where BBP did not work. In 1995 random sample surveys from all eight program areas showed an under-five mortality rate of 54 per 1,000 live births versus a national rate of 118 per 1,000 (Pradhan et al. 1997). Communities with three to four years of association with BBP showed contraceptive prevalence substantially above the national average—between 35 and 62 percent of married women of reproductive age versus 29 percent nationally (Pradhan et al. 1997). Moreover, in contrast to national statistics that showed a method mix dominated by sterilization, spacing methods represented more than 90 percent of contraceptive use in program areas. This was due at least in part to the fact that BBP provided regular and convenient access to spacing methods, especially pills, Depo-Provera, and condoms.

Over time it became evident that the most durable and effective user groups were those managed by women. These groups were better at loan recovery and evolved into women's savings and credit groups. Each began by developing rules for operation and participation; selecting a president, treasurer, and secretary; and establishing interest rates, minimum deposits, and other financial parameters. One hundred percent of the money in the savings funds came from participants' own contributions—no seed money was provided by the project. Women used loans for a variety of purposes, including buying pigs or goats to breed, raise, and sell, and producing vegetables for sale.

Interestingly, monitoring of the savings and credit groups indicated that some of the groups were making loans for costs related to health care, particularly referrals to hospital facilities for emergencies or complications—up to 15 percent of loans in some groups. Some of the close links between women's assets and health were beginning to emerge.

At the same time, World Neighbors and BBP staff were reflecting on the outcomes of the 1994 International Conference on Population and Development and considering the implications for their work. Consequently, in 1996 World Neighbors commissioned a reproductive health needs assessment and embarked on a process of institutional and programmatic learning to better define reproductive health as a social as well as clinical concept, and to clarify its links with women's and communities' social and economic development.

FINDING OUT WHAT WOMEN WANT

Findings from a qualitative study in the BBP program areas indicated that enormous potential existed for an integrated, multifaceted program (Haberland 1996). The study also uncovered extensive reproductive health needs that were not fully recognized and that would not be remedied through the program as it was then designed. Women's reproductive health needs were, as in most settings, determined by social factors such as women's relative lack of power in intimate relationships, multiple sexual partnerships, and violence against women in the home. While health services such as family planning and antenatal care were clearly needed, they would not address women's lack of bargaining power in sexual relationships or the many reasons—such as limited, if any, say in financial decisions—that kept some from seeking services altogether.

For example, most women were aware of the benefits of antenatal care and assisted delivery, yet they were not receiving these services, resting adequately after birth, or receiving postpartum care. As one woman stated, "If we don't work, we don't eat." Infertility was also of concern to women. A woman who did not bear children did not benefit from an important source of social respect. One woman explained that a further social consequence of infertility was polygamy: "After six of my babies died [as a result of miscarriages], I told my husband to remarry." In the needs assessment, a number of women expressed their feelings about polygamy:

> We feel sorrow. But if we try to prevent it, our husband will hit us.

> We can't leave our husbands, we have children.

> Men are bringing so many wives, this is a kind of discrimination.

RTIs (including STIs and HIV) were yet another problem. Two factors emerged as barriers to women seeking RTI diagnosis and treatment. First, they did not perceive that the symptoms indicated a serious condition. Perhaps more important was the stigma attached to RTIs. Some of the reasons women were uncomfortable seeking services for RTIs were directly related to clinic services, including lack of female providers in one site and lack of privacy in a number of the clinics' counseling areas.

The risk of STIs, including HIV, was shaped by common patterns of sexual networking, including men visiting prostitutes, polygamy, and extramarital sex. The risk was further compounded by sexual trafficking—the sale of women and girls who were forcibly brought or lured to other countries or cities as part of the sex trade.[3] One woman described a young girl whose husband sold her in Bombay for approximately US$220 when she was six months pregnant. Another talked about a woman who "sent her daughter to work" in New Delhi, a euphemism for having forced her to work in the sex trade. The women also described physical abuse by their partners. When the researchers encouraged discussion about what women or others might do to combat domestic violence, the overwhelming sense was that nothing could be done. "She cannot send her husband to police custody because she needs him tomorrow . . . She needs to maintain the relationship."

Women's limited access to contraception and lack of sexual decisionmaking authority resulted in multiple pregnancies, many of which were unwanted. These pregnancies led to a range of other obstetric and gynecologic problems, including unsafe abortion and uterine prolapse. The high incidence of uterine prolapse and its effects on women's capacity to function were not widely known to BBP staff before the 1996 assessment. In addition, because women had not been aware that anything could be done to alleviate the problem, they did not bring it to the attention of service providers. The few women who came to providers for related care were treated for infection, if necessary, and provided with a vaginal pessary (a ring-shaped rubber device that fits around the cervix and helps support the uterus).

In the discussions with members of the women's savings and credit groups conducted as part of the qualitative study, some expressed views critical of prevailing gender disparities. As one woman noted, "[Women] should be equal." Women also reported that involvement in the groups increased their autonomy: "Previously my husband would not let me go anywhere, and now he does." Women's remarks highlighted the connections between reproductive morbidity and mortality and underlying social factors, such as domestic violence, sexual trafficking, and sexual networking patterns. Yet there was limited understanding of what could be done to address these underlying factors at the program level. As one staff person noted, "We have to change the social structure . . . how do we do that?"

RESPONDING TO WOMEN'S CONCERNS

BBP and its partners already had the foundations of a better way to address the issues underlying women's reproductive and sexual health. The existing savings and credit groups provided a means of empowering women. Further, there was clear enthusiasm among senior BBP staff for reorienting its programs. The health coordinator (a senior nurse) and program advisor—who were trusted by clinic staff of the BBP NGOs and members of the surrounding communities—were prepared to help health and community development staff understand the reproductive health issues women faced, as well as their social antecedents. Steps were taken at three levels.

- Clinic level: BBP ensured that female service providers were available at each clinic and designed private rooms for consultations; clinic personnel were trained to upgrade their skills; reproductive health services were improved and expanded throughout the BBP area; and staff were trained to refer cases they could not manage themselves.
- Community level: New women's savings and credit groups were formed; there are now 52 across the BBP area. Capacity building and other activities are being conducted with all of the new and existing groups.

- NGO level: Staff and board members at all eight BBP NGOs were trained in reproductive health and gender issues. Organizational and management capacity is being fostered, and the facilitation skills of the 23 clinic and community development staff members are being strengthened.

FIRST STEP: TRAINING OF TRAINERS

Senior auxiliary nurse-midwives and community organizers from several BBP NGOs participated in a week-long training session organized by World Neighbors.[4] The training made use of the women's own comments from the needs assessment and applied principles of participatory learning. One objective of the workshop was to explore the ways in which reproductive health goes beyond biomedical definitions. For example, one exercise (called the problem tree) identified the causes and consequences of specific reproductive health and gender concerns (see Box 1).[5]

Participants sorted the "root" (causes) cards from several of the trees according to whether the causes were biomedical, social, or both. During discussion, participants recognized that many social issues that contribute to poor reproductive health are outside the scope of clinical services, especially as they were currently configured. The social context variables that contributed to poor reproductive health were not well appreciated by staff, not directly acknowledged in exchanges with clients, and not acted upon. Participants also commented that there were many similarities among the various tree trunks (in other words, different reproductive health problems had similar causes).

A second workshop objective was to provide participants with the skills to conduct similar workshops with other staff and board members, as well as with the women's savings and credit groups. For this reason, the participatory learning exercises were repeated numerous times during the workshop, first as a learning experience in terms of content for participants and to introduce the exercise; then, replicated and facilitated by the participants, as an opportunity for them to practice using the exercise so they could later conduct it with other staff or women's groups. In addition, the World Neighbors trainers developed 16 drawings depicting key reproductive health problems for use with nonliterate groups.

Participants were engaged in the training, but they were intimidated by the number of issues and the complexity of the underlying causes of reproductive health problems. When discussing what they could do about the problems they had identified and analyzed, they focused primarily on narrow, more tangible clinical responses, rather than on the social issues they had already identified as root causes. The trainers therefore carried out exercises that helped participants prioritize issues and make plans to address them.

Box 1. Roots and fruits: The "problem tree" exercise

This exercise is used to help participants identify the connections between the underlying causes and various consequences of a problem.

Materials: Poster-size sheets of paper (one for each problem to be discussed), markers, tape, two stacks of colored cards (each stack a different color).

Instructions to trainers:

1. Sketch a tree with roots and branches on each poster sheet and tape the sheets to the wall. Label each trunk to represent a specific problem.

2. Ask participants to analyze the root causes of the problem represented by the tree and to write them on cards of one color, one cause per card. Tape these to the roots of the tree.

3. Ask participants to write the consequences of the same problem, using cards of another color. Tape these cards along the branches of the trees, as the fruit.

   A sample problem tree generated to analyze RTIs is illustrated below:

Roots:	Fruit:
Lack of appropriate services	Itching
Lack of private and appropriate counseling	Infertility
Infection caused by health service providers (iatrogenic)	Giving birth to an unhealthy child
Lack of condoms	Pain in pelvic area
Lack of reproductive health knowledge	White discharge
Unsafe delivery	Burning sensation during urination
Unprotected sex	Ulcer
Lack of hygiene	Spontaneous abortion
Bad customs (social evil)	Weight loss
Poor economic status	Cervical cancer

4. Facilitate discussion about the connections made during the exercise. While participants may not always come up with the "correct" answers, these discussions among the entire group—versus didactic corrections from the facilitators—can clarify almost all misinformation.

"Bean-wise pairwise ranking" was one such exercise: The "root" (causes) cards or actual problems from the problem tree exercise were placed in a vertical column and systematically compared to one another. If there were ten cards, the card at the top was compared first to the one below it, then in succession to each following card. For each comparison, participants asked, "Which of these two is more important in our community/program?" A bean (or some other marker) was placed next to the more important issue. After the first card had been compared to all nine cards below, the second was compared to the eight below it, then the third to the seven below it, and so forth. The issue that collected the most beans was ranked first, that with the second highest score was ranked second, and so forth.

The final exercise led to the development of action plans. Small groups of participants from specific communities employed a simple planning format (described in Box 2) to address their two highest-priority reproductive health issues.

Box 2. Illustrative action plan

Each of the small groups developed action plans to address their two priority issues. The sample below illustrates one group's plan to address deficiencies in family planning services. A few of the interventions (adult literacy, promotion of girls' education, and street dramas) seek to address some of the underlying contextual issues that may hinder use of services, rather than merely focusing on the supply and promotion of contraceptives. Nonetheless, the plans did not stray far from more predictable, NGO-conceived, -controlled, and -implemented interventions, illustrating the struggles many of the groups faced in grappling with more fundamental concerns and in working with the women's savings and credit groups as agents of change. Finally, while it appears that the majority of interventions proposed are an expansion of pre-existing activities, the staff demonstrated that they understood directly their relation to reproductive health. This was one of the hoped-for outcomes of the workshop: to help staff understand the connections among the various activities they already undertake.

Issue	What are we doing now?	To what extent are we doing it (are we doing it with everyone?)	What could we do if we did not have resource constraints?	What will we do in the next year with existing resources?
Family planning	Adult literacy	5 literacy classes	38 adult literacy classes	15 adult literacy classes
	Distribution of contraceptives	Clinic and 47 depo points	Clinic and 84 depo points	Clinic and 55 depo points
			Expand the clinic to offer contraceptives that require more advanced technical inputs (IUD, Norplant®)	
	Education about birth spacing	At 47 depo points and with four women's savings and credit groups	Educate women about spacing at 84 depo points and with four women's savings and credit groups	Educate women about spacing at 55 depo points and with four women's savings and credit groups
			Street drama	Two dramas in schools
	Education about importance of girls' education	Discussion of importance of girls' education at monthly women's group meetings	Discuss importance of girls' education with 38 women's groups	Discuss importance of girls' education with 17 women's groups

The participants needed time and further discussion to develop action plans that responded to the analysis they had carried out. Accustomed as they were to working only through clinical services, some groups still focused exclusively on what could be achieved in the conventional way. For example, most of the small groups chose family planning—BBP's flagship service—as their priority. Further, most of the suggested interventions focused on increasing the supply of contraceptives or educating community members about the benefits of family planning, even when it was clear from the exercises that women were already interested in spacing or limiting births but often did not have the economic or social resources to access services or to persuade partners. When such narrowly conceived plans were presented, the larger group was able to offer a helpful critique.

In the months following the workshop, participants implemented their workplans and conducted awareness sessions in their communities for the board and staff (including clinic staff) of each of the BBP NGOs and for affiliated women's savings and credit groups. The individuals who attended these sessions identified priority issues for the coming year that included both social and biomedical problems. Uterine prolapse and girls' education were two high-priority issues on the agendas of the participants.

In response to issues raised in the needs assessment and highlighted in the training-of-trainers workshops, similar changes in reproductive health service delivery were planned for all eight BBP clinic sites. In contrast, community work would be tailored based on women's self-identified priorities. The senior BBP and World Neighbors staff prepared to support the entire process with ongoing monitoring and technical assistance.

CHANGES IN REPRODUCTIVE HEALTH CARE DELIVERY

By and large, clinic staff were eager to implement new ideas and provide better services. All clinics made efforts to increase the comfort of clients. Responding to a new understanding of women's need for privacy, they hung curtains or relocated the room where counseling sessions were held. Separate, private spaces were also created for delivery. To respond to women's desire for female service providers, additional staff were recruited and deployed to assure that there was at least one female clinic assistant or auxiliary nurse-midwife in every site.

In the first year, BBP clinical program staff also responded to the reproductive health concerns women had expressed in the needs assessment and reoriented and expanded their services accordingly. BBP staff organized two-day "gynecological" camps, in which an obstetrician/gynecologist and support staff traveled to remote locations and offered a full range of reproductive health services, including antenatal care, general pelvic exams, pregnancy testing, and management and referral of uterine prolapse and infertility cases. RTI management services were also available. At the camps, women would be asked about their medical history, current symptoms, and other issues, and treatment would be provided presumptively. Partner treatment was also recommended. When necessary, women would be referred to well-equipped facilities in Banepa or Kathmandu for sample collection and testing.

Clinic ledgers were revised to reflect this broader approach and to include reproductive health problems such as RTIs and uterine prolapse. Acknowledging that women were concerned about unwanted pregnancy and that unsafe abortion was widespread, BBP staff developed a referral relationship with the Marie Stopes clinic, a trusted and reputable provider of menstrual regulation in Kathmandu.[6] Staff also established a referral relationship with Dhulikhel Hospital in Kavre District (about 17 kilometers from Bahunipati) for treatment of infertility and for vasectomy and other more complicated reproductive health care procedures.

COMMUNITY-BASED WORK: A FOCUS ON WOMEN'S SAVINGS AND CREDIT GROUPS

Work on the social and economic underpinnings of reproductive health problems was principally accomplished through the women's savings and credit groups. This provided an easy means of gaining insight into women's priority needs, as well as a means to influence the wider community on such subjects as maternal health, alcoholism, girls' education, and domestic violence. Although the savings and credit groups were initially intended for narrowly specified economic purposes, they had become an important source of solidarity and empowerment. Now they would also serve as an arena in which women could express themselves and deal with sensitive subjects.

As part of this strategy, the BBP NGOs organized additional women's savings and credit groups, increasing the total number from less than ten to 52. These groups underwent training similar to that given to NGO staff and identified the following priorities:

- Uterine prolapse
- Maternal health
- Alcoholism
- Gender violence
- Girls' education
- Women's low status

The savings and credit group members are addressing these issues with technical support from BBP. Use of services among members is promoted simply by having these sensitive subjects more widely and actively discussed. For example, the group that placed a priority on spacing and limiting childbearing encouraged its members with two or three children to use Depo-Provera. One of the groups that sought to improve maternity care wanted to help women who needed emergency obstetric care. When BBP staff told them about a women's group in another village that was successfully making loans for obstetric emergencies, the group set aside a special fund for such cases. These funds were segregated by the president of the women's group and not deposited in the bank, so that they could be easily accessed in a crisis.

Some of the new groups are focusing on improving drinking water and irrigation, which, according to the women, saves time, allows them to grow kitchen gardens and fruit, improves health and cleanliness, increases agricultural and livestock fodder production, and increases prestige. At first glance these issues do not appear to be reproductive health concerns per se, but they were the strategies chosen by some of the groups. Respecting these choices is part of the philosophy of the program and the partners involved, and builds needed trust between women and the BBP NGOs. Moreover, addressing these issues often creates some of the preconditions necessary for improving reproductive health.

Other groups are seeking to bring about social change. Women in the group that placed a priority on girls' education made a commitment to ensuring that their own daughters, at least, would go to school. The group that identified increasing literacy as its goal promoted attendance at an NGO-sponsored literacy class. Other groups, concerned about gambling, began confronting the men in the communities directly.

Subjects that previously were rarely if ever discussed, such as alcoholism, trafficking in girls, sex work, and gambling, were beginning to be aired through this process. In some instances, women were even beginning to think of ways they could address these concerns directly. Several groups were concerned with alcohol consumption, which they linked closely to poverty. As one woman stated during the needs assessment, "Men go and drink and women don't eat." In response, some of the women's groups sought to decrease alcohol consumption by curbing its sale. However, making and/or selling alcohol generates income for some other women, so the solution was not straightforward from a women's welfare perspective. Staff agreed that they had to help find alternative sources of income for these women. In contrast, in other villages drinking alcohol is considered part of life. Some of the loans taken by women in the savings and credit group were used to purchase grain, which they used to make and sell alcohol; a few groups allow women to secure loans for the express purpose of alcohol production.

Trafficking and commercial sex work are subjects of extreme sensitivity but also have extreme consequences. Although sex trafficking was too sensitive a topic to make it onto the women's official list of priorities, women in one village—from which girls are often bought for sex trafficking—felt they should begin to do something. When young sex workers came back to the village to visit their families, the women tried to convince them to stay in the village rather than go back to India. The most important outcome is that women have begun to talk about the practice.

RESULTS

Just a few years after developing their workplans, both the clinic staff and the women's groups have begun to leave their mark on health and gender conditions in their villages.

Increased Use of Reproductive Health Services

The number of women who receive reproductive health services in the eight project sites has risen substantially. The data presented in Table 1 include services provided via the clinic, gynecological camps, and other community outreach services, but do not include other curative health services.[7] The change is striking: The overall number of reproductive health visits increased 83 percent between the first year and the second. In the second year 70 percent more clients were treated for RTI/STIs, there was a 50 percent increase in visits for uterine prolapse, a 600 percent increase in the number of clients treated for urinary tract infections, and a 63 percent increase in antenatal care visits; postpartum care visits increased from none to 251.

Some of this change is due to the gynecological camps. Nineteen have been organized in 11 locations throughout the area; during each camp, the female obstetrician/gynecologists saw between 44 and 241 women ages 15–70.

More complicated reproductive health problems are also being addressed through explicit referrals. In the first two years of the project, 45 women came to the clinics for menstrual regulation and were referred to Marie Stopes. Several infertile couples have been referred and are being treated, and one vasectomy client has had his procedure successfully reversed.

In some sites, there is still a lack of information about and access to needed services. For example, during a monitoring visit at a particularly remote site, BBP and World Neighbors staff spoke with several women who were in need of treatment for uterine prolapse but still did not know about the pessary and referral services available at the clinic.

One of the members of a women's savings and credit group was pregnant but did not know about the need for tetanus immunization. An NGO staff member said that her responsibility to the women's group was "providing Depo services," and the community organizer for the women's group said that her job was "to help the group do the accounting," and that tetanus was not her responsibility. Central BBP staff subsequently worked with the NGO staff to broaden their understanding of their roles.

Women Judge Their Progress

Sustainable changes in the social factors that underlie poor reproductive health are multiply determined, slowly achieved, and difficult to measure. BBP and World Neighbors are using traditional service statistics to monitor the program's effects. However,

Table 1. Number of clients provided with reproductive health services, by type, 1997–98 and 1998–99

	Year 1 July 1997–June 1998	Year 2 July 1998–June 1999[a]
Uterine prolapse	173	260
Reproductive tract infection	174	276
Sexually transmitted infection	38	84
Infertility	11	0
Postpartum hemorrhage	65	71
Urinary tract infection	22	155
Incomplete abortion	4	0
Antenatal care	935	1,525
Postpartum care	0	251
Delivery	95	63
Pregnancy test	0	89
Miscellaneous[b]	103	194
Total	1,620	2,968

[a] By the time of the 1999 data collection, an additional NGO had been added. This NGO was not included in the 1998–99 totals here in the interest of comparability with the 1997–98 data.
[b] Includes irregular menstruation, breast problems, vesicovaginal fistula, fibroids, and so forth.

they recognize that these data provide only a partial indication of the progress of the women's initiatives. Hence, they are moving beyond conventional data mechanisms to innovative participatory techniques that involve local staff and women in assessing their own progress (Caudill 2000).

One such technique is an exercise that uses *mana*, a local measure for dry goods such as spices and beans. Metal mana cups vary in size: 1/8, 1/4, 1/2, 3/4, and full mana. Participants are asked to rank their progress on a particular issue on the "mana scale." For example, if a group feels that it is only beginning to make progress on an activity, it ranks itself at 1/8 (tiny/emerging). A ranking of 1/2 denotes that progress is greater but still incomplete; and full is self-sustaining. While this technique is subjective, it enables women to set clear goals and identify how much progress they feel they have made toward achieving them.

For example, one women's savings and credit group focused on maternal health, an issue that had received no attention in their community. A year after the group began its work, one traditional birth attendant (TBA) had received training in safe delivery practices. However, the women scored themselves at the lowest level of progress (1/8 mana), explaining, "Many should be trained. We have babies in the village and this can save lives. The TBA should use the safe delivery kits." A woman from another women's savings and credit group offered a similar comment: "We're not even at 1/2 mana, now we are learning. For [full] mana, all pregnant women would have antenatal checkups. . . . We've just started going to the health post for checkup and delivery."

A group that had prioritized spacing births and limiting childbearing rated itself according to the prevalence of Depo-Provera use among its members. Because all group members with two or three children were using Depo-Provera, the members gave themselves 3/4 mana. To reach full mana, the members felt that women who want to delay their first birth or space their second should face no barriers to doing so.

The mana evaluations are particularly useful for the women's savings and credit groups that are taking on more difficult social and economic issues. A group working to promote girls' education felt it had made important inroads in increasing girls' school attendance. One commented, "Previously we were not sending our girls to school, they did the housework, and so on. Now we think the girls should go to school." Another added, "I have five children, now sons and daughters both go." But the group agreed it still had a long way to go, ranking its progress at 1/4 mana. A full mana for them, they explained, required girls' being educated as professionals, such as nurses or teachers. Another group also ranked itself at 1/4 mana in terms of girls' education. As one member commented, "We all send our daughters to school now. To reach [full] mana, our daughters should all be able to pass the school-leaving exam."

Two groups working on literacy felt they were making "tiny/emerging" progress toward their goals. As a member of one group explained, "At the beginning there were many participants [in the BBP-sponsored literacy class], but by the end there were only seven or eight left. Only a few women go for classes. If we scored full mana, everybody [in the group] would read and write." A woman from another group commented, "A literacy class was started once by [BBP] but we didn't learn much. Some of us only know how to write our names." Both groups rated themselves at 1/8 mana.

Women from a number of the newer groups reported that the most important effect of their efforts had been reducing the amount of time spent fetching water. One explained, "With water nearby, we have time for rest, and with rest we can have good health and discussions like this." When discussing irrigation, another woman noted, "We can plant winter crops. From those we have mustard and don't have to buy oil and wheat. So we can save money and that money can be used for education for our children." A third echoed this sentiment, saying, "Because of the vegetable production our income has increased and our families are healthy." Nonmembers from richer households have also perceived a change in women's situation, reporting, "The members' incomes are rising. . . . Before they used to come to us to ask to borrow grains and vegetables. . . . Nowadays they have it themselves."

The results were mixed for those groups attempting to address highly charged issues such as sex trafficking and male behavior. In the village where women discouraged two young women from returning to their foreign sex work, one girl decided to stay in Nepal; the other returned to India. Because this is a newer site, BBP is following the women's lead and is not taking this issue on institutionally until rapport and trust are built with the village.

Women view gambling, a male practice, as expensive and unproductive, a drain on a family's meager income. Those women's groups that tried to reduce gambling in their villages achieved mixed results. In one site a member reported, "Now there is no more gambling." In another site, women went together to the place where the men gambled and tore up all the cards; when one of the women got home, she was beaten by her husband. Working on these highly charged problems will thus require deeper analysis of the short- and long-term returns and drawbacks of different strategies, as well as discussion about the human rights issues involved.

Despite these difficulties, women are beginning to discuss sensitive social issues and, by doing so, are beginning to reshape the norms surrounding them.

Changes Among Women: Assessing Effects

While results related to specific social and reproductive health initiatives are preliminary, savings and credit group members report an increased sense of confidence and capacity, as well as:

- Fewer feelings of isolation;
- A sense of unity and power with the other members;
- Confidence in themselves to be a member of the group, express their own ideas in public, meet with outsiders, and manage their funds;
- Freedom from fear of debt and moneylenders, and of their in-laws and husbands; and
- A sense of hope for the future with dreams of increased well-being for themselves and their families.

This sense of control and the belief that one can change the status quo are prerequisites for beginning a process of social change. Even at this early stage, for example, women note, "As a group we can approach the NGO and village development committee [VDC, a locally elected government body] for resources. . . . Before the group formation, it wasn't like that."

The groups have created respectable roles and activities for women in communities where women's social mobility remains limited. Men's support of the groups has also increased with time. In general, husbands do not complain or punish their wives for participating and paying dues. Some women indicated the need to work with men directly and to increase men's awareness both of the inequities women face and of men's role in reproductive health and well-being. Indeed, with the assistance of the NGOs, some of the groups are organizing events on particular topics, such as the rights and responsibilities of women and men, to which they invite their husbands.

At the same time, some groups feel they still have a long way to go. In Dhap, women scored themselves at 1/2 mana toward their goal of being able to gain independent access to external material, financial, and other resources. One member summed up the group's situation: "The power is in our brain, but we are still too small for a full mana. We can go to the VDC for resources but we have not gone yet. The VDC chairman doesn't look at us. We put him in that post, we elected him, and we can approach him."

LOOKING FORWARD

BBP has expanded reproductive health services in Nepal to respond to poor rural women's expressed needs. More women are seeking care and are being treated for a wider range of reproductive health problems. More women's savings and credit groups have been organized, and almost all of these groups are acting as change agents in their villages, often tackling difficult social issues. The BBP program has sought to empower women to take action to improve their reproductive health, in addition to providing neglected reproductive health services through their clinics, in the community, and through special camps and explicit referral arrangements.

The program continues to develop and refine its activities and to expand to other World Neighbors sites in Nepal, such as Ramechhap District and three districts in the Terai. Training is being planned to assist staff in helping women address some of the more sensitive issues in their communities, such as gender violence. Staff will also receive further training in topics that will help them assess needs, plan projects, and evaluate progress. Building the capacity of the local BBP NGOs and the women's savings and credit groups to plan, implement, and evaluate their activities is an ongoing priority.

Staff of BBP and World Neighbors are encouraged by the progress of their integrated approach to reproductive health, and their experiences are yielding lessons that call for thoughtful reflection:

It is possible to address the root causes of women's poor reproductive health. The women's savings and credit groups have begun to identify, prioritize, and change social practices that have negative health consequences, and to reduce the social and economic barriers to women's achievement of sexual and reproductive health. These include action on such issues as access to nonfamilial funds for women in obstetric emergencies, sending girls to school, decreasing workloads, and challenging men's prerogative to spend scarce family income without women's consent. However, some of the issues (e.g., challenging male behavior where there is a threat of violence) require greater management and technical assistance (in the form of time, patience, political sense, and specific skills) than BBP realized. While women should not be dissuaded from taking action on such issues as gambling or gender violence, programs must be careful not to take on more than they can adequately support.

Working in an integrated manner on livelihood, health, environmental, and reproductive health issues requires a realization that reproductive health may not be women's first priority. While women's groups can be a powerful force for change in matters of reproductive health, cooperating organizations must respect their key areas of interest and reasons for existing. As was the case for many of the women's savings and credit groups, these interests—which often relate to livelihoods and workloads—are often not about what most consider to be reproductive health per se. Nevertheless, these issues are often at the root of many reproductive health problems. Local access to safe drinking water decreases a woman's workload, protects her health, and thus creates some of the preconditions necessary for good reproductive health. Together with efforts to redress deficiencies in clinical services, broad-based action to address the root causes of poor reproductive health can have a mutually reinforcing effect.

An important element of the program is building the capacity of women's groups to change the status quo. The participatory exercises and evaluation tools allow participants to identify what they view as problems in their communities as well as possible solutions. This approach is mirrored by a finance scheme that is grounded solely in women's own savings. No external start-up funds are provided; rather, group members save their own money and use these pooled resources for loans. Membership in such a group appears to have a positive effect. Women noted changes in their confidence, sense of agency, and hope for the future. As one recounted, "Before, we could not speak with outsiders; we used to bow to men. But being with the group, we can talk." Another explained, "If one is trying to push alone it's difficult, but if many push together, it can be done."

Transformation of women's sense of agency is a powerful force for change in a variety of domains. A woman who is able to better her livelihood is also more confident about her ability to challenge social norms. One who is able to speak up for herself in public is in a better position to do so in other realms—for example, in protecting her sexual and reproductive health. Learning about and challenging gender inequities can have

Reproductive Health and Women's Savings and Credit in Nepal   413

profound effects on a woman's agency and, ultimately, far-reaching effects on her well-being. As one woman reflected: "Now I feel men and women are equal. I feel I am more clever than before. We have revitalized ourselves."

Acknowledgments

The authors thank the Ford Foundation, the William and Flora Hewlett Foundation, and the Summit Foundation for their support of the World Neighbors integrated program in Nepal. Without their vision and encouragement, this effort would not have been possible. We thank Michael Koenig, whose guidance and foresight were key to the development of this project. We acknowledge the local NGOs that are now part of BBP, and especially those that participated in the participatory action assessment: Mahankal Swasthya Sewa Sanchalan Samiti and Indrawati Jana Sewa Samiti. We are especially grateful to the staff who have been key to making this project happen both in the clinics and the communities. We also thank Mohan Dhakal, Tanka Gurung, Shanta Jirel, Bishnu Pratap Khadka, Prem Moktan, and Hari Bahadur Thapa for their assistance with the participatory research.

Notes

1   The data in this and the two following paragraphs are from Pradhan et al. (1997).

2   While BBP no longer operates in the town of Boudha, its activity in and around Bahunipati increased dramatically over the past 20 years. It now serves an estimated 160,000 people in 48 villages.

3   In addition to the permanent sale of girls and women to traffickers, girls were also sold for shorter periods of time (e.g., to work for two or three years as sex workers in New Delhi or elsewhere, after which they would return home). The communities did not consider this to be trafficking because it was for a limited time.

4   For more details on the content of the training session, see Caudill 1998.

5   "Problem tree" exercises are also used in the ReproSalud project, described in Chapter 20.

6   While abortion is illegal, menstrual regulation is permitted by the government in some areas, such as Kathmandu (it is not permitted in the BBP area). Menstrual regulation is provided up to ten weeks following a missed menstrual period. Marie Stopes (headquartered in Great Britain) is a nonprofit, international network of providers of menstrual regulation and reproductive health care in resource-poor settings.

7   The total number of visits for all services was approximately 17,000 in 1997–98 and 18,500 in 1998–99.

References

Caudill, Denise (ed.). 1998. *Responding to Reproductive Health Needs: Participatory Approach for Analysis and Action, A Report and Training Guide on Experiences in Nepal.* Oklahoma City, OK: World Neighbors, Nepal.

Caudill, Denise. 2000. "We tried to measure ourselves and find we have progressed!" participatory impact assessment of the integrated program in reproductive health, Nepal. Oklahoma City, OK: World Neighbors, Nepal.

Central Bureau of Statistics. 1995. *Women in Nepal: Some Statistical Facts.* Kathmandu: Central Bureau of Statistics.

Haberland, Nicole. 1996. *Gender and Reproductive Health: A Needs Assessment of Women's Concerns in Rural Nepal.* Oklahoma City, OK: World Neighbors, Nepal.

Pradhan Ajit, Ram Hari Aryal, Gokarna Regmi, Bharat Ban, and Pavalavalli Govindasamy. 1997. *Nepal Family Health Survey 1996.* Kathmandu and Calverton, MD: Ministry of Health (Nepal), New ERA, and Macro International Inc.

UNAIDS and WHO. 1998. "Epidemiological fact sheet on HIV/AIDS and sexually transmitted diseases: Nepal." Geneva: UNAIDS and WHO.

UNICEF. 1998. *The State of the World's Children 1998.* Oxford, UK: Oxford University Press.

Contact information

Jagdish Ghimire
South Asia Area Representative
Tom Arens
Area Representative 1971–99
World Neighbors
P.O. Box 916
Kathmandu, Nepal
telephone: 977-1-54-66-88
fax: 977-1-53-87-56
e-mail: info@wnsa.org.np

Catharine McKaig
Reproductive Health Coordinator
World Neighbors
4127 NW 122nd Street
Oklahoma City, OK 73120 USA
telephone: 405-752-9700
fax: 405-752-9393
e-mail: cat@wn.org

Denise Caudill
Consultant
International Health and Development
2200 Dublin Road
Oklahoma City, OK 73120 USA
telephone: 405-755-6258
fax: 405-755-6218
e-mail: denisecaudill@cs.com

Mobilizing Communities to End Violence Against Women in Tanzania

Lori S. Michau, Dipak Naker, and Zahara Swalehe

The northwest corner of Tanzania, site of East Africa's Lake Victoria, is home to approximately six million people originating from numerous tribes living in urban centers, like Mwanza, as well as in rural communities. As is true in many settings, gender inequity in this region (known as the Lake Zone) is institutionalized from an early age. Girls are less likely to be sent to school than boys, and early marriage and childbearing are the norm. Nationally, the median age at first marriage for women is 17, and almost half of all girls are mothers by the age of 18 (Bureau of Statistics [Tanzania] and Macro International 1997; Tanzania Planning Commission 1992). Women are seen as the property of men, primarily their husbands or fathers, and, as such, have little power over their own bodies or lives. Women's lack of power, particularly in sexual relationships, leaves them vulnerable to violence and the myriad health problems that arise from abuse. In Mwanza town, HIV rates peak at 20 percent for women ages 25–34 (Borgdorff 1994). The prevalence of sexually transmitted infections among women attending antenatal clinics in that city has been documented at 37 percent (Grosskurth et al. 1995).

In 1996 two organizations—*kuleana*, a dynamic, rights-based organization with a focus on children, and the African Medical Research Foundation, a health service delivery organization—joined forces to address problems related to sexual health in Mwanza by focusing broadly on their root causes. Their joint initiative, known as Jijenge!, sought to analyze and confront gender inequity and promote change as a matter of women's rights. This chapter discusses Jijenge!'s evolution from a broad-based women's health and rights project to a tightly focused campaign to combat one of the most damaging manifestations of women's subordinate status—gender violence, particularly women's subjection to violence within the family.

BEGINNING WITH A BROAD WOMEN'S RIGHTS AGENDA

Jijenge! began with a bold sexual health, rights-based approach. Its focus on sexual health meant moving beyond the traditional biomedical conceptualization of health toward a more comprehensive analysis of the social and economic factors affecting women's well-being, including power imbalances in relationships, violence, and double standards for women and men. Jijenge!'s rights-based approach was founded on the belief that women are equal to men and that individuals, communities, and governments are accountable for treating them accordingly. This approach is in stark contrast to the traditional welfare perspective, in which women depend on men and the community at large for kindness, favors, or goodwill. The approach created a legitimate channel for placing women's issues on the agenda for social change. Jijenge! developed three program components to address its broad agenda:

- *Providing information and clinical services for women.* A clinic provided basic reproductive health services, including confidential and voluntary HIV testing, sexual health counseling, contraception, and diagnosis and treatment of sexually transmitted infections. The counseling that accompanied these clinical services focused on helping women identify and address the root causes of poor sexual health in their own lives.
- *Training community workers to create more gender-sensitive service agencies.* Participatory training workshops on gender, women's rights, violence, and sexual health were designed for police officers, teachers, health service providers, church groups, and social welfare staff to enable them to reorient their workplaces toward more woman-friendly practices.
- *Changing gender attitudes in communities.* To stimulate public debate about critical issues affecting women's lives throughout Mwanza, a range of community-based activities was planned, including community theater, booklet clubs, radio programs, murals, community meetings, exhibitions, and distribution of learning materials.

A NEW FOCUS ON VIOLENCE

After six months of operation and monitoring, Jijenge! staff organized a workshop to reflect on their experiences. A common concern emerged: The broad-based promotion of women's health and rights was a daunting task for many members of the community. The project's sweeping approach failed to help community members understand the new language of rights, discuss relevant issues, or offer sufficiently compelling reasons for change. In addition, it threatened to alienate those members Jijenge! needed as allies. Staff struggled to remain focused amidst the wide range of women's rights issues on the agenda, and partner groups were confused by and pessimistic about such an overarching call for change. Some women were fearful of participating in Jijenge! activities because its broad agenda represented a radical departure from existing ways of life. As Celestina Nyenga, Jijenge!'s community awareness coordinator, said: "People heard all the different rights and felt like it was too much; women were making too many demands."

To prioritize and narrow the initiative's focus, staff discussed the various issues emerging in their work in the clinic, training program, and with the community. One issue came to the fore: violence against women, including sexual violence. Many men were unapologetic about the use of force to get their way:

If a woman doesn't want it [sex] there is no way out, just rape.

When we see a daughter of someone has completed primary school, we start to seduce her as she has grown [old] enough to cook.

A woman in the community remarked:

You might have been beaten by your husband badly, all the body is painful but he will order you to cook ugali [porridge]. During the night he will say, "Turn this way," demanding [sex] and you have to do it.

Indeed, violence was commonplace in the lives of many women in and around Mwanza. Girls and women often faced physical assault if they resisted offering domestic, economic, or sexual services to husbands or other males in the family. Many women were subjected to female genital cutting and forced sex. Many reported having been chased from their own homes, mostly by their partners. Women recounted facing public and private humiliation, and, fearing threats of violence, had to accede when they were refused food or money for medical care.

Staff noted that despite its prevalence and serious consequences, gender violence was generally dismissed as a "domestic issue," or a matter of tradition, culture, or human nature—and therefore considered inappropriate for public discussion. The acceptance of—or at least ambivalence toward—violence had permeated the collective psyche, resulting in shame, stigma, and silence. Community members held back from supporting women experiencing violence, and from confronting violent men:

When you refuse to have sex, you are beaten badly and no one is going to support you. Normally men say, "I have paid [dowry] for your body." Even if you go to your parents' house, they will send you back.

We women have so many responsibilities. If you go into the village you will cry. Women are grazing cows, fetching water, looking for firewood, and raising children. It is so much work.

If a goat is lost you are beaten. Just the day before yesterday I met one woman crying and asked her what was wrong. She replied, "I'm tired, I was beaten up and threatened with a machete." We shouldn't fool each other. When are we women going to be free?

A Jijenge! clinician observed:

Women are brought up not recognizing violence because they are taught before marriage that they will face such things. Men are socialized that they have ultimate power. Now the problem is that women and men fail to see the impact of the violence on women's lives, especially their health.

Jijenge! staff also found that public institutions, which tended to be overextended and undersupported, perpetuated the cycle of violence and social ostracism. Women were often subject to blame and ridicule from social welfare workers, representatives of the legal system, religious leaders, and health care providers who were prepared to deal only with the biomedical aspects of women's health. This prevented women who were abused from seeking necessary legal protection, social and emotional support, and medical treatment. As Jijenge! counselor Pelagia Lugeleka noted: "Women feel afraid to report violence because they won't be listened to and if they do report, they know they will return home and experience even more."

Furthermore, lack of local institutional support severely limited the staff's ability to suggest constructive solutions to the violence clients faced. Verdiana Kamanya, another Jijenge! counselor, said:

As a counselor I was not comfortable because the options I was suggesting to women would not really work out. For example, she may choose to go to the police or social welfare services but then goes there expecting support and instead experiences teasing or an interrogation. She becomes discouraged and withdraws again.

By the end of the workshop, the staff decided that the idea of women's rights and health means little to women if their daily lives are circumscribed by the threat of violence. They agreed that personal safety and control over the integrity of one's body were fundamental precursors to positive sexual health and the realization of other human rights. Jijenge! decided to reorient its programs under one theme: ending violence against women.

FOSTERING A NEW AND SUSTAINABLE
ANTI-VIOLENCE VALUE SYSTEM

Staff realized that meaningful effects would be achieved only if the community accepted a new value system that embraced the goal of ending violence against women. At a grassroots level, as well as within key institutions, the primary task was to create an environment supportive of changed attitudes regarding violence. In the words of Verdiana Kamanya:

> Women alone can understand their problem and know what they should do about it. But because of how society is, she won't be able to make the changes if the people and environment don't support changes or her right to make them.

Jijenge!'s goal was to create a single, potent anti-violence message that would reach large numbers of people across social strata. The plan was to expose individuals and communities to messages and images developed to encourage personal reflection, spark public debate, and bring about change.

To prepare staff, Jijenge! organized a training workshop and discussion series. Both activities strengthened staff understanding of violence, extended their ability to analyze its effects on women's health and lives, and informed their programmatic response. Staff agreed that Jijenge!'s health care program would continue providing the usual medical and counseling services while exploring the issue of violence with clients. The capacity-building program would also continue its established activities but would focus the content of its education and training on violence. The community awareness program would launch a two-part effort: (1) a municipal awareness campaign; and (2) an intensive and sustained pilot project to create lasting change in the community of Igogo. The remainder of this chapter focuses largely on the community awareness efforts, with a particular focus on activities in the Igogo pilot area.[1]

THE IN-DEPTH PILOT PROJECT IN IGOGO

Igogo is a low-income, semiurban community of approximately 4,000 families within Mwanza. Its population comprises a number of tribal groups, including several that practice female genital cutting. As is true in many traditional communities, Igogo's leaders have the power to refuse or foster entry of intervention efforts. Jijenge! staff knew that these "gatekeepers" were the bridge to a successful community-based project.

Building a Network of Community Leaders

Jijenge! staff identified 19 community leaders, three of whom were women. The group included the community health officer, the community development officer, the village representative, several elders, and the ward secretary. After meeting with each individually, Jijenge! staff brought the leaders together for a three-day training workshop to explore their perceptions of and feelings about violence against women. While some of the men struggled with the potential personal effects of change, the workshop provided a nonadversarial environment that allowed many of them to consider other views and engage in discussion.

The process resulted in an endorsement of the anti-violence intervention and in the formation of a volunteer community interest group to guide it. Several of the community leaders who had attended the training workshop volunteered to join the group and recruit other members. Through the community interest group, several prominent community members became responsible for supervising the project in Igogo and for organizing activities to promote awareness about gender violence.

Jijenge! staff worked with the community interest group—seven women and three men ages 17–42—to draw community maps so that no part of Igogo would be neglected. The maps also identified common meeting areas so that group members could talk informally with street leaders about preventing violence—including informing them about upcoming events and getting feedback on project activities. Weekly, and then biweekly, support sessions for members of the community interest group continued for approximately one year. The sessions provided information about violence and rights, as well as technical assistance to help group members solve problems, plan activities, and facilitate discussions among community members. During these sessions, community interest group members discussed questions and issues they were encountering in their work, including how to respond to resistance and ambiguous attitudes—such as when men asserted that the project was "teaching women to misbehave, and to disrespect their husbands"—or what to do after learning that a friend was being abused by or abusing other family members.

The community interest group was highly visible within Igogo. For most, membership afforded status and respect, which served as an incentive to invest time and effort. Initially a few members requested financial compensation or incentives (e.g., bicycles) but a clear policy was maintained and only small per diems for workshops were given. Two members decided to leave the group because of the policy and new individuals were recruited. In 1998, two years after its inception, the group is still a vibrant force in Igogo and its members are seen as advocates to turn to when a community member is in crisis.

How the Igogo Community Views Violence in the Home

To create a sound basis for the development of interventions, Jijenge! conducted a needs assessment in Igogo. Assisted by the community interest group, staff conducted in-depth interviews with ten female and eight male community members and seven focus-group discussions (two female-only, two male-only, and three that were mixed) to obtain a deeper understanding of community attitudes about domestic violence, the perceived prevalence of violence, and opinions of women's rights. Members of the interest group, who could easily bring large numbers of people together, recruited participants for the research.

The needs assessment found significant community willingness to deal with violence. There was, however, resistance from some, particularly men, who accused Jijenge! and the community interest group of trying to impose new views.

The needs assessment revealed that some men feared change. They voiced anxiety and anger that women's needs were being discussed rather than their own. Some reacted strongly to the idea of sharing power and seeing women as equal. Some men could not conceive of equality and thought that removing violence would give women control over men. Men commonly made statements such as, "Jijenge! now wants to put women in control," "Watch out or you'll become the woman!" and "They will expect us in the kitchen next!" These comments revealed that violence was used to ensure women's submission in the home and maintain rigid gender roles.

Women's views were sometimes ambivalent. Some thought violence was a cultural norm, and even interpreted it as an expression of affection: "Some women like beating because after they are beaten they get gifts as an apology, so they feel they are loved." Others expressed a conditional acceptance of violence: "I guess it is okay to beat a woman who has been warned by her partner several times if she does not change."

There was resistance to bringing what was considered "private" out into the open. Before intervention activities could begin, therefore, staff invested considerable effort trying to convince men of the legitimacy of publicly discussing violence and women's rights, often framing the issue within the context of family harmony. With the support of the community interest group and respected men in the community, much of the resistance was diffused, and violence in the home was established as a subject that was appropriate for public discussion.

Staff were then ready to begin the intervention. On the basis of the needs assessment, they developed several community awareness activities, described below.

Out From Behind Closed Doors: Facilitating Debate and Discussion

Jijenge! employed several strategies and media outlets to encourage community members to discuss violence against women, as described below.

Impromptu discussions. To stimulate public dialogue on violence, community interest group facilitators began impromptu discussions with people gathered in busy public places throughout the town, including the bus stand, markets, and ferry ports. The facilitator asked thought-provoking questions, such as: "Do women experience violence in this marketplace?" and "Do you think violence is acceptable behavior?

Why or why not?" In one such discussion a market vendor responded, "Men touch us like we are tomatoes," a comment that sparked hours of lively debate.

Community theater. A common domestic violence scene was enacted in front of an audience—which typically included between 500 and 2,000 spectators. The drama was stopped at key points and audience members were encouraged to give their opinions or even to join in the drama as a family member, neighbor, elder, or other character. Jijenge! collaborated with the Mahagama Theater Group, an established troupe of actors who had put on plays about social issues in the past. Together, they developed a short drama that highlighted domestic violence and opportunities for intervention. Several members of Jijenge!'s staff, as well as community members, were trained in acting techniques and participated in the drama with the troupe.

In one skit, a young man married a woman after paying dowry to her parents. After living together for several months the young man began coming home drunk and subjecting his wife to physical and verbal abuse. At this point the actors would clap loudly and begin drawing the audience in with questions such as, "Does this happen in our community? Why?" or "What do you think she should do?" After a brief discussion, the actors would resume the drama and the woman would seek help from friends, family members, neighbors, and local leaders—all of whom placed the responsibility for abuse on her, suggesting that she try to be a better wife, try not to provoke her husband, or learn to live with the abuse. At this stage, the actors would stop again and ask the audience, "Is the woman to blame?" or "Do you agree with the advice she has received?" An audience member who disagreed would be given the opportunity to jump in and act out an alternative behavior or express a different opinion in character. For example, a participant might show ways that the woman could protect herself when her husband comes home drunk, or what a friend, neighbor, community leader, or parent might do if asked for help, or how a friend of the abuser could encourage him to end the violence. At the end of the play, learning materials were distributed and a brief discussion was held about what the community can do to prevent domestic violence.

Special public events. Events that combined education on violence and women's rights with fun and games were held on International Women's Day and on World AIDS Day. For example, on World AIDS Day, a program on sexual abuse and violence against children, particularly girls, was held at a local primary school. A video—*Karate Kids,* by Street Kids International—was shown, in which animated characters tell the story of how girls and boys can be forced into sex work. After each show, Jijenge! staff led separate discussions with teachers and children about how to keep children safe from abuse.

Story booklets. In a booklet on domestic violence—*Stop Violence Against Women at Home!*—a woman recounts to friends her experience of being abused by her husband, and the husband recounts the incident to other men. In the booklet, women offer their views on how violence affects them and assert their belief that they have a right to be safe in their homes: "For me, too, violence takes away my dignity and self-respect," and "We have a right to live in a safe and respectful environment—everyone does!" From the male perspective, nonviolent men explain to the abusive man the consequences of violence for women and children and offer suggestions on how to deal more appropriately with anger. In one vignette, a community elder says to the husband, "But John, your wife is an intelligent human being. You should discuss issues with her, not beat her." Later, he suggests, "For me, when I am very angry, I take time out and when I return later, I feel calmer and ready to [talk] with my wife." The booklet also offers guidelines to facilitate its use in groups, schools, and homes.

Booklet clubs. These single- and mixed-sex groups were established by word of mouth on 18 streets in Igogo. Each group initially drew close to 50 women and men. They met weekly or every other week (depending on the availability of participants) for 1–2 hours, with a community interest group facilitator present.[2] Over the course of six to eight sessions, the clubs discussed the issues of violence and rights, using the pocket-sized booklets *Girls and Women Have Rights!* and *Stop Violence at Home!* as discussion guides. The booklets and discussion guides gave facilitators confidence and alleviated their fears about speaking in front of groups on controversial topics. At the same time, both the content and the participatory methods used by the booklet clubs were new and challenging for all involved. One community interest group member observed, "The way we are conducting sessions in booklet clubs in a participatory way took time for people to cope with, as they were expecting us to teach them."

Posters. The *Take Action!* poster portrayed a street scene with individuals recalling how their behavior changed in order to end violence. Messages on the poster, communicated by women and men, included: "We've found a new way—instead of fighting we talk about our problems," "When my partner says no, I don't force her to have sex," "When I hear violence at my neighbor's house I gather other people and we go help," and "Don't go home angry! Calm down before you return home."

Both the posters and booklets were widely distributed to other nongovernmental organizations, health centers, businesses, schools, religious groups, and government agencies. The materials were also distributed at each of the public events and discussions described above, giving community members something tangible to refer to during and after these events.

Radio programs. Igogo residents were also exposed to radio programs that explored different types of violence (e.g., domestic violence, rape, sexual harassment, and female genital cutting), their causes and consequences, and ways to prevent them. The programs, broadcast throughout the Lake Zone, were produced in a variety of formats, including interviews, roundtable discussions, and personal narratives.

Murals. Five-by-five-foot murals were painted on eight storefronts and walls throughout Igogo. Using informal language, the murals posed questions about the validity of resorting to violence during an argument or participating in sexual harassment on the street. Several murals also used a fictitious couple to depict positive relationships. In one, a couple speaks to the community about their relationship: The woman proudly states, "My partner and I decide together when to have sex," and the man backs her up, proclaiming, "It's true!" Another shows a couple embracing, with the man saying, "I don't hit my partner, we talk about our problems instead."

Intervening in the Cycle of Violence: Watch Groups and Working with Men

The public discussions and media messages helped Jijenge! begin to change the community's value system regarding violence against women. To actually stop violence, however, these emerging values needed more active support and direction.

In effect, there was virtually no support for victims of violence. Community members viewed the courts and legal system as inaccessible and expensive, and people did not intervene in other couples' "business." To create a system of community support for victims of domestic violence, the community interest group recruited 16 volunteers who were committed to developing a watch group to provide support and intervention services. As was the case with the community interest group itself, the involvement of men was deemed crucial; six members of the watch group were men. Two male members spoke about their motivation:

> *After attending a seminar from Jijenge! then I understood the meaning of violence against women and got the motivation to come back to teach others.*

> *I feel bad when a woman is being violated. When I heard there are people who are stopping violence I was glad and joined the group.*

To prepare the watch group, Jijenge! held a three-day interactive workshop on violence prevention. Using the framework of women's rights, the sessions encouraged participants to reflect on their own experiences, deepen their understanding of the causes and consequences of violence, and offer practical steps to end violence. The watch group then began distributing Jijenge! print materials, promoting involvement in the booklet clubs, and documenting domestic violence on each Igogo street, using forms to record any violence they witnessed or that was reported to them.

Igogo homes are built close together. Residents share communal courtyards, in which they cook, do laundry, and attend to other chores. The family spends a great deal of time in this communal space—privacy is minimal, and neighbors commonly know intimate details about one another's relationships and families. As a result, community members are often aware of families who are experiencing domestic violence.

Watch group members believed in the importance of ending the silence around domestic violence and felt they needed to take action. They began offering assistance to women experiencing violence, speaking privately to the woman and/or man involved about the violence and available support services, or seeking assistance from the *balozi* (block leaders),[3] many of whom had participated in Jijenge! workshops. If watch group members witnessed an act of violence, they sought support from others in the group or community and intervened collectively, when appropriate. In extreme cases (e.g., if a woman's life was in danger) they alerted the police. Any action was carefully balanced against concerns for the privacy and safety of the woman experiencing violence and the safety of watch group members. Seeing community members move from talking about violence to acting to stop it created an increasingly supportive climate for women, and an increasingly uncomfortable one for male perpetrators of violence.

The added responsibilities associated with the watch group were time-consuming for local leaders, who already had to fulfill many supportive roles in the community. Hence, it was difficult for the *balozi* or watch group members to find time to follow through with all the needs that were surfacing, particularly as community expectations rose. A member of the community interest group explained: "Women are expecting to get more support from us, they want us to intervene or escort them to the social welfare agency, but we are just volunteers. It is difficult to find time."

It was becoming clear that changing men's behavior is critical to stopping violence against women. Indeed, there were even requests for workshops from men interested in resolving conflicts, improving family harmony, and learning more about women's rights, increasingly the subject of conversation among community members. Some of these men had been suspicious of the project early on. In response, Jijenge! conducted three-day participatory workshops for men that discussed gender roles, cultural practices affecting women's lives, sexual health, status, violence against women, and women's rights as human rights.

Some of the men who participated were argumentative, despite the fact that they were attending of their own accord. There were often a few men in each group

who were particularly vocal or disruptive. The female facilitator would talk privately
with them to encourage productive participation. A shift in approach from women's
rights to family harmony[4] also facilitated constructive participation. Useful exercises
included asking men to specify how violence negatively affected intimate relationships and the family in general. Another strategy was to ask participants to discuss
human rights, at which point they tended to think of their own. When a facilitator
asked whether these rights were applicable to both men and women, the men often
had a hard time defending their applicability to men alone. Controversy was more
likely to arise over women's right to initiate sex or to make autonomous decisions,
rather than their right to be free from violence.[5]

These forums were useful in encouraging reflection on topics that are not generally discussed, particularly among men. Most importantly, they offered a direct means
to reach men, to increase their understanding of the implications of abuse, and to help
them develop strategies to confront violence in their own homes and communities.

While the community leaders sought to change attitudes and values, the Jijenge!
project also continued to provide services and collaborate with existing institutions
serving women. These activities are described below.

Sexual Health Services Aimed at Reducing Violence

Clinicians and counselors at the Jijenge! clinic continued discussing the root causes of
reproductive health problems with clients, but with an eye toward reducing violence
toward women. They recognized that violence in the home is manifested in ways
beyond physical injury. Further, they knew that the threat of violence can prevent
women from asserting themselves in a relationship, protecting themselves from disease, or seeking health care. For example, if a woman requested treatment for a sexually transmitted infection, the clinician would explore how the infection was contracted
by addressing, for example, the sexual and social dynamics leading to transmission
such as lack of negotiating power in a relationship over when to have sex, partner
refusal to use condoms, or multiple sex partners. Clients had the option of seeing a
counselor for further discussion or support in developing necessary skills for communication, negotiation of condom use, and safer sex practices.

This gender-oriented approach to service delivery was groundbreaking in Mwanza
and the Lake Zone and was in great demand. Women traveled to the clinic from other
regions in the Lake Zone, even crossing the border from Kenya and Uganda, having
heard about Jijenge! through word of mouth or radio programs. As a female client
from Kenya said:

After hearing about Jijenge! services, I decided to come here. The services are good, everyone is treated equally, they listen to your problems and give full information. I was cared for better than at other places.

Women and men, individually and as couples, sought additional counseling independent of clinical services as they attempted to build mutually respectful, non-violent relationships. The sexual health and HIV counselors also told women about outside services that were available for victims of violence and made appropriate referrals to police stations, social welfare agencies, hospitals, and courts. To help women secure acceptable treatment, the counselors reviewed their rights as part of making the referral. When necessary, they provided written introduction or referral notes for clients to take to the appropriate agency. In some cases (e.g., during one-time hospital visits or during the prosecution of their cases in court), the counselors accompanied clients to the agencies and served as their advocates. Counselors also encouraged clients to keep them informed of their cases and maintained contact with other service providers as clients moved through the system.

Making Changes to End Violence

The existing service agencies in Mwanza did not have the capacity or perspective needed to provide appropriate assistance to women. Jijenge! worked with selected individuals and groups to improve this capacity. The aim was to enable service agencies to make changes that would increase women's safety and health. Two major activities were conducted to accomplish these goals.

Changing the perspective of service institutions. Jijenge! identified the police department, the social welfare department, a women's group within the Catholic church, health service providers, and partner nongovernmental organizations working on HIV/AIDS as having both the need and the potential for change. A few individuals from each organization were invited to participate in the Jijenge! training program. A series of three-day workshops fostered personal reflection about sexual health, women's rights, and violence, as well as an examination of these issues in the workplace and the community. Each organization also developed a plan of action for its workplace, and the training coordinator subsequently provided onsite assistance to participants as they carried out their plans. This training-of-trainers approach worked well with those groups that were independently motivated to explore the issue of violence and make changes within their work environments. However, the workshops had less effect on larger agencies, such as the police and social welfare departments, where the participants lacked the power to overcome entrenched institutional structures and widespread unfamiliarity with or hostility toward concepts of gender and rights.

Internship program. An internship program oriented reproductive and maternal health service providers from the government and private sector toward more women-centered services that addressed the root causes of women's poor sexual health. Working side by side with Jijenge! clinicians and counselors, interns observed consultations with clients. They were exposed to and practiced listening skills, open-ended questioning, respectful and educational communication, and confidential record keeping. Over 80 interns from the Lake Zone were trained. One intern, a public health nurse, reported, "I can now talk with a woman or client in such a way that they can explain their problem freely."

PRELIMINARY ASSESSMENT

It is difficult to measure change in personal behaviors that have multiple determinants and may be manifested in myriad (and even contradictory) ways. Anecdotal evidence from staff, the community interest group, volunteers, and other community members indicates that there is now greater openness in questioning and discussing violence. As one shopkeeper commented, "Things are changing. In past days it was in some ways difficult to even speak on women's rights and violence against women, but nowadays people are discussing these issues freely." A male community member stated, "People are now asking themselves if it is true that women really do have a right not to be beaten." And a member of the watch group reported, "Street leaders are congratulating us because cases of violence have decreased these days."

Celestina Nyenga, who headed the Igogo program, reflected on its progress:

> The awareness campaign has helped people, especially women, to have courage and words to speak out about the violence. At the beginning of the project, while talking of violence or rights during the focus groups, women would hide their faces behind their khangas [a printed cloth commonly worn by women]. But now women are stronger, they are willing to speak and are gaining confidence.

Slowly, attitudes toward gender violence show signs of change, as women and men learn to behave differently toward one another. One watch group member remarked, "There were some men who were cruel to their wives, not sharing responsibilities in the families, but now they have started helping their wives."

The testimony of shopkeepers and residents in Igogo suggests that the murals have been effective at stimulating people to think about gender violence. As women in the community observed:

People started to discuss the mural, some said it is true what they say about violence against women, while others say it is wrong. People were thinking that violence is beating only, and they were not aware of other types of violence.

I feel proud to have messages on women's rights and violence [on my shop] because I myself did not know that women and men are equal in the sense of human rights. I thought that men are more important than women.

As a woman, I feel very happy to have such a message on my shop. I would like to have it forever. I feel now it is time for us as women to fight for our rights and the violence against us.

Two men in the community made the following observations:

Most men read the message and make comments like "Jijenge! has started to build up women. Women nowadays are more aware of their rights. We should be more careful."

At the beginning people were shocked. They would look at the mural and just leave. Now they discuss [it]. Many people also request that the murals be painted on their homes to educate their family and other people.

There has been an observable shift in people's willingness to intervene against violence. A watch group member told of a couple fighting outside their home: "People said, 'This is violence!' and they stopped the fight and supported the woman so she would not get any more injuries." Women and men reported that they were more willing to address violence since the Jijenge! project began, as they feel there is a greater sense of community responsibility. As another watch group member described it: "Together they agreed that as community members they can end the violence."

Even the training efforts with the police have begun to pay off, as illustrated by the experience of one member of a community interest group who was taking a bus home when a man started harassing her:

He said I was a prostitute and other bad things. I went to the police station and said what had happened. A female police officer told two policemen in civilian clothes to go with me to get the man. We found him and told him he was needed at the police station. The man started laughing and said that he had only been kidding and I shouldn't have taken him seriously. I told him that it was serious and that he had embarrassed me in front of all those people.

The police officers with me told him he had to come. At the police station the female police officer told him that sexual harassment was not a joke and locked him up. The next day he was sent to the local court. Those elders heard the case and fined *him 30,000 shillings [approximately US$35]. The man promised he would never repeat the behavior and now, every time I see him, he respectfully greets me as his sister.*

LESSONS LEARNED

Meaningful behavior change is a gradual, long-term process. Service provider organizations and donor agencies need to recognize that the introduction of new ideas and hoped-for changes in behavior take time. Program strategies and timelines need to take into account the fact that individuals and communities go through various stages to process and internalize information, reflect on the advantages of any proposed change, and build confidence and support before practicing alternative behaviors. This is especially true when addressing an issue such as violence, which requires individuals to question and adjust fundamental beliefs about themselves and their relationships. Unrealistic short-term expectations can demoralize staff and community members. While Jijenge! had originally planned to spend six months in Igogo, ultimately one and a half years were necessary to responsibly and effectively begin to address violence in the community.

Behavior change and public dialogue are more likely to be fostered if anti-violence messages are received from a variety of sources over a period of time. The discussion of ideas in a wide range of public forums is key, particularly in the context of a poorly developed communication/media sources. Recruiting broad-based support from various parts of the community lends credibility and influence to new ideas. Encouraging community members to raise the issues themselves increases acceptance. As community awareness coordinator Celestina Nyenga commented:

> *The more people in the community who are talking about violence and feel it is wrong, the safer women become. Abusers are aware of this changing social climate and fear that their violent behavior may now bring sanctions against them.*

The rights-based approach to women's sexual health may be too diffuse; identifying tangible priority subjects such as violence in the home may be more effective. Although the concept of women having basic rights was new, its application to a specific issue that the community felt strongly about resonated for many people. Jijenge! staff found that while promoting a broad spectrum of rights was overwhelming and alienating, focusing on one tangible issue and discussing women's rights within that context was effective and empowering. Once people, particularly women, identified violence as a legitimate problem, they were motivated to find a solution; for many, the idea of rights was part of the solution. Nyenga explains:

> *Talking about all of the different women's rights with people who are unfamiliar scares many women. But if you talk about violence against women and emphasize that*

women have a right to live without violence, then they feel that rights protect them instead of endanger them.

Bringing topics deemed "private" into the public sphere is possible and necessary. Women and men are willing to talk about domestic violence but need sustained support, including support from community leaders, to engage in public discussion and debate. Many community members remarked that at first, discussing violence makes things worse because it forces women to identify with the pain in their lives. Facilitators of the community projects must understand this situation and support women to move forward and take action to change their situations.

Addressing men separately as well as in mixed-sex groups is crucial. Working with men is critical if progress is to be made in preventing gender violence. Jijenge! used messages directed at men in its community awareness efforts, as well as in men-only workshops. Key strategies included using nonviolent men as role models in information materials, engaging community leaders and elders in fostering a new value system, and encouraging communication and discouraging abuse in intimate relationships.

Endorsement from influential figures in the community, both male and female, and the development of a more formal system of support for women, are critical. In Tanzania, where power is hierarchical and entrenched, it was essential for Jijenge! to have the support of other prominent, established organizations and community leaders.

Service providers at all levels—teachers, police, health workers, and community members—need to be sensitized to the issue of domestic violence and given tools to identify it and take action against it. Community-level efforts are especially important where the service-delivery sector is undeveloped. It is essential to look beyond institutional service providers to local and traditional governing bodies. This is particularly true in resource-poor settings, where official government services are often weak or nonexistent. Community leaders are often the first source of assistance for women and can have tremendous influence on public opinion.

Staff and community volunteers need sustained support and opportunities to build skills and confidence when working on controversial issues. It is important to provide forums for staff and volunteers to internalize the issues, reflect on their effects in their own lives, and recognize and draw strength from the changes they experience as they facilitate similar changes in the lives of others.

AFTERWORD

The Jijenge! project's current priorities include improving health service delivery within municipal and government institutions. An extensive training program for health service providers at a maternal and child health clinic will culminate in the development of a training guide for health care providers in the Lake Zone. While Jijenge!'s sexual health center has closed, the Igogo group continues to be involved in many activities, including creating and conducting community role-plays about violence and human rights. Support to the group of volunteers in Igogo continues, and Jijenge!'s program on violence, now more specifically focused on female genital cutting, is reaching new communities. The Jijenge! project is also working closely with a new organization, Kivulini, which is dedicated to preventing violence against women in Mwanza.

In efforts to build on and advance lessons learned at Jijenge!, the authors have established Raising Voices, a new project that develops programmatic tools and forms partnerships with organizations working at the community level to prevent violence against women and children. We developed *Mobilizing Communities to Prevent Domestic Violence: An Organizational Resource Guide*, which translates the concept of communities organizing against violence into practical strategies that organizations can use as they confront domestic violence. We are currently working with partner organizations in Kenya, Tanzania, and Uganda to implement the approach embodied in this document.

Acknowledgments

Many thanks to Celestina Nyenga, Rose Bwibo, Verdiana Kamanya, Levina Mosha, Clara Mayala, Pelagia Lugeleka, Gladness Oluto, and Emmy Mangweha for their commitment to women's rights and for their assistance in compiling materials for this chapter. Thanks also to Marco Tibasima, whose accomplished artwork put a public face on Jijenge!'s ideas.

Notes

1   A number of the interventions, such as the health services and capacity-building programs and several of the awareness-raising efforts, were implemented on a larger scale in urban Mwanza.

2   Because these groups proved to be too large to permit useful discussion, the facilitators began breaking them down into smaller groups. When possible, additional community interest group members were recruited to lead the additional groups; when no facilitators were available, the participants were encouraged to take copies of the booklet, which included a discussion guide, and lead their own small groups.

3   *Balozi* are official neighborhood problem-solvers. They are generally older men and women who command substantial respect.

4   Successfully confronting domestic violence within the framework and language of family harmony is also discussed elsewhere in this book. See, for example, Chapter 20.

5   The issue of male victimization in violence was rarely raised during the sessions.

References

Borgdorff, Martinus Willem. 1994. *Epidemiology of HIV-1 Infection in Mwanza Region, Tanzania.* Amsterdam: Royal Tropical Institute.

Bureau of Statistics (Tanzania) and Macro International. 1997. *Tanzania Demographic and Health Survey 1996.* Calverton, MD: Bureau of Statistics and Macro International, Inc.

Grosskurth, Heiner, Frank Mosha, James Todd, Ezra Mwijarubi, Arnoud Klokke, Kesheni Senkoro, Philippe Mayaud, John Changalucha, Angus Nicoll, Gina ka-Gina, James Newell, Kokugonza Mugeye, David Mabey, and Richard Hayes. 1995. "Impact of improved treatment of sexually transmitted diseases on HIV infection in rural Tanzania: Randomised controlled trial," *Lancet* 346(8974): 530–536.

Tanzania Planning Commission. 1992. *National Population Policy IV.* Dar es Salaam: President's Office.

Contact information

Lori S. Michau
Dipak Naker
Raising Voices
P.O. Box 6770
Kampala, Uganda
telephone: 256-41-531-186
fax: 256-41-531-249
mobile: 256-71-839-626
e-mail: rvoices@igc.org
www.raisingvoices.org

23

Protecting and Empowering Girls: Confronting the Roots of Female Genital Cutting in Kenya

Asha Mohamud, Samson Radeny, Nancy Yinger, Zipporah Kittony, and Karin Ringheim

More than two million girls each year—or approximately 5,500 every day—undergo genital cutting, the partial or total removal of the female external genitalia (see Box 1). It is estimated that some 100 million females, the great majority of whom live in Africa, have been subjected to this practice.[1] Genital cutting is considered part of a larger rite of passage from childhood to adulthood, and circumcision rituals have played cultural, social, and even economic functions viewed as important in the societies in which they are conducted. By regulating sexuality, female circumcision is believed to prevent girls' promiscuity, preserve virginity, promote cleanliness, and improve fertility, thereby increasing the chances that a girl will marry and improve her family's economic status. By means of the ritual surrounding circumcision, communities integrate youth into the local "moral order," and educate their children about sex in the context of preparing them for adult life. As a social and cultural occasion, the initiation ceremony provides the father with an opportunity to exhibit his wealth and increase his status in the community, and gives girls an opportunity to receive social recognition. The process often involves a period of isolation; preparation by an elder; spiritual cleansing; physical rituals such as bathing, shaving of hair, and/or genital cutting; offerings, prayers, and blessings; and a celebration with traditional food, dress, music, and dance. Finally the girl is welcomed back into society with changed status.

Genital cutting itself, however, can have serious health consequences. Short-term complications include hemorrhage, wound infection, urine retention, shock, sepsis, and even death. Long-term complications include scarring; cysts; obstructed labor, which can lead to perineal lacerations, bleeding and infection, possible brain damage to infants, and fistula formation; and sexual and psychological problems. In the Central African Republic, Egypt, and Eritrea, the only countries for which such data are

---

Box 1. Defining female genital cutting

The World Health Organization classifies FGC into four broad categories:

- Type I or clitoridectomy (also called "sunna"): Removal of the clitoral hood with or without removal of part or all of the clitoris.
- Type II or excision: Removal of the clitoris together with part or all of the labia minora.
- Type III or infibulation: Removal of part or all of the external genitalia (clitoris, labia minora, and labia majora) and stitching/narrowing the vaginal opening, leaving a small hole for urine and menstrual flow.
- Type IV or unclassified: All other operations on the female genitalia, including:
  - Pricking, piercing, stretching, or incision of the clitoris and/or labia;
  - Cauterization by burning the clitoris and surrounding tissues;
  - Incisions to the vaginal wall, scraping ("angurya" cuts) or cutting ("gishiri" cuts) of the vagina and surrounding tissue; and
  - Introduction of corrosive substances or herbs into the vagina.

Source: World Health Organization 2000.

---

available, one million women have suffered the adverse health effects of female genital cutting (FGC). (Carr 1997).

In addition, while there is no published evidence linking FGC with increased risk of HIV, hepatitis B, and other blood-borne diseases, the theoretical links are compelling (World Health Organization 2000). Transmission may result from the use of nonsterile instruments to perform the procedure, often in group settings, and in repeated cutting before labor and restitching after delivery. Likelihood of transmission may also be increased as a result of a higher incidence of wounds and abrasions during sexual intercourse (Kun 1997).

Over the past decade, there has been increasing recognition among many African governments, women's organizations, and the international community that FGC harms women's health and violates their bodily integrity and human rights. The World Health Organization (WHO) has consistently and unequivocally advised that FGC, in any of its forms, should not be practiced by any health professional in any setting—including hospitals and other health care establishments (WHO 1982, 1993). Calls for protection of women and children or eradication of harmful traditional practices have been articulated by a number of international agreements.[2]

The Cairo Programme of Action, which regards FGC as a fundamental violation of basic rights and as a practice that seeks to control women's sexuality, calls on governments to "urgently take steps to stop the practice" and to provide treatment, education, and counseling (United Nations 1995, paragraphs 7.35 and 7.40). The Beijing Platform of Action identifies FGC as a form of sex discrimination that begins early in life (United

Nations 1996). Governments that are signatories to these two documents are responsible for protecting girls and women against harmful traditional practices, including FGC. Bolstered by these commitments, a growing number of advocacy and public education programs are seeking to raise awareness about the health and social implications of FGC and, ultimately, to eliminate the practice.

Maendeleo Ya Wanawake Organization,[3] a national grassroots women's organization committed to improving the health and well-being of Kenyan women (hereafter referred to as Maendeleo), was the first group—governmental or nongovernmental—to mount a major campaign against FGC in Kenya. Despite official political opposition to the practice, the path to changing people's attitudes and behaviors about such a sensitive issue was neither clear nor straightforward. Along the way, Maendeleo and its partner, the Program for Appropriate Technology in Health (PATH), learned what worked and what did not. They delved deeply into the values and traditions that underlie the circumcision ritual. This chapter describes the experience of Maendeleo and PATH in four districts in Kenya.

FEMALE GENITAL CUTTING IN KENYA

It is estimated that female circumcision is carried out in half of the districts in Kenya. The Kenya Demographic and Health Survey estimates that at least 38 percent of Kenyan women ages 15–49 have undergone some form of FGC (National Council for Population and Development, Central Bureau of Statistics [Kenya], and Macro International 1999). The figure is probably an underestimate, however, because it does not include the North Eastern districts, where the prevalence of FGC is believed to be 100 percent.

During the colonial era, missionaries and colonial doctors attempted to outlaw the practice, arguing that it was dangerous, unnatural, and un-Christian. In a backlash against colonialism, however, pro-independence Kenyans viewed the campaign against FGC as an assault on their self-determination and cultural heritage. Despite an intense post-colonial debate, the government of newly independent Kenya did not establish specific laws or programs to curb the practice. Nonetheless, the unquestioning acceptance of FGC had begun to wane. Some Christian families, particularly Protestants, followed church proscriptions and ended the practice within their families.[4]

By the late 1980s, a few women's groups and health organizations in Kenya were speaking out against genital cutting. In 1990, President Daniel arap Moi publicly stated that FGC should be abandoned, saying, "I will not allow children to die while I am the leader of this country."[5] Kenya was also a signatory to the documents resulting from the 1994 Cairo and 1995 Beijing conferences. Although Moi's position on FGC was not made into law, some tribal chiefs complied and banned the practice in their communities. As a result, some families abandoned the practice, but others began circumcising their daughters surreptitiously (e.g., late at night without a public ceremony). Still others, concerned that the practice might soon be prohibited outright, began to circumcise their female children at an earlier age. The trend was toward earlier circumcision by health care providers performing less-extensive types of the procedure (Types I and II).[6] Overall, however, the prevalence of FGC had fallen very little (Maendeleo Ya Wanawake Organization 1991).

In response to this problem, leaders of Maendeleo met with representatives of the Program for Appropriate Technology in Health. PATH had been providing technical assistance to Nigeria's National Association of Nurses and Midwives on an anti-FGC project in that country. With support from the Wallace Global Fund,[7] Maendeleo staff visited the Nigerian project and attended the 1990 conference of the Inter-Africa Committee on Harmful Traditional Practices. These experiences strengthened Maendeleo's commitment to mobilize its grassroots membership to work toward elimination of FGC in Kenya.

LEARNING ABOUT THE ISSUE

By 1991, Maendeleo and PATH had selected four districts (Kisii, Meru, Narok, and Samburu), reputed to have high prevalence of FGC, in which to develop and test an intervention to eradicate the practice.[8] To guide the intervention design, project staff began with quantitative and qualitative community studies to learn more about the communities themselves and the role of circumcision in community life (Maendeleo Ya Wanawake Organization and PATH 1993a, 1993b).

Community Characteristics and Circumcision Practices

The studies showed that the districts varied significantly. Each had its own majority ethnic group and mix of religions, including Catholic, Protestant, independent churches, traditional religions, and, to a lesser extent, Islam. Female literacy rates ranged from 9 percent in Samburu to 66 percent in Meru. Marriage customs, which provide an indication of women's autonomy, also varied. The percentage of women who reported selecting their own spouse (as opposed to their parents' making the choice for them) ranged from 10 percent in Samburu to 83 percent in Meru.

The prevalence of FGC was high, although a slight declining trend at younger ages emerged. Virtually 100 percent of women over 50 years of age had been circumcised, while 78 percent of 15–19-year-olds reported having been circumcised. Meru District had the lowest rate (73.5 percent), while virtually every woman in Kisii was circumcised. Circumcisions took place during the months of April, August, and December, coinciding with school holidays and harvest time. Most circumcisions took place in the village, at the initiate's house, or in the bush. A few procedures (5.2 percent) took place in health centers or hospitals. Procedure type varied from excision of the clitoris to infibulation, the most severe form of FGC.

The rites surrounding the circumcision are described as a time of joy, gift-giving, and festivity at home and in the community, with visitors, feasting, dancing, special privileges, and an abundance of good food. Girls are given special treatment, showered with gifts (e.g., new clothes, ornaments), and granted favors (e.g., separate rooms from the uncircumcised, the right to tease those who are younger and uncircumcised, and permission to loiter without being reprimanded by parents).

In Samburu and Narok, circumcision is followed by marriage, usually on the same day. Marriage is a "dream come true" because the girl receives wedding presents and her family receives dowry and recognition. For girls from well-to-do families, celebrations can last longer than a week. The longer the celebrations, the more gifts a girl can request and receive.

Community Attitudes Toward FGC

According to a baseline survey of a random sample of 1,365 women ages 14–60 a majority of women (63 percent) in the four districts favored continuation of FGC, while 37 percent opposed it (Maendeleo Ya Wanawake Organization and PATH 1993b).[9] Older women tended to support infibulation. Two-thirds (63 percent) of all women planned to circumcise their own daughters. Among the benefits of the practice, they cited: (1) its value as a marker of girls' transition to adulthood, including their maturing sexual attitudes and practices; (2) enhancement of girls' marriage prospects; (3) promotion of respect in the community for parents in exchange for having instilled good cultural values in their daughters; and (4) the belief that circumcised girls tend to "make better, more obedient wives." Although many community members reported knowing of a few women in their community and of Kenyan tribes who do not circumcise, they viewed such people as "deviants who are copying Western cultures" and "cowards" whose daughters were "dirty" (Maendeleo Ya Wanawake Organization and PATH 1993a). Such mothers were often isolated from other community members as a form of punishment.

In focus groups, girls themselves tended to assert that circumcision was a good practice that should be continued, although they were more likely to favor less drastic forms of the procedure. They mentioned that it provided them with the opportunity to (1) be recognized by peers; (2) socialize with boys who would eventually marry them; (3) prove their bravery and readiness to experience pain (such as they might endure in childbirth or during other hardships); and (4) show their parents that they would do anything for them. They also said that circumcised girls feel superior, since they receive information on boy–girl relationships during the healing period. The majority of girls feared that if they refused circumcision, they would be cursed by their parents, ostracized by the community and their peers, and, worst of all, not get married. They believed that uncircumcised girls develop physical problems, including an overgrown malodorous clitoris, difficult childbirth because of a narrow birth canal, and, in some cases, mental problems.

A few girls (both circumcised and uncircumcised) did not want the practice to continue, characterizing the procedure as humiliating, painful, and traumatic. These girls insisted that there was no difference between the attitudes, practices, and aspirations of circumcised and uncircumcised girls. They argued that other mothers—not their peers—harbored negative opinions of uncircumcised girls. They added that girls from communities that do not practice circumcision get married and are highly educated, respected, and maintain a measure of independence from their parents and from community influences; in addition, they are seen as Christians whose parents are progressive and conscientious. The girls admitted, however, that members of their own communities do not share their views and that those who refuse to be circumcised are looked down upon and isolated as outcasts.

Fathers in the four districts expressed a range of attitudes toward the practice. Some stated that FGC was a tradition that represents negative values. Some who defended the practice felt that circumcised women tend to be more reserved and submissive, whereas uncircumcised women are overly sexy and unclean, lack moral values, and "tend to be rude, bossy, do not behave according to the cultural norm, and disrespect their age mates, parents, and elders in general."

Boys in the four districts felt strongly that the practice should continue. Most stated that they would not marry uncircumcised girls, who they claimed were dirty, childish, disrespectful, aggressive, overly sexy, ignorant, nonconformist, cowardly, and a curse to the community. Some boys regarded circumcised girls as "good wives," who, having received training in preparation for the rite of passage, "know their place in the community." A minority of boys disagreed with this view, saying that they admired uncircumcised women because they are independent and make better wives.

Perceptions of Health Risks of FGC

The baseline survey had found that 80 percent of circumcisions had taken place in group settings. In 71 percent of these cases, a single blade was used to circumcise all participants.

Scarring, hemorrhage, infection, urinary retention, painful intercourse, and perineal tears were reported. Not surprisingly, the severity of complications increased with the more severe types of circumcision. For example, infibulation was more likely to be associated with difficult childbirth, perineal tearing, and hemorrhage than were less severe forms. Only 18.5 percent of women interviewed reported that they had no complications.

Despite these circumstances, many mothers did not associate difficult childbirth, painful intercourse, anemia, or even septic wounds with circumcision. In fact, they believed the operation eased childbirth. Even when mothers were aware that FGC had harmful effects, they still felt inclined to support what they perceived as a good tradition.[10] A few mothers who understood the health effects of FGC expressed a strong desire for the practice to be discontinued. They felt that it was outdated, meaningless, dehumanizing, contrary to religious teachings, and an abuse of human rights and dignity.

Many girls seemed to be weighing mixed messages about the health risks of FGC. Many were aware of the potential consequences, including septic wounds, scarring, and death resulting from excessive bleeding. However, some expressed uncertainty about whether these problems actually occur; and for most girls the existence of such problems did not outweigh their desire for the practice to continue. Further, the majority of girls in Kisii felt that the type of circumcision (Type I) they had undergone was not serious enough to warrant alarm, especially since most had been circumcised by health care providers.

Many men attributed the negative consequences of FGC to witchcraft, bad luck, and other supernatural powers. Boys were generally aware of the health problems associated with FGC, but nevertheless supported the practice. A few boys who opposed the practice argued that after circumcision many women cannot reach orgasm.

Decisionmaking: Who Are the Custodians of Culture?

Many women stated that, even if they wanted circumcision to be discontinued, they were not in a position to enforce its eradication. First, they lacked information to convince men of the dangers of FGC. Moreover, many women stated that men and elders are the custodians of culture and should make the decision to continue or stop the practice. Women felt that FGC could be eradicated if men dictated it. Paradoxically, most fathers interviewed cited women as the biggest barrier to the eradication of FGC, saying that their wives enjoyed and looked forward to the circumcision, as it was a time for them to dance and entertain their friends. Some fathers who opposed the practice stated that they went along with it to prevent marital discord.

While some men and boys stated that women are the main perpetrators of FGC and declared that they would support an eradication campaign spearheaded by women, data on decisionmaking about FGC at the family level showed that men as well as women are implicated in the continuation of the practice and that girls have less say, particularly in Kisii, Narok, and Samburu.[11] It is difficult, however, to isolate the influence of family members, or even of the family unit, on the practice. As a Maendeleo official said:

> The tradition of female circumcision is so deeply entrenched in the culture, and decisions regarding the practice are not made by individuals. In addition to the father, the mother, and the girl, we have the community and the extended family system. This makes it difficult for one individual or family to decide on its own without pressure from others.

STEP ONE: PROMOTING HEALTH AND CHALLENGING FEMALE GENITAL CUTTING

Armed with the information from the baseline studies, staff of Maendeleo and PATH understood that to change deeply rooted perceptions, beliefs, and behaviors about FGC, they had to engage members of the communities in a far-reaching examination of their perceptions. They developed a three-part strategy:

- Raise awareness about the harmful effects of female genital cutting;
- Develop a strategy to promote a positive image of uncircumcised girls; and
- Develop an alternative rite of passage for girls that would replace initiation by cutting.

Garnering Community Support

Over the next five years, Maendeleo staff worked with community members to help them evaluate their own traditions and identity. Staff knew that challenging a deeply entrenched tradition could lead to feelings of anger and betrayal; indeed, staff from the Family Planning Association of Kenya reported being whipped during an anti-FGC campaign in Meru District. They also knew that people would cite the goal of opposing "foreign interference" to defend circumcision customs (Kenya Family Planning Association 1995). As one high school girl told project volunteers, "I just feel that circumcision should be continued because it is part of our culture. We should not be influenced by Western cultures." To minimize opposition, project staff organized district-specific and national-level workshops, involving a minimum of 50 participants each, at which they reviewed findings of the community studies with chiefs, elders, religious leaders, government officials, health personnel, local volunteers, and women leaders and sought their input on the design of follow-up activities.

Initially, community members, including some local health officials, asked Maendeleo why elimination of FGC was more critical than other community needs such as treatment of malaria, which is rampant during the rainy season. Staff focused on the health consequences of FGC, using anatomical models with removable parts showing normal genitalia, different types of FGC, and complications such as perineal tears and scarring of the vulva. Many participants were surprised to hear some women admit that they had suffered health complications or sexual problems.

The workshops succeeded in promoting discussions among members of the community. One or two vocal supporters of eradication could always be found among many wary members, most of whom were fascinated to hear their feelings. For example, at a workshop in Meru some of the elders reminded the group that "in [the village of] Njuri Necheke, elders resolved to reject the practice of FGC in 1956" and supported Maendeleo's efforts to revive their pledge. Indeed, the majority felt the community should be educated about the risks of FGC. On the other hand, most people were unable to fathom not circumcising their own daughters. "An uncircumcised Kisii!" "An uncircumcised Samburu!" The mere idea of girls not being circumcised brought disbelief, distress, and rounds of giggles.

The workshops ultimately had some positive effects. Community members began questioning cherished traditions, and chiefs and district officials gave their approval for educating all community members about the consequences of FGC. Maendeleo was thus able to continue the dialogue, organizing one-day seminars and group discussions for various stakeholders. In the few communities where tribal leaders were not consulted from the beginning, initial opposition to the project and delays in implementing activities occurred. Eventually, Maendeleo obtained leaders' support in all sites, even if the leaders did not make clear pronouncements about eradication.

Creating a Strong Staff and a Clear Plan

To implement its educational programs, Maendeleo organized district teams composed of a coordinator, medical officer, educational officer, field workers, volunteers, and local leaders (teachers, elders, local government officials, and nongovernmental organization representatives). PATH and Maendeleo co-organized a series of training workshops to strengthen the teams' communication skills and ability to interpret the research findings, as well as to teach methods of participatory change and guided group discussion. Each team developed specific strategies for their community (outlined below) and was provided with ongoing monitoring and assistance.

Developing Materials and Crafting Messages for Particular Audiences

With guidance from PATH and using the formative research results, a group of staff, artists, and community volunteers developed a set of educational materials that addressed the health consequences of FGC. To demonstrate how girls are cut (and stitched) during FGC Types I–III, a plastic anatomical model was purchased for each district. The model was carried from place to place until a wood-carver was hired to make additional models.

To transmit educational messages, staff and community volunteers crafted poems aimed at parents, booklets for girls and boys, posters for the general community, and an information sheet for religious leaders, policymakers, teachers, and journalists. Six months were required to field-test, modify, and produce the materials. In addition to distributing the materials, volunteers found other ways to disseminate information (e.g., literate daughters were encouraged to read their booklets to their mothers). Equipped with targeted educational materials, the district coordinators and volunteers began organizing activities such as dramas, debates, workshops, and individual discussions.

Each district selected a target audience based on prevailing attitudes and patterns of decisionmaking regarding circumcision. For example, in Kisii both mothers and fathers were implicated in the decision to circumcise girls, so Kisii District teams focused on parents and recruited and trained a 42-member women's group to join the campaign. Because it appeared that more and more procedures in Kisii were being performed in health posts, health care providers became another important audience there. (Because the majority of girls in Kisii undergo circumcision before age ten, they were considered to have little potential effectiveness as advocates for their own well-being.)

In Meru, where girls are circumcised at older ages and have some say in decisionmaking, the district team reached out to both parents and girls.

In Narok and Samburu, fathers make most of the decisions to circumcise; however, because the men were not receptive to messages encouraging eradication of FGC and circumcision takes place at an older age (it is closely linked with the marriage ceremony), project staff used the education of girls as the entry point. Staff promoted keeping girls in school as a way to delay both circumcision and marriage. The girls were also educated about the harmful effects of the practice and encouraged to refuse genital cutting. The project also reached out to the great number of out-of-school boys in Samburu and Narok (who are being initiated into warrior status) with information about the practice in order to curb their insults and promote respect for uncircumcised girls.

Because both Protestant and independent Christian denominations showed higher disapproval rates for the practice than other denominations, project staff worked with denominational leaders of these churches to educate their congregations about the harmful effects of the practice and to reinforce the fact that it is contrary to their religious beliefs.

STEP TWO: CONFRONTING THE LIMITS
OF THE HEALTH ARGUMENT

Maendeleo had accomplished its most immediate goals: sensitizing the community and fostering discussion. However, its efforts were not convincing people to change their behavior, at least not in the ways intended. Indeed, simplistic messages about the health complications of FGC prompted some families to take their daughters to health care providers for the procedure. Government statements opposing the practice resulted in parents' circumcising their daughters at a younger age. As one parent explained, "Once a girl is circumcised, there is no turning back and the government cannot do anything!" Others abandoned the traditional public celebrations and began to have their daughters surreptitiously circumcised at night.

People who were persuaded in principle often lacked the courage and wherewithal to abandon the practice. Even the staff of Maendeleo had difficulty at times responding to questions they received, such as "What if my father and ancestors curse me?" "If I say I will marry an uncircumcised girl and my father does not agree, who will ask the girl's hand for me?" and "Why are you against female circumcision and not male circumcision—they are practiced for the same reason!" (Interestingly, male circumcision was seen as more painful and difficult than female circumcision, and thus boys were perceived as more courageous than girls.) Furthermore, Maendeleo staff and volunteers began to note passivity in the community in response to the same negative messages about female genital cutting.

For two years, the project messages had dealt primarily with the health implications of FGC and had sought to debunk myths about uncircumcised girls, but they had not directly addressed underlying beliefs about women, their sexuality, and their genitalia. Faced with their failure to bring about behavior change, staff sought a deeper understanding of these belief systems and how they perpetuate FGC in the four districts. Reviewing the literature on FGC, the project's baseline research, and their own experience in the field, the group came to an important realization. Wherever FGC was practiced, it drew on powerful spiritual, religious, sociological, hygienic, and aesthetic beliefs, indoctrinating members of society into the practice without explicitly addressing fundamental beliefs about female sexuality and the need to control it. Underlying these rationales were fears about oversexed girls losing their virginity and shaming their families and negative perceptions of the clitoris as being ugly, dirty, and capable of growing to unsightly proportions, having the power to blind midwives, and causing death to husbands and fathers and abnormalities in infants. Against this backdrop, genuine concerns and fears arose about the fate of uncircumcised girls. Families who did not agree with these views found that their daughters forfeited the right to identify with members of their age group, their ancestors, and even the human race (Mohamud, Makalou, and Feinberg 1997).

Project leaders began to understand that simple messages such as "FGC has negative health consequences" would not lead to behavior change because they did not address the community's concerns and fears about uncircumcised females. As a result, Maendeleo and PATH set about restructuring the entire program. Project staff and volunteers needed to see themselves principally as facilitators of behavior change. To this end, project staff developed a new set of messages and strategies that dealt with how people form and maintain belief systems, particularly those underlying attitudes toward sexual health, gender, and power. Six new discussion guides emerged:

- The first guide explores how traditions start and evaluates their contemporary relevance. As an example, the facilitator asks why men always sleep by the door. Participants generally have no response, and the facilitator explains that in the past men had to be ready to jump out the door and protect the village from attack. The facilitator then goes on to address a cultural myth about uncircumcised women—that midwives who deliver their babies will go blind. Participants are asked how many blind midwives can be found in the Luo community, which does not practice circumcision.

- The second guide helps participants acknowledge that some traditions can be harmful. It begins with a discussion of early marriage and son preference, the harmful consequences of which are less obscured by myth, and then goes on to discuss FGC.

- The third focuses on sexuality, including a comparison of how females and males are affected sexually by the genital cutting involved in circumcision.

- The fourth guide explores why rites of passage exist and whether they still represent the same transition in a girl's life.

- The fifth examines gender inequities in education and in the law, asking, for example, what rights have been violated when a girl has been raped, forcefully circumcised, or withdrawn from school.

- The sixth guide advocates for change at multiple levels, starting with an individual commitment not to circumcise one's daughter and extending out toward family, community, and country.

With a clearer conceptual focus and redesigned discussion guides, Maendeleo developed specialized outreach and awareness initiatives for four audiences: students and teachers, health care providers, religious leaders, and role models/peer educators (see Box 2).

Box 2. Specialized initiatives for target audiences

Students and teachers. Because young people often adopt new ideas and practices quickly, the project reached out to students, eventually concentrating on three schools per district. In each school, staff selected and trained eight teachers on FGC issues and a variety of related topics, including gender, human rights, the importance of girls' education, interpersonal skills, and how to communicate with parents and withstand social pressure. The main goal of the training was to help teachers change students' attitudes and behavior (e.g., abandoning the idea of circumcision as a prerequisite for marriage, or intervening against the circumcision of their siblings). Many teachers took steps to institutionalize anti-FGC education. For example, in Samburu and Narok, girls were kept in school during the holidays to help them avoid circumcision and early marriage. During this time, they participated in anti-FGC seminars and other peer education activities, sharing their experiences as uncircumcised girls.

Health care providers. A survey in Kisii of 55 health care providers—some of whom perform circumcision and many of whom also manage FGC-related complications and give prophylactic tetanus toxoid shots—found that a substantial majority were not in favor of the practice. Only 15 percent claimed they had circumcised their own daughters (Abwao, Mohamud, and Omwega 1996). Project staff organized workshops to help providers sort through the conflicting values that emerge from their different roles as parents, community leaders, and health care providers. They discussed whether circumcision violates the Hippocratic oath ("first do no harm"). After these sessions, four of the 40 participating providers identified themselves as circumcisers and declared that they would no longer perform the operation. The 40 participants also developed a statement calling on their coworkers to stop circumcising girls and on the Ministry of Health and professional associations to take a stand against the practice. Finally, project staff developed a poster: A mother is holding her daughter's hand and trying to hand money to a nurse. The nurse pushes the money away and says, "I am a health care provider. I do not earn [money] from circumcision. Do not circumcise girls."

Religious leaders. Project staff carried out FGC workshops for religious leaders in all four districts, highlighting theological arguments against the practice (e.g., that baptism replaced circumcision as an identification mark for males, that there is no mention of female circumcision in any religious documents, and that certain denominations formally oppose the practice). The facilitators encouraged the religious leaders to pledge that they would not circumcise their own daughters, and that they would oppose FGC within their extended families, congregations, and communities. Religious leaders helped develop a poster for religious parents. The poster shows a little girl kneeling in prayer and saying, "God, give my parents the wisdom to protect me from circumcision."

Role models/peer educators. To expand the project's capacity, staff developed a peer outreach strategy. Although adolescents and men are involved, women are the backbone of the peer program. The project provides three days of training on issues surrounding FGC, interpersonal communication and counseling, decisionmaking, conflict mediation, and peer outreach techniques. These women then reach out to other mothers, first within their extended families and then in the wider community. An important focus of discussion has been on deliberate decisionmaking, because sometimes both parents are opposed to FGC but allow their daughters to be subjected to it simply by not taking action or withstanding pressure from extended family.

PROMOTING POSITIVE ASPECTS OF CULTURE: DEVELOPING NEW RITES OF PASSAGE

One intention of the original project plan was to develop alternative rites of passage for girls to replace initiation by cutting. However, this intention had not been well thought out and therefore had not been implemented. Maendeleo staff still believed that alternative rites of passage had great potential to save girls from circumcision.

They sought to design an alternative that both empowered and protected girls, combining the best of modern and traditional sexuality education and celebrating young women's passage to adulthood—without cutting their genitals. The remainder of this chapter describes Maendeleo's experience promoting this innovative alternative.

Project leaders prepared by looking closely at the rite of passage. They found that the custom in the four districts is similar to that found in many other settings across Africa, and that it is disappearing in urban settings but remains common in rural areas. Traditionally, circumcision and the rite of passage marked readiness for sexual activity and marriage. Although marriage in these communities is now generally delayed a few years while girls continue their schooling, the ceremony is still associated with sexual maturity. Hence, girls receive mixed messages about sexuality—on the one hand they are expected to avoid pregnancy and remain in school; on the other they are told that once they are circumcised, they are mature. Indeed, girls often engage, whether willingly or not, in sexual activity outside of marriage, frequently without protection from pregnancy or infection.

In Kisii and Meru, both boys and girls undergo elaborate rites of passage that include celebrations and the cutting of genitals. Young people receive messages about respecting themselves, their parents and grandparents, community members, and peers. Girls receive guidance about relationships with the opposite sex and how to avoid situations that may lead to unwanted sexual relations or incest. Girls also learn that their behavior is being monitored by peers, parents, grandparents, and the community at large.

A mother looks forward to her daughter's rite of passage ceremony because it is the culmination of multiple achievements: She has raised her daughter successfully and she can display her organizational skill and wealth by hosting family, friends, and prospective in-laws in her home. For fathers, it is a time to show off their daughters and their wealth, and to negotiate with prospective in-laws for bride price. For grandparents, it is a time to ponder how far the family has come, to hand down ancestral teachings, and to feel proud of the new generation following in their footsteps.

Despite the prevalence of traditional attitudes toward circumcision ceremonies, not everyone in the two communities shared these views. Some suggested that the ceremonies have become prohibitively expensive and a source of tension between families trying to impress each other. Some families had abandoned the ceremony and were simply having the circumcision done on an individual basis in a hospital or by a health professional in their homes. Some parents opted for less severe forms of circumcision or faking the practice.[12] When asked, some community members recommended that circumcision and related ceremonies should simply be allowed to die out.

Maendeleo knew that there was significant support for initiation ceremonies, but had no strong mandate to establish variations of existing rites. The project staff sought to achieve three goals:

- Allow parents who have already stopped circumcising to come "out of the closet";
- Provide a "way out" to families educated by the project who are undecided or afraid of community pressure; and
- Establish a strong noncircumcising community alongside the traditional community.

In anticipation of fears that the project's goal was to instigate a "foreign" strategy, the initiative was designed to emphasize the relevance of the new ritual to the community and to build on existing traditions. Staff gathered ideas from mothers, girls, community leaders, and fathers through both individual and group meetings. They asked what sorts of information girls needed, who should serve as seclusion sponsors and teachers, what kinds of gifts girls should receive, what types of celebration the community should have, and who should participate. Questions were also asked about rituals such as washing all or part of the body or cutting hair. In Meru, responses to these questions gave reason to hope that changes could be made. The following section details the experience of that district, as well as the subsequent experience of other districts.

Recruitment of Families for Alternative Rites of Passage

The project team approached women who had either already stopped circumcising their daughters and wanted to declare their position publicly, or were knowledgeable about the harmful effects of the practice yet still hesitant to stop it on their own. Three mothers, one of whom had volunteered with the project since its early days and all of whom had participated in the peer educator training, came forward. These women recruited additional families, creating the first cohort of 30 circumcision-age daughters. To avoid family conflict during the recruitment process, one of the ground rules for participating in the program was that both parents (where applicable) had to agree with the decision not to circumcise their daughter. Thus, women who wanted to have their daughters initiated through the alternative rite had to convince their husbands to participate. At the same time, these women were staking out new roles for themselves as custodians of the culture.

Drawing on the community's input, the team designed a program that included all aspects of the traditional coming-of-age ceremony—seclusion, information sharing, and celebration—except cutting the genitalia. The alternative ceremony was called "Ntanira Na Mugambo," or "circumcision by words." In August 1996—less than one year after Maendeleo and PATH outlined their strategy for alternative rites of passage—the 30 girls experienced Meru's first such ritual.

The Ritual in Meru

Traditionally, newly circumcised girls were separated from the community, kept in a hut, fed, and instructed on various issues of family life during one week of healing. As the first step in the alternative rite, the mothers decided to have their daughters go through a similar period of seclusion—a week of intensive instruction, guidance, and counseling on modern family life skills and traditional wisdom.[13] The content of this instruction is rooted in accurate information about their bodies (e.g., male and female reproductive anatomy, menstruation, conception, and prevention of pregnancy, sexually transmitted infections including HIV, and FGC). The guidance is oriented around issues such as sexuality, dating, consequences of adolescent pregnancy, marriage, family relations, self-esteem, decisionmaking, and girls' rights to education and good health. As one of the project coordinators explained, "During seclusion we teach them about respect, how to behave, the challenges of being a woman, about relationships with men, and many, many other things."

Each girl also has a sponsor, typically aunts or godmothers who have informal after-dinner talks with the girls in groups and individually. These discussions focus on positive aspects of the culture, such as respect for elders and parents and various religious teachings. Girls and their sponsors also write and rehearse anti-FGC songs and dramas in preparation for the coming-of-age ceremony and celebration.

The first ceremony was hosted at the district chief's compound. While 15–30 people generally attend traditional ceremonies of well-to-do families, over 500 people attended the new ceremony. The chief opened the ceremony, and the district officer issued a statement of support: "Cultures you cannot change overnight. But we have to accept that society is dynamic and must change. Such change does not come on a silver plate." After receiving gifts (such as dresses, hats, shoes, and cosmetics), the girls performed songs, recited poetry, and danced. Mothers, fathers, younger sisters, and members of the community were invited to participate in the dancing and feasting, to celebrate "circumcision by words," and to condemn cutting. Mothers also received gifts from community members and families whose ceremonies they had attended in the past. Community members who had attended out of curiosity later joined in the celebration—in essence sanctioning the occasion. Finally, the 30 girls were given certificates of "community wisdom"—reinforcing messages on respect and how to avoid unwanted sexual relations—and were declared mature, marriageable, and acceptable to society.

The first alternative rite was a success for the peer educators, for the mothers, for Maendeleo Ya Wanawake Organization, and for PATH. But the main beneficiaries were the girls. They had been defended by their fathers and brothers as well as by their mothers, they had been trained, and they had been honored. As one 14-year-old graduate said, "I feel I am mature now. I feel more courageous. I was taught how to cope with situations. I am very proud indeed."

Maintaining Community Support in Meru

Earlier community studies had found that uncircumcised girls desperately needed to find at least one other uncircumcised girl and her family in the community to help them overcome isolation and stigma. Families who participated in the first alternative ceremony, along with community supporters, thus became the nucleus of a support group. Members agreed to work with each other to ensure that well-meaning community and extended family members did not overturn the families' decisions, and to advocate for and recruit additional families for subsequent ceremonies.

For the most part, community response has been extraordinary. Because members of the community participated in the conceptualization, development, and implementation of the project, they identify strongly with its goal. Males (largely fathers and brothers) have publicly supported the new tradition. Some boys have expressed their support for the program and have promised to protect girls threatened with circumcision. In a recent seminar for boys, every participant declared that he would no longer consider female circumcision a prerequisite in a marriage partner. Endorsement has also come from religious leaders, particularly those within Protestant denominations, who felt that the approach supported their own religious convictions and teachings that had fallen by the wayside. As one pastor said, "We fully support stopping this practice. God does not support such things."

There was also skepticism about the new ceremony, as well as outright opposition. The father of one of the girls who participated in the new ceremony said: "We were to face some problems with neighbors, parents, especially grandparents. I called them and told them that I needed to make a decision and that they have to accept what I have decided because it is within my family" (Tuju 1997).

More troubling were the objections of groups opposed to sexuality education and from those who supported the continuation of FGC. These groups spread malicious rumors about the program, stating that the alternative rite promotes sexual activity among adolescent girls, forces girls to drink blood under oath, involves injecting contraceptives into the girls' clitorises, is counter to the culture and traditional practices of the community, and is sponsored by foreigners who do not care about the interests of the community. Some people, presumably unaware of President Moi's position on FGC, threatened to take the matter to the president.

A campaign was launched to dispel the rumors and explain to community members what actually happened during the seclusion. In this way, the girls themselves became important public voices. Graduates of the program testified about what they had learned, and a series of awareness campaigns and discussions was organized. On one occasion, six circumcised girls and one mother were invited to observe the alternative seclusion. The girls and the mother not only gave a favorable report to the community about the instruction being offered, but asked that the seclusion training be extended to circumcised girls and called upon community members to enroll their circumcised daughters (Ntaniro Na Mugambo 2000). The realization that Kenyans, not foreigners, were behind the program made it easier for people to support it.

Meru's first ceremony gained much attention, and afterward Maendeleo started receiving inquiries from enthusiastic individuals and groups wanting to participate in a similar program. Within a year 200 families from 11 locations in Meru had participated. The program continues to gain popularity throughout the district.

Alternative Rites of Passage in Other Districts

The alternative rites of passage have been introduced in other districts in Kenya, including Kisii, Narok, and Nyamira. Each district has tailored the rite of passage to its distinct culture. In Kisii District (which has the highest prevalence of FGC, early ages of circumcision, and more health care provider involvement in the practice), two types of initiation ceremonies were implemented: one following the Meru style with formal training and coming-of-age ceremonies for 50–90 girls, the other offering home-based ceremonies for one or two families. In the latter type, the girl is secluded in a relative's home while the family's home is decorated with flowers and banana tree leaves and food is prepared for the guests. The girl is carried back to her mother and accepted into the home by her father or another male family member. Everyone feasts and dances, and both mother and daughter receive gifts. Sexuality education was not included in most home-based ceremonies, which involved very young girls.

The close association of FGC to girls' status is central to the approach in Narok District. The Masai of this region do not traditionally conduct rite of passage ceremonies for girls, and the project staff had already been organizing seminars for girls during the school holidays to delay early marriage, circumcision, and withdrawal from school. After the Meru and Kisii experiences, the team adopted the Meru educational curriculum followed by feasting and celebrations attended by community members and government leaders. Because of the low levels of education in Narok, girls' education is one of the key project messages in this district.

Because of intermittent banditry, droughts, and the migratory nature of residents of Samburu District, FGC eradication efforts were more difficult to initiate in this area. However, the project has continued to provide institutional support to help girls delay circumcision and marriage while continuing their education. In some cases, for example, girls have run away from home to escape circumcision and early marriage; Maendeleo volunteers and project staff have pooled resources to place these girls in boarding schools and have sought to reconcile the girls with their families.[14] In addition, Maendeleo continued to explore the possibility of using the alternative rite of passage to discourage FGC and provide reinforcement to families that had chosen not to circumcise their daughters. With the support of the Narok field staff, a few Samburu families resolved to adapt the approach and succeeded in mobilizing a few others. Their first ceremony was held in April 2001.

Effects of the Alternative Rites of Passage

Maendeleo continues to expand the new rites of passage to other communities. By December 2001, five years after the first ceremony, 5,500 girls in the target districts had experienced the alternative rite of passage without circumcision.[15] This number represents 20 percent of the total population of girls ages 10–19 in Kisii, Meru, and Narok.[16] The fact that only eight of the girls who participated in an alternative rite were later confirmed to have been circumcised underscores the strength these girls and their families have gained from the alternative rite and the support of others who chose not to circumcise.[17]

Initiates report that the training has helped raise their self-esteem and ability to resist community pressure. In addition, initiates in all participating districts continue to form support groups, consolidating their new role as public stakeholders in community culture. In Meru, site of the first ceremony, one of the first activities of the support group took place during the marriage of one of the girls. The initiates and their families gathered at the church to demonstrate that uncircumcised girls are marriageable.

The original group of Meru trainers has now formed an independent nongovernmental organization named after the alternative rite of passage—Ntanira Na Mugambo ("circumcision with words" or "bringing to age with advice"). Their support group for initiates works to end FGC and promote girls' rights; they see their role as protecting, defending, and supporting all girls within the community, whether or not they are threatened with circumcision.

NATIONAL POLICY ACTIVITIES

In addition to its activities in the four districts, Maendeleo carried out a limited national policy effort around FGC. Activities included training staff at key ministries, working with the Kenya Medical Association on a position statement for its membership, training media professionals and successfully encouraging them to increase reporting about FGC, and working with women parliamentarians to educate other parliamentarians on the practice. According to a content analysis of newspaper articles published over the last seven years, nearly one-third of the coverage on eradication of FGC in Kenya has been generated by or concerned with the Maendeleo/PATH collaboration (Bahemuka, Owiti, and Njoka 2000). One member of parliament from Narok who had initially opposed the project in his community (noting that as a custodian of culture, he could not support an initiative that might undermine strong Masai traditions) later appeared on a Maendeleo videotape asserting that he did not circumcise his daughters. In addition, Attorney General Amos Wako appealed to all Kenyans "to support the fight against circumcision of girls" (*Sunday Nation* 1994). The advocacy initiative created support and visibility for Maendeleo's activities both within and outside Kenya, and led many other agencies to begin including efforts to eradicate FGC in their programs. In December 2001 President Moi declared a national ban on FGC. The current chair of Maendeleo, Zipporah Kittony, called the President's declaration "a wonderful directive. Our girls must have a say in whatever they want to do with their lives. The old practices must be discarded" (Agina 2001).

PROJECT EFFECTS

The alternative rites of passage, together with ongoing educational and policy activities, have contributed to demonstrable behavior change. A project evaluation found a significant decline in the overall prevalence of FGC, from 90 percent of women and girls ages 14–60 at baseline (Maendeleo Ya Wanawake Organization and PATH 1993b) to 82 percent in 1999 (Olenja 2000).[18] Since the majority of women undergo FGC in early adolescence, the drop in age-specific prevalence provides a clearer indication of the project's effects. Among girls ages 14–19, prevalence declined from 78 percent in 1992–93 to 56 percent in 1999—an average drop of nearly 4 percentage points per year over the six-year life of the project.[19] The percentage of women favoring the discontinuation of FGC rose from 37 percent to 53 percent (Olenja 2000). Although men were not interviewed during quantitative baseline surveys, findings from men during the evaluation were comparable to those of women, with less than half (49 percent) favoring continuation of the practice. Similarly, mothers' intentions to circumcise their daughters fell from 67 percent to 29 percent. Data collected in nonproject sites within the same districts also showed a decline in FGC prevalence. The research-ers believe that this was due to spillover effects from project-generated media mes-sages, as well as from limited activities directed at behavior change and advocacy implemented in some of the other villages (e.g., in Tharaka, alternative rites of passage were vigorously introduced by a former Maendeleo official who received initial training through the project). A strong indication that the alternative rites of passage did have an effect is that 34 percent of women who said they would not circumcise their daughters claimed they were influenced in reaching this decision by the new approach. The major-ity of those opposed to FGC now agreed with a primary message of the project, that FGC is a violation of women's and girls' human rights.

The evaluation also indicated that community members are more knowledgeable about FGC's effects on health and sexuality than they were before the intervention. Re-spondents agreed that FGC has negative effects on women's sexuality, has lost its signifi-cance as a rite of passage, does not prevent promiscuity and infertility, and that uncircumcised females behave the same as circumcised females. Of particular importance is that out of 430 unmarried male adolescents, 55 percent favored marrying uncircumcised females. They cited having learned that much of what they previously believed about female cir-cumcision was false (e.g., that uncircumcised girls are infertile or have complications dur-ing delivery). They also stated that uncircumcised girls might be better partners.

Adult male respondents were also asked what they learned from the project. Out of 813 males who responded to this question, 59 percent reported learning that they should not circumcise their daughters, 42 percent that FGC has never been practiced in many Kenyan communities, and 30 percent that many Kenyan communities have stopped circumcising their daughters.

On the other hand, the use of health care providers to perform FGC is on the rise in Kisii District. This is particularly true in nonproject areas, where health care providers performed nearly one-third of all circumcisions in 1999, compared to 7 percent in 1992–93. In the remaining districts, where circumcision is generally per-formed at a later age, such "medicalization" remains far less common. The authors speculate that in the parts of Kisii District where project activities have not been imple-mented, parents may have heard about the health consequences of FGC, and their good intentions may lead them to turn to health care providers to make the practice safer for their daughters. A decision to abandon FGC emerges when parents and girls become convinced of the broader harmful dimensions of the practice, including the fact that it violates girls' human rights. The trend toward medicalization and the will-ingness of health care providers to perform the procedure remain major challenges for the project, whose staff and resources cannot reach everyone in each of the districts.

CONCLUSION

Female circumcision will disappear only as quickly as individuals grapple with its underlying cultural and ethical dimensions,[20] including those related to gender and sexuality. Efforts to combat the practice must extend beyond narrowly focused messages about health consequences and acknowledge the positive aspects of the rituals in which circumcision plays a part. In this way, people can become more conscious of how traditions are born and maintained, and of which aspects are positive and which are detrimental. Although part of Maendeleo's success depended upon a shared vision and successful collaboration with an international organization, the effort must come from within society and must involve the local community—including men—at every stage.

Change—which a few years ago seemed elusive—is taking place, and girls and women are assuming roles as co-custodians of a culture that can protect and empower them. One 20-year-old girl described how she felt to be one of the first young Kenyans to experience an alternative rite of passage:

> It is very important to me because some of the things I learned in the seminar I never knew before. It is a rite of passage which I need also to enjoy as others enjoy. It is an achievement, if I may say!

Acknowledgments

We dedicate this chapter to our dear friend and colleague, Leah Muuya, who died in December 2000. Leah worked for Maendeleo Ya Wanawake Organization for 20 years and was instrumental to the conceptualization and success of the project documented here.

Many people contributed to the success of this project. We thank the Maendeleo and Ntaniru Na Mugambo coordinators Aniceta Kiriga, Michelina Lengewa, Jeria Kerubo Moragia, Jerusha Mubishi, Flora Kawanja Nthiga, Nancy Ogega, Agnes Pareiyo, and Agnes Yapan, who provided excellent leadership in the design and initiation of alternative rites of passage. Maendeleo national and district leaders, field workers, and volunteers dedicated themselves to promoting adolescent girls' right to education and advocated against FGC. Peer educators—women, girls, boys, teachers, and religious leaders—conducted outreach door to door and through their institutions.

PATH staff, including Stella Abwao, Carol Corso, Beth Crane, Michelle Folsom, Joan Haffey, Robert Sharp, Donna Sutton, Anne Wilson, and Margot Zimmerman, assisted us with project conceptualization, design, technical assistance, and fundraising. The comments of Karin Ringheim of PATH strengthened the chapter.

The project would not have been possible without the support of donor agencies and the vision and dedication of their program officers, including Susan Rich of the Wallace Global Fund, who conceptualized and funded this project while advocating for other donor support; Adisa Douglas of the Public Welfare Foundation; Shira Saperstein of the Moriah Fund; and Mary Ann Burris of the Ford Foundation. Finally, we thank the many other donors, including the Threshold Foundation, Save the Children Fund, Australian Aid for International Development, and the United Nations Development Fund for Women, who contributed to the support of project activities.

Notes

1   These figures may be underestimates. National surveys conducted in six African countries (Central African Republic, Egypt, Eritrea, Ivory Coast, Mali, and Sudan) found that nearly 30 million women over the age of 15 had undergone some form of genital cutting, while an additional 21 million girls under age 15 were estimated to have undergone cutting or to be likely to undergo genital cutting in the near future.

2   Convention on the Elimination of All Forms of Discrimination Against Women (1979); Convention on the Rights of the Child (1989); World Conference on Human Rights (1993); International Conference on Population and Development in Cairo (1994); and World Conference on Women in Beijing (1995).

3   "Maendeleo ya wanawake" is Kiswahili for "women's development."

4   Among women ages 15–49 in Kenya, 65 percent identify themselves as Protestant, 28 percent as Catholic, and 5 percent as Muslim (National Council for Population and Development, Central Bureau of Statistics [Kenya], and Macro International 1999). The prevalence of FGC is 36 percent among Protestants, 44 percent among Catholics, and 28 percent among Muslims (special tabulations of Demographic and Health Survey results by Rod Knight of Principia International).

5   In more recent years, in speeches made while touring districts where female circumcision rates are high, President Moi has reiterated his opposition to FGC.

6   The trend toward earlier circumcision is apparent in most countries that practice FGC. For example, in Mali the median age for genital cutting for women ages 45–49 was 8.8 years, compared to 4.3 years among women ages 15–19. In Egypt, medical professionals performed the procedure on 55 percent of respondents' daughters while doctors or nurses/nurse-midwives had circumcised only 17 percent of respondents. The shift to less extensive cutting is evident in Eritrea, where 91 percent of women ages 45–49 had been infibulated (Type III) compared with 81 percent of 20–24-year-olds (Carr 1997).

7   Then called the Population Crisis Committee.

8   Financial support for the project was provided by the Wallace Global Fund, PATH, the Ford Foundation, the Public Welfare Foundation, the Moriah Fund, the Threshold Foundation, the United Nations Development Fund for Women, and Australian Aid for International Development.

9   Key factors associated with opposition to the custom were education (women with secondary education were four times more likely to disapprove of FGC) and religion (Protestants and independent Christian denominations were twice as likely as Catholics to disapprove).

10   Concerns about health risks motivated some families to seek a health care provider to perform the procedure; others took their daughters to a health post for a tetanus inoculation before arranging to have FGC performed at home by a health care provider.

11   While there was variation among the districts, overall 39 percent of decisions regarding FGC were made by both parents. Fathers made the decision 27 percent of the time, and mothers were the sole decisionmaker in only 9 percent of cases overall, and did not participate in the decisionmaking at all in 43 percent of cases. Girls' participation in decisionmaking was highly variable, with 1 percent deciding in Samburu, 11 percent in Kisii, 13 percent in Narok, and 53 percent in Meru.

12   Some critics of FGC criticize faking the practice on the grounds that it may reinforce people's perceptions that the custom is acceptable and is continuing unchallenged.

13   Initially, Maendeleo and PATH staff carried out the seclusion training for girls. They later trained a team comprising schoolteachers, nurses, mothers, and local government officials to carry out the training.

14   Early work by Maendeleo in Samburu led to the establishment of a community-based organization supporting girls' education and the elimination of FGC.

15   PATH and Maendeleo have also assisted other organizations who want to provide opportunities for girls to participate in an alternative rite of passage, including the Seventh-day Adventist Church and the Federation of Women Groups. In December 2001, nearly 1,000 girls participated in an alternative rite of passage in Gusii District. Maendeleo trained 450 girls, while the Federation of Women Groups and the Seventh-day Adventist Church trained 280 and 250, respectively. Involving other organizations in conducting alternative rites of passage ceremonies increases sustainability, as demand for these alternative rites now exceeds the staff capacity and financial resources of the PATH/Maendeleo collaboration.

16   This calculation is based on projections of 1989 census data.

17   Most of the eight girls who were later reported to have been circumcised had undergone the procedure before the alternative rite of passage. They had either concealed their circumcision status from project staff or were permitted by local staff to participate in the alternative rite of passage (Radeny 2001).

18   The evaluation was based on interviews with 1,237 randomly selected women ages 14–60, 1,220 men, and 180 youth in school.

19   The intervention began in mid-1994, and the evaluation was conducted in early 1999.

20   It is particularly important to address the ethical dimensions of FGC with health care providers in order to help them reconcile their medical ethics and cultural beliefs, stop circumcising their own daughters and the daughters of others, and take action against the practice.

References

Abwao, Stella, Asha Mohamud, and Edna Omwega. 1996. "Health workers' knowledge, attitudes, and practices regarding female circumcision in Nyamira District," unpublished report submitted to the Basic Support for Institutionalizing Child Survival project by the Program for Appropriate Technology in Health (PATH) and Seventh-day Adventist–Rural Health Services. Washington, DC: PATH.

Agina, Ben. 2001. "Kibaki backs stand," *East African Standard,* 13 December, p. 2.

Bahemuka, Judith Mbula, Lilian Awuor Owiti, and John Murimi Njoka. 2000. "Final evaluation of MYWO FGM eradication project." Nairobi: University of Nairobi.

Carr, Dara. 1997. "Female genital cutting: Findings from the Demographic and Health Survey program." Calverton, MD: Macro International Inc.

Kenya Family Planning Association. 1995. Personal communication with the FGC program coordinator during a National Advisory Committee Meeting for Seventh-day Adventist–Rural Health Services, Nyamira, Kenya.

Kun, Karen E. 1997. "Female genital mutilation: The potential for increased risk of HIV infection," *International Journal of Gynaecology and Obstetrics* 59(2): 153–155.

Maendeleo Ya Wanawake Organization. 1991. "Harmful traditional practices that affect the health of women and their children in Kenya," background paper. Washington, DC: PATH.

Maendeleo Ya Wanawake Organization and PATH. 1993a. "Qualitative research report on female circumcision in four districts in Kenya," unpublished report. Washington, DC: PATH.

———. 1993b. "Quantitative research report on female circumcision in four districts in Kenya," unpublished report. Washington, DC: PATH.

Mohamud, Asha, Kalle Makalou, and Madeline Feinberg. 1997. "Towards elimination of female genital mutilation: Mobilizing health professionals and the community in Nyamira District," final report to the BASICS Project for USAID contract no. HRN-6006-Q-00-3032-00. Washington, DC: USAID.

National Council for Population and Development, Central Bureau of Statistics (Kenya), and Macro International. 1999. *Kenya Demographic and Health Survey 1998*. Calverton, MD: Macro International.

Ntaniro Na Mugambo. 2000. "Interim report submitted to PATH, Washington, DC." Washington, DC: PATH.

Olenja, Joyce. 2000. "Evaluation report on eliminating the practice of female genital mutilation: Awareness raising and community change in 4 districts of Kenya," draft report. Washington, DC and Nairobi: PATH and Maendeleo Ya Wanawake Organization.

Radeny, Samson. 2001. Personal communication.

Sunday Nation. 1994. 6 November.

Tuju, Rafael. 1997. Interview conducted for videotape *Rite of Passage*. Nairobi: Maendeleo Ya Wanawake Organization.

United Nations. 1995. "Programme of Action of the International Conference on Population and Development, Cairo, Egypt, 5–13 September 1994," in *Report of the International Conference on Population and Development*, UNDoc.A/CONF.171/13/Rev.1. New York: United Nations.

———. 1996. "The Beijing Declaration and the Platform for Action, Fourth World Conference on Women, Beijing, China." UNDoc.DPI/1766/Wom.112-113. New York: United Nations.

World Health Organization. 1982. *Female Circumcision: Statement of WHO Position and Activities.* Geneva: World Health Organization.

———. 1993. "Female genital mutilation: World health assembly calls for elimination of harmful practices," press release WHA/10. Geneva: World Health Organization.

———. 2000. "Female genital mutilation: Fact sheet no. 241," revised June. Geneva: World Health Organization.

Contact information

Asha Mohamud
Regional Director, Africa Youth Alliance Project,
    Program for Appropriate Technology
    in Health (PATH)
PATH Uganda
Plot 62, Kiira Road
(opposite the Uganda Museum)
P.O. Box 10370
Kampala, Uganda
telephone/fax: 256-41-530-863
e-mail: amohamud@path-dc.org

Zipporah Kittony
Chairwoman
Maendeleo Ya Wanawake Organization
Maendeleo House
Monrovia Street #4
P.O. Box 44412
Nairobi, Kenya
telephone: 254-2-222-095
fax: 254-2-225-390

Samson Radeny
Program Officer
PATH Kenya
3 Ole Odume Road
Nairobi, Kenya
telephone: 254-2-577-177/189/180
fax: 254-2-577-172
e-mail: sradeny@path-kenya.or.ke

Contributors

NAHLA ABDEL-TAWAB, formerly host country advisor, Population Council, Cairo, is an independent consultant in Egypt.

NAPOLEON AMOYEN is lecturer, Social Research Office, Ateneo de Davao University, Philippines.

TOM ARENS, formerly area representative for World Neighbors in South Asia, is retired.

DEBORA BOSSEMEYER is clinical training advisor, Clinical Services Office, JHPIEGO, Baltimore, MD.

AYŞEN BULUT is professor and head, Family Health Department, Istanbul University Institute of Child Health.

FRANCISCO CABRAL is vice president, Reprolatina, Campinas, Brazil.

LUCELLA CAMPBELL is senior program advisor, International Planned Parenthood Federation/ Western Hemisphere Region, New York.

DENISE CAUDILL is a consultant specializing in participatory evaluation in community health and development.

CHRISTIANA COGGINS, a researcher in reproductive health, is a consultant to the Population Council, the New Mexico Department of Health, and the University of New Mexico.

MARILOU COSTELLO is program associate, International Programs Division, Population Council, Manila, Philippines.

JUAN DÍAZ is senior associate, Population Council, Campinas, Brazil.

MARGARITA DÍAZ is president, Reprolatina, Campinas, Brazil.

MAJ-BRITT DOHLIE is a supervision specialist seconded to the PRIME II Project from EngenderHealth, New York.

CHRISTOPHER ELIAS is president, Program for Appropriate Technology in Health, Seattle, WA.

ADENIKE O. ESIET is executive director and co-founder of Action Health Incorporated, Lagos, Nigeria.

SHARON FONN is associate professor, School of Public Health, University of the Witwatersrand, Johannesburg, South Africa.

CECILIA GARCÍA-BARRIOS is director of educational developments in health, Ministry of Health, Mexico.

SARASWATI GAUTAM is health coordinator, World Neighbors Integrated Program in Reproductive Health and Development, Nepal.

LAURA GHIRON is research associate, Department of Health Behavior and Health Education, University of Michigan School of Public Health, Ann Arbor.

GÜLBIN GÖKÇAY is professor of pediatrics, Family Health Department, Istanbul University Institute of Child Health, Turkey.

BAOCHANG GU is deputy secretary-general and director for international cooperation, China Family Planning Association, Beijing.

ALESSANDRA C. GUEDES is program officer, Sexual and Reproductive Health, International Planned Parenthood Federation/Western Hemisphere Region, New York.

NICOLE HABERLAND is program associate, Gender, Family, and Development Program, Population Council, New York.

ANGELA HEIMBURGER, formerly regional staff associate for Latin America and the Caribbean, Population Council, Mexico City, is a consultant in international reproductive health.

JUDITH F. HELZNER is director, Sexual and Reproductive Health, International Planned Parenthood Federation/Western Hemisphere Region, New York.

CHARLOTTE HORD is director of policy, Ipas, Chapel Hill, NC.

DALE HUNTINGTON is senior associate, Population Council, New Delhi, India.

DENNIS I. IFENNE is senior lecturer and consultant, Department of Obstetrics and Gynecology, Ahmadu Bello University Teaching Hospital, Zaria, Nigeria.

ANRUDH JAIN is senior director, Policy and Regional Programs, International Programs Division, Population Council, New York.

ZIPPORAH KITTONY is chairwoman, Maendeleo Ya Wanawake Organization, Nairobi, Kenya.

MARLINA LACUESTA is professor, Social Research Office, Ateneo de Davao University, Philippines.

MERVIN LAMBEY, formerly director of evaluation and resource development, Belize Family Life Association, is now executive director, Society for the Promotion of Education and Research, Belize.

ANA LANGER is regional director for Latin America and the Caribbean, Population Council, Mexico City.

B. NDUGGA MAGGWA is regional director, Population and Reproductive Health Program, Family Health International (East and Southern Africa), Nairobi, Kenya.

MARIA YOLANDA MAKUCH is researcher, Center for Research on Maternal and Child Health, Campinas, Brazil.

DIANA MEASHAM is a consultant to the Population Council, on the staff of the Department of Obstetrics, Gynecology, and Reproductive Sciences and the AIDS Research Institute of the University of California, San Francisco, and a doctoral student in reproductive epidemiology at the University of California, Berkeley.

SUSANA MEDINA is coordinator of the Gender-Based Violence Program, PLAFAM, Caracas, Venezuela.

LORI S. MICHAU is a founder and co-director of Raising Voices, Kampala, Uganda.

ERIN MIELKE is program manager for quality improvement, EngenderHealth, New York.

ASHA MOHAMUD is regional program director, Behavior Change Communication Component, Africa Youth Alliance, Kampala, Uganda.

W. HENRY MOSLEY is professor of population and family health sciences, Bloomberg School of Public Health, Johns Hopkins University, Baltimore, MD.

NIRMALA MURTHY is president, Foundation for Research in Health Systems, Bangalore, India.

GOPAL NAKARMI is program coordinator, World Neighbors Integrated Program in Reproductive Health and Development, Nepal.

DIPAK NAKER is a founder and co-director of Raising Voices, Kampala, Uganda.

HACER NALBANT is sociologist, Family Health Department, Istanbul University Institute of Child Health, Turkey.

LAILA NAWAR is regional advisor, West Asia and North Africa, Frontiers in Reproductive Health Program, Population Council, Cairo, Egypt.

EZZELDIN OSMAN is professor of obstetrics and gynecology, Mansoura University, Egypt, and executive director, Egyptian Fertility Care Centre.

PERTTI PELTO is emeritus professor of anthropology, University of Connecticut, and a freelance research consultant based in Pune, India.

SAMSON RADENY is senior program officer, Program for Appropriate Technology in Health, Nairobi, Kenya.

LAKSHMI RAMACHANDAR is a doctoral student in medical anthropology at the Key Centre for Women's Health in Society, University of Melbourne, Australia.

SAUMYA RAMARAO is program associate, International Programs Division, Population Council, New York.

KARIN RINGHEIM is senior program officer, Program for Appropriate Technology in Health, Washington, DC.

DEBBIE ROGOW is editor of the Population Council series *Quality/Calidad/Qualité* and an independent consultant.

ANATOLE RUKONGE, formerly director of the EngenderHealth Program with the Public and Family Planning Association of Tanzania, is medical director, St. Gasper Hospital, Itigi, Singida Region, Tanzania.

BONNIE SHEPARD is senior program manager, François-Xavier Bagnoud Center for Health and Human Rights, Harvard School of Public Health, Boston, MA, and senior consultant to the Latin American program of Catholics for Free Choice.

OLADAPO SHITTU is head, Department of Obstetrics and Gynecology, Ahmadu Bello University Teaching Hospital, Zaria, Nigeria.

RUTH SIMMONS is professor, Department of Health Behavior and Health Education, University of Michigan School of Public Health, Ann Arbor.

LYNNE STEVENS is a consultant, psychotherapist, and educator in the field of gender-based violence.

ZAHARA SWALEHE is clinical trainer, Jijenge! Project, African Medical and Research Foundation, Mwanza, Tanzania.

DIANA SZATKOWSKI is a Ph.D. candidate in medical anthropology, Columbia University, New York.

KHIN SAN TINT is senior researcher, Women's Health Project, School of Public Health, University of the Witwatersrand, Johannesburg, South Africa.

JANET MOLZAN TURAN is reproductive health specialist, Family Health Department, Istanbul University Institute of Child Health, Turkey.

AKHILA VASAN is research associate, Foundation for Research in Health Systems, Ahmedabad, India.

GRACE WAMBWA is program manager, EngenderHealth, Nairobi, Kenya.

CORINNE WHITAKER is senior program officer for Africa, International Women's Health Coalition, New York.

BEVERLY WINIKOFF is director, Reproductive Health Program, International Programs Division, Population Council, New York.

SUSAN WOOD, formerly program director, International Women's Health Coalition, New York, is an independent consultant.

NANCY YINGER is director of international programs, Population Reference Bureau, Washington, DC.

HALA YOUSSEF is assistant professor of public health, Cairo University, Egypt.